Ethics in Nursing

Cases, Principles, and Reasoning

FOURTH EDITION

Martin Benjamin
Professor Emeritus, Department of Philosophy,
Michigan State University

Joy Curtis
Professor Emerita, College of Nursing, and
Ombudsman Emerita, Michigan State University

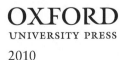

OXFORD
UNIVERSITY PRESS
2010

OXFORD
UNIVERSITY PRESS

Oxford University Press, Inc., publishes works that further
Oxford University's objective of excellence
in research, scholarship, and education.

Oxford New York
Auckland Cape Town Dar es Salaam Hong Kong Karachi
Kuala Lumpur Madrid Melbourne Mexico City Nairobi
New Delhi Shanghai Taipei Toronto

With offices in
Argentina Austria Brazil Chile Czech Republic France Greece
Guatemala Hungary Italy Japan Poland Portugal Singapore
South Korea Switzerland Thailand Turkey Ukraine Vietnam

Published by Oxford University Press, Inc.
198 Madison Avenue, New York, New York 10016
www.oup.com

Oxford is a registered trademark of Oxford University Press

Library of Congress Cataloging-in-Publication Data
Benjamin, Martin.
Ethics in nursing : cases, principles, and reasoning /
Martin Benjamin, Joy Curtis.— 4th ed.
p. ; cm.
Includes bibliographical references and index.
ISBN 978–0–19–538022–4
1. Nursing ethics. I. Curtis, Joy. II. Title.
[DNLM: 1. Ethics, Nursing. WY 85 B468e 2010]
RT85.B39 2010
174.2—dc22
2009018900

9 8 7 6 5 4 3 2 1

Printed in the United States of America
on acid-free paper

For our grandchildren

Nora and Lucas
Emma, Julia, Sabrina, Thomas, and Matthew

PREFACE

The changes in this edition reflect important developments in nursing, ethical theory, and nursing ethics. First, facts, figures, and references have been updated throughout. Second, the total number of cases has been expanded from 53 to 64. Of these, 15 are entirely new and 22 are updated to reflect current practice. Among the new topics raised by cases in various chapters are care of SARS patients and others during deadly epidemics or disasters, care of elderly persons contemplating suicide, work with nonphysician health care providers, independence of nurses in advanced practice, supervising unlicensed personnel, and workplace violence (which includes an entirely new section in Chapter 6). New cases in the Appendix address such issues as responsibility for dirty hospitals, payment for patients with Alzheimer's, and the effects of health care funding on nursing care decisions. Third, Chapter 2, "Unavoidable Topics in Ethical Theory," has been significantly revised and expanded. The emphasis in earlier editions on selecting a comprehensive ethical theory has been replaced by an explanation and defense of *moral pluralism*, the view that there are, and always will be, conflicts between good and important ethical values and principles. The chapter includes, in addition, a new section on the ethics of care and an expanded discussion of reflective equilibrium as a method of moral reasoning. As revised, the chapter is a much better fit with, and guide to, our analyses of cases in subsequent chapters that, from the first edition, have assumed the truth of moral pluralism. Fourth, the addition of a subtitle, "Cases, Principles, and Reasoning," provides an accurate characterization of the book as a whole. Starting with *cases* based on real life, we draw on relevant ethical *principles* and careful *reasoning* in thinking them through. Though much has changed in this edition, the principal aim of the book remains the same: to provide practicing and student nurses with a useful introduction to the identification and analysis of ethical issues that reflects both the special perspective of nursing and the value of systematic ethical inquiry.

A number of people have contributed to this edition. Students in our courses at Michigan State University and, most recently, students in the nursing program at Mills College, have provided useful suggestions and continuing inspiration for updating and improving the book. Nurses, nursing faculty, and other health care providers from across the country have helped us to identify new topics and issues. We have benefited, too, from several colleagues affiliated with Michigan State University's Center for Ethics and Humanities in the Life Sciences, particularly Leonard Fleck, Tom Tomlinson, and Hilde Lindemann. Marilyn Rothert, former Dean of the Michigan State University College of Nursing, made numerous useful suggestions for this as well as earlier editions. Howard Brody, long-time friend, colleague, and now Director of the Institute for the Medical Humanities of the University of Texas Medical Branch at Galveston, helped with the Suggestions for Further Reading, as did David Boersema of Pacific University and Rodger Jackson of Stockton College.

Special thanks go to Jason Curtis for solving various computer problems and to Bruce Curtis and Hilary Arthur for invaluable assistance in proofreading.

Thanks as well go to Zubin Abraham for help with files and computers. Finally, we appreciate the support of Peter Ohlin and the assistance Molly Wagener of Oxford University Press, and the efforts of Anupama Gopinath who capably oversaw the transformation of our typescript into a book.

M.B.
J.C.
Oakland, California
East Lansing, Michigan
September 2009

PREFACE TO THE FIRST EDITION

The aim of this book is to provide practicing and student nurses with an introduction to the identification and analysis of ethical issues that reflects both the special perspective of nursing and the value of systematic philosophical inquiry. Discussions of general and theoretical points are, wherever possible, grounded in and illustrated by their application to specific nursing situations. The text includes 30 actual cases, which are discussed in some detail. In addition, Appendix D contains a set of 11 case studies for further practice in ethical analysis and reasoning.

The book begins with an account of the nature of moral dilemmas and outlines the philosophical skills and understanding necessary for addressing them systematically. Next, Chapter 2 provides an introduction to basic ethical principles and the complex relationships between ethical, legal, and religious considerations in the nursing context. Then, through a series of ten case studies, Chapter 3 focuses upon ethical issues involving nurses and clients. Chapter 4 discusses complications that arise due to the unclear nature of the relationship between nurses and physicians. In Chapter 5 we turn to ethical dilemmas involving relationships among nurses. Finally, Chapter 6 examines the extent to which nurses ought to be concerned with the nature and direction of institutional and public policy.

Throughout the book, our emphasis in discussing individual cases is to illustrate the application of ethical analysis and reasoning and the importance of thinking for oneself. Where we come to conclusions on particular points therefore, we do not intend readers to accept them without carefully examining our reasoning. The importance of critically analyzing the reasons given for various positions applies to our arguments no less than to those of others. Readers may or may not agree with our analyses of particular cases, but if they come to their conclusions by applying some of the methods, principles, and distinctions that we have stressed, our purpose will have been fulfilled. As a recent report on *The Teaching of Ethics in Higher Education* put it: "The test of the teaching of ethics is not whether students end by sharing the convictions of their teachers, but whether they have come to those convictions by means of the use of skills that might have led in other directions and may do so in the future" (Hasting-on-Hudson, The Hastings Center, 1980, p. 61).

Unless otherwise noted, all cases presented in the text were obtained from practicing nurses as part of a 1978 research study on nurses' perceptions of ethical dilemmas. The study was based upon one-hour, structured, tape-recorded interviews with a sample of 40 practicing baccalaureate-educated nurses in Michigan's lower peninsula. The distribution of the principal employment settings of the nurses who participated in the study closely approximated the percentage distribution of all active registered nurses in Michigan whose highest degree was in baccalaureate nursing: there were 28 hospital nurses, 5 community health nurses, 3 nursing school faculty, 2 school nurses, 1 nursing home nurse, 1 office nurse, and no private duty, occupational health, or self-employed nurses. While the cases developed from these interviews do not raise all possible ethical issues in nursing, they offer a fair sampling of the ethical dilemmas that frequently recur in nursing practice. Names and places have been changed to insure confidentiality but, wherever possible, the nurses' actual words have been retained.

We want to express our gratitude to the nurses who participated in this study as well as to a number of others who helped us in preparing this book. Isabelle K. Payne, Dean of the College of Nursing at Michigan State University, and Suzanne Brouse, Maureen Chojnacki, Marilyn Rothert, and Linda Beth Tiedje read the manuscript and made suggestions about the nursing aspects. Lewis Zerby and Thomas Tomlinson, of the Department of Philosophy, suggested helpful changes with regard to the philosophical aspects. Linda Henlotter, a graduate assistant in the College of Nursing, helped conduct the interviews of practicing nurses, and Stanley Werne, a graduate assistant in the Department of Philosophy, helped compile the list of further readings and made suggestions about the manuscript. Though they are too numerous to mention by name, we also want to express our thanks to students in our team-taught course in Ethics in Nursing who helped us evaluate the clarity and relevance of the manuscript and encouraged us to complete it.

We are grateful, too, to Michigan State University for an M.S.U. Foundation Grant, which supported the survey of nurses, and an All-University Research Grant, which helped in the preparation of the manuscript. Finally, thanks are due to three people who provided special assistance. JoAnn Wittick, of the Medical Humanities Program, cheerfully and skillfully typed the manuscript. Bruce Curtis, of the Department of American Thought and Language, made line by line stylistic improvements. And Jeffrey House, of Oxford University Press, offered detailed criticisms and useful suggestions which helped us strengthen some of our arguments and made certain sections clearer and more concise.

M.B.
J.C.
East Lansing, Mich.
January 1981

CONTENTS

CASES

Ethics in Nursing

1

Moral Dilemmas and Ethical Inquiry

1. MORAL DILEMMAS IN NURSING

Advances in medical knowledge and technology, together with social and political changes, have raised a number of well-publicized moral dilemmas for patients, physicians, and policy makers. Less well publicized, but no less important, are the troubling conflicts that arise for nurses in these changing circumstances. As an example of the sort of dilemma created by the special role and responsibilities of nursing, consider the following case.

1.1 Withholding Troublesome Details

Mary Evans, a new urology clinic staff nurse with more than three years of oncological experience in a different institution, learned during a postoperative prostatectomy visit with Luis Vasquez and his wife, Geneva, that they both believed Dr. John Lampson had told them he "got it all." They had been greatly relieved by the good news, but added that the whole ordeal—diagnosis, surgery, and troublesome after-effects—was a nightmare. They agreed that they had trouble sleeping and were still terribly nervous. Even though they were dealing with tough issues, including Luis's incontinence, they were happy the surgery was successful.

As Mary could see from Luis's records, their belief that Dr. Lampson "got it all" could be questioned. Luis had come through the prostatectomy well, and the pathology report indicated the cancer was localized. His lymph nodes and seminal vesicles were clear. His postoperative prostate-specific antigen (PSA) level was less than 0.01 (indicating removal of almost all prostate cells). However, the cancer was judged to be moderately aggressive and extended to some margins of the resected prostate gland (incision edges); that is, he had "positive margins." In Mary's experience, other patients with similar pathology reports had chosen to begin additional treatment (hormone and radiation) within six months after surgery.

(Continued)

3

Troubled, Mary decided to discuss the matter with Dr. Lampson. When they met, Mary said that she had seen Luis and Geneva Vasquez during a follow-up visit. Mary told Dr. Lampson she needed to know what he had told the Vasquez couple about Luis's condition so that she might be more open and supportive with them. She said the couple appeared not to understand the pathology report concerning the positive margins since they thought Dr. Lampson had "got it all."

Dr. Lampson, who was not Luis Vasquez's long-standing physician, said he had informed Luis and his wife that the surgery had been successful, that he had discussed the pathology report, and had given them a copy. He added that just because some of the cancer extended to the margins of the resected prostate gland, it did not necessarily mean the surgery was unsuccessful. He said he had a "good success rate" in similar cases, and that the best course was to leave well enough alone. To him, postoperative issues were worry enough for Luis and Geneva. Should Luis's PSA rise (indicating a recurrence of the cancer) in the next 18 months or so, he would encourage him to begin hormone treatments to control the cancer. Moreover, he insisted, if Mary took any action to bring the issue of the positive margins to Luis's or Geneva's attention at this time, he would consider that inconsistent with the patient's well-being and inconsistent with her role as a nurse. Dr. Lampson's tone, though not hostile, was self-assured and disapproving.

Mary later sought her nurse manager's counsel. The nurse manager acknowledged that acceptable medical practice in prostate cancer included various treatment methods, but whatever course followed was usually selected jointly by a patient and his doctor. After agreeing that Dr. Lampson's position presented Mary with a dilemma, the nurse manager advised her to avoid a messy confrontation by complying with his directions. If this sort of thing really bothered Mary, the manager said, she would in the future shift Mary to a different clinic so she would not be in contact with Dr. Lampson's patients.[1]

In this case, a nurse faces a difficult moral dilemma. Strictly speaking, a dilemma is a situation requiring a choice between what seem to be two equally desirable or undesirable alternatives. Students sometimes find themselves in a dilemma when they have to choose between two highly rated, interesting courses that are scheduled at the same time. One might face a dilemma in deciding whether to go out in a heavy rain to bring in a bicycle or to let it become a bit more rusty: neither alternative, getting soaked or the bike's getting rusty, is desirable, but there is no way to avoid both. These, however, are not moral dilemmas. In a moral dilemma, each alternative course of action can be justified by fundamental moral rules or principles. The nurse who believes that she is duty-bound both to preserve life and to reduce suffering may be confronted with a dilemma when preserving life involves prolonging suffering or when suffering cannot be reduced without increasing the likelihood of shortening life. Choosing either seems to violate an ethical principle, yet the choice must be made.

The moral dilemma in "Withholding troublesome details" centers on the choice Mary Evans must make between bringing the troubling matter of "positive margins" to the attention of Luis and Geneva Vasquez or supporting their comforting, but not completely accurate, belief that Dr. Lampson had "got it all." On the face of it, each course of action could be grounded on fundamental principles.

Mary's informing Luis that there were still traces of the cancer at the edges of the resected prostate gland could be defended by appealing to Mr. Vasquez's right, as a competent adult, to an accurate, detailed account of the results of his surgery. This right, it may be argued, is based on the right to self-determination, which is itself based on the respect owed to all persons by virtue of their capacity for informed choice and reflection. If he were fully and accurately informed, he might, like other patients Mary knew with similar pathology reports, now choose to begin additional hormone and radiation treatment within six months after surgery. Moreover, Mary Evans could also maintain that her withholding troubling, but important, details seriously compromises the integrity of the relationship between Luis and her, thus diminishing her personhood as well as Mr. Vasquez's.

On the other hand, Mary's acting in accord with the wishes of Dr. Lampson could also be supported by an appeal to moral principle. Dr. Lampson indicates that Luis and Geneva Vasquez have just undergone a terrible ordeal—a "nightmare"—and they are still terribly nervous. In withholding certain details of the resected margins, he is hoping to spare them further, probably quite unnecessary, anxiety. Despite the positive margins, Dr. Lampson's experience in similar cases leads him to believe that a recurrence of the cancer is quite unlikely. The reduction of pain and suffering is not only a general, moral imperative; it has long been a cornerstone of both medical and nursing morality. Perhaps, this is what Dr. Lampson meant when he said that any attempt by Mary to bring the issue of positive margins to the attention of the patient or his wife would be inconsistent with Luis's well-being and inconsistent with her role as a nurse. The latter, too, can be construed as a moral appeal if we assume that Mary Evans has some sort of moral obligation to the profession and to the hospital, as well as to the patient, to act in accord with the special role—that of a nurse—she has voluntarily assumed.

How, then, should the nurse resolve the dilemma? Perhaps, her initial inclination to inform the patient of his "positive margins" can no longer be defended. After all, can she disregard the wishes of Dr. Lampson? He is a good person and seems as concerned with the patient's well-being as she is. If she still has some reservations, perhaps the wise thing to do is to take the head nurse's advice and try to avoid such situations in the future, but to go along in this instance. But what if she is right, after all, and Dr. Lampson, though well intentioned, is wrong? If so, wouldn't it be either immoral or cowardly of a nurse not to fulfill her moral obligation to disclose the troubling details of the surgery to Mr. and Mrs. Vasquez?

What can Mary Evans appeal to in making her decision? Many people think codes of medical or nursing ethics should be able to resolve such problems. In the next section we will see to what extent this is so.

2. ETHICAL CODES: USES AND LIMITATIONS

Codes of professional ethics are often a mixture of creeds and commandments. As creeds, they affirm professional regard for high ideals of conduct and personally commit members of the profession to honor them, thus constituting a sort of oath of professional office. The opening sentence of the Preamble to the International Council of Nurses (ICN) Code of Ethics (revised in 2006) states that "Nurses have four fundamental responsibilities: to promote health, to prevent illness, to restore health and to alleviate suffering."[2] This is a statement of creed. As commandments, codes of professional ethics provide a set of prescriptions designed to regulate conduct in more specific situations. For example, the same ICN Code states that "the nurse holds in confidence personal information and uses judgment in sharing this information."

As creeds, codes of nursing ethics provide a valuable reminder of the special responsibilities incumbent upon those who tend the sick. Nurses often deal with people who, because of their illness or injury, are especially vulnerable and must depend upon the professional's special knowledge and skills. Hence, it is important that the nursing profession formulate and adhere to high ideals of conduct in order to assure the public that individual nurses will not exploit their advantaged position.

As sets of commandments, codes of professional ethics have two principal functions. First, they provide an enforceable standard of minimally decent conduct that allows the profession to discipline those who clearly fall below the minimal standard. In 1978, for example, the *New Yorker* reported that some nurses were being paid by antiabortion groups for the names of women who had had abortions. Members of these groups then proceeded to harass the women with abusive phone calls when they returned home from the hospital.[3] Such conduct on the part of the nurses, regardless of the strength or correctness of their views on abortion, clearly violated provisions of nursing codes that were in effect—basic provisions that continue in those same revised codes in the twenty-first century. Their conduct violates both the provision of the ICN Code stating that "The nurse holds in confidence personal information and uses judgment in sharing this information" and Provision 3.2 (Confidentiality) of the 2001 American Nurses Association (ANA) Code for Nurses, which holds that "Associated with the right to privacy, the nurse has a duty to maintain confidentiality of all patient information. The patient's well-being could be jeopardized and the fundamental trust between patient and nurse destroyed by...the inappropriate disclosure of identifiable patient information."[4]

A second function of the commandments in codes of professional ethics is to indicate in general terms some of the ethical considerations professionals must take into account in deciding on conduct. Thus, as indicated above, privacy and confidentiality are important considerations. So too are maintaining one's own professional competence and safeguarding patients from the incompetent, unethical, or illegal practice of others.

It is a mistake to think that all a conscientious nurse needs in order to deal with the moral dilemmas that arise in nursing is an adequate code of ethics coupled with a healthy measure of common sense. To demonstrate the limitations of ethical codes, we need only to try to resolve Mary Evans' moral dilemma in "Withholding troublesome details" by appealing to the ICN Code or the ANA Code.

Parts of the ICN Code for Nurses can be cited to support each alternative in Mary Evans' dilemma. For example, a decision to disclose the troublesome details of Luis Vazquez's condition to him and his wife can be based on the provisions of the ICN Code that hold that "The nurse ensures that the individual receives sufficient information on which to base consent for care and related treatment" and "The nurse carries personal responsibility and accountability for nursing practice...." Thus, it could be argued that the ICN Code requires Mary Evans to inform the patient that traces of cancer remained on the margins of his resected prostate gland and that he may, as a result, want to consider beginning additional hormone and radiation treatment within the next six months. Moreover, because Ms. Evans carries personal responsibility for what she does, she, and not the head nurse or the doctor, must make the final decision.

On the other hand, one can also cite provisions of the ICN Code to support the opposing position. For example, the Code also states that nurses have a responsibility to "alleviate suffering" and that they sustain "a cooperative relationship with coworkers in nursing and other fields." It could, therefore, be argued that the Code requires that Mary Evans not inform Luis Vasquez of the troubling details of his surgery, since this may, as Dr. Lampson believes, create additional worry for the already anxious patient and his wife and seriously strain the cooperative relationship she is supposed to sustain with the physician and, perhaps, the nurse manager as well.

To interpret this Code in a way that supports one or the other of Mary Evans' choices would be controversial and would require a considerable amount of supporting argument. Moreover, the usefulness of the Code as a straightforward guide to the resolution of moral dilemmas is significantly diminished by the need for such interpretations.

The source of the difficulty is not so much this particular code but the very idea of attempting to codify, in a simple yet consistent and comprehensive way, all of the precepts one needs to resolve dilemmas in a field as morally complex as nursing. Any such attempt will be caught on the horns of a difficult dilemma. If the code is to be simple, comprehensive, and acceptable to all nurses, it will be so abstract and general that it cannot, without significant interpretation, be applied to many specific problems. Such codes may gain widespread acceptance before their use in actual situations, but only because their abstractness allows people holding opposing views to mask their differences by silently interpreting the code in accord with their favored positions on various issues. When the code is then appealed to in dilemmas like that facing Mary Evans, the hitherto submerged differences in interpretation rise to the surface, and those who are engaged in the dispute must go beyond the code itself in order to resolve them. If, on the other hand, one tries to draft a very specific, concrete code aimed at anticipating all of the moral problems that can arise, one encounters three significant problems. First, the code will not be able to avoid controversial precepts and hence will be unlikely to win widespread acceptance. Second, it will probably fill many thick volumes, and thus lose the advantages of brevity and simplicity. And third, no matter how detailed it is, such a code will always be incomplete if its aim is to give unambiguous guidance in all possible situations. Therefore, neither a brief, simple code nor a long, detailed one will both offer clear guidance and attain widespread acceptance.

Before accepting this argument about the limitations of codes of professional ethics, let us briefly examine the ANA Code for Nurses. The ANA Code, together with its extensive interpretive statements, is much more detailed than the ICN Code. Still, Mary Evans cannot use it in a more or less mechanical way to resolve her dilemma. Provision 1.1, Respect for Human Dignity, says that "A fundamental principle that underlies all nursing practice is respect for the inherent worth, dignity, and human rights of every individual. Nurses take into account the needs and values of all persons in professional relationships." This is a good principle and good advice. But the problems in this case are that the needs, values, and rights of Luis and Geneva Vasquez are not crystal clear and that Mary Evans and Dr. Lampson have different values and interpret them differently. And the principle itself provides no way of resolving it.

Reading further, one might think that Provision 1.4, The Right to Self-Determination, might decisively settle the matter in Mary's favor. It reads:

> Respect for human dignity requires the recognition of specific patient rights, particularly, the right to self-determination.... Patients have the moral and legal right to determine what will be done with their own person; to be given accurate, complete, and understandable information in a manner that facilitates an informed judgment; to be assisted with weighing the benefits, burdens, and available options in their treatment, including the choice of no treatment; to accept, refuse, or terminate treatment without deceit, undue influence, duress, coercion, or penalty; and to be given necessary support throughout the decision-making and treatment process. Such support would include the opportunity to make decisions with family and significant others and the provision of advice and support from knowledgeable nurses and other health professionals. Patients should be involved in planning their own health care to the extent they are able and choose to participate.

Dr. Lampson might well agree with this provision, but at the same time appeal to the last sentence to defend his decision not to inform the patient and his wife of the troublesome details of his surgery. Given their psychological state and the likelihood of his "good success rate" in such cases, he might argue that this part of the Code requires "leaving well enough alone."

Even if, contrary to fact, the ANA Code unambiguously directed Mary Evans to bring the issue of "positive margins" to the attention of Luis and Geneva Vasquez, it would conflict with Dr. Lampson's strong belief that she not do so. He, too, is motivated by ethical considerations. Why therefore should *he* now alter his position? He is not a nurse and the ANA Code is not his code. Why, then, should we think that certain provisions of a nursing code settle the matter for all parties to the situation? If, in this event, Mary Evans is unable to do more than simply recite the relevant sections of her professional code of ethics, she will make little headway in bringing the issue to a satisfactory resolution. She must also be able to set out the *reasoning* or *arguments* underlying these sections. And they are not part of the Code itself; all that can be found in the Code are the *conclusions* of those who had a hand in drafting it.

Furthermore, as Robert M. Veatch has cogently argued, neither nurses nor doctors can reasonably expect a code of ethics drafted by members of their respective professions to be the last word on ethical issues in health care. Most of these issues involve and affect patients, their families, and the public as well as doctors and nurses. And it is hard to see why patients and families should feel themselves bound, ethically, to courses of actions devised solely by health professionals. "An ethic that professionals base on their own consensus of what their role entails has no ethical force," Veatch writes, "at least with nonprofessionals. It is doubtful such a standard can be called an ethic at all."[5] Ethical disagreements in nursing often involve parties who have no special obligation to uphold the rules or ideals of nursing. And the ANA Code has no purchase on doctors or patients and their families if their views run contrary to those embedded in the Code.

Our aim has not been to denigrate the ANA Code and its Interpretive Statements—indeed, as codes of professional ethics go, it is among the best—but rather to demonstrate the limitations of any code of professional ethics as a resource for resolving difficult moral dilemmas in health care. That any code will be limited in this way can be explained in part by an examination of the most basic question of philosophical ethics.

3. THE FUNDAMENTAL QUESTION OF MORALITY

Ethics, understood here as a discipline whose roots go back to Socrates in the fourth century B.C.E., is an attempt to formulate and justify systematic responses to the following questions: What, *all things considered*, ought to be done in a given situation—*and why*? It is the unrestricted frame of reference indicated by the phrase "all things considered" that limits the usefulness of ethical codes and makes ethics such a difficult subject.

Many questions about what a person ought to do raise no ethical questions because they are limited to a certain context where a definite framework establishes various rules and roles that provide unambiguous direction. Thus, suppose that a person is playing checkers. At various points in the game, she may ask herself, What should I do? Assuming that the question is bounded by the rules of the game and motivated by a desire to win, it is not an ethical one. The answer will be determined solely by appeal to the rules and strategies of checkers. Similar questions that arise *within* various clearly defined occupational or familial roles may be answered in the same way. But now suppose that we expand the account of the circumstances of our checker-player to include that her opponent is her six-year-old son, who is just learning the game. Here, the question of what move she ought to make in a given situation is more complex. Of course, if she wants to disregard the fact that her opponent is a beginner and her child, she may proceed as before. But if she considers that her opponent is her son and that he is just learning the game, she will want to play with much less competitive vigor than if he were someone like herself. Her task here is a ticklish one. Because she presumably wants to help develop her son's skills and knowledge without crushing his spirit and enjoyment of the game, she must play reasonably well (otherwise he would not learn to play well himself) but not too well (otherwise his confidence would be dealt a severe blow). So, as this simple example shows, determining what one ought to do, *all things considered*, is more complex than determining what one ought to do within a more narrowly circumscribed frame of reference. And as with the combined roles of checker-player and parent, so too there can be tension between what one ought to do as employee, health professional, citizen, parent, spouse, and so forth, when these roles overlap.

Consider, for example, a driver who approaches an intersection at 3:00 A.M. as he is taking his pregnant wife, whose labor has begun, to the hospital. The light is red, and there are no other cars in sight. Should he wait until the light turns green or proceed through the intersection? As a law-abiding citizen, he has a duty to wait, but as a husband taking his wife to the hospital, it could be argued, he has a duty, after checking for traffic, to continue. Thus, the question arises as to what, all things considered, he ought to do. And this *moral* question requires that the framework of inquiry go beyond a simple appeal to the ordinary requirements of drivers and husbands, respectively.

Ethical issues about whether one ought or ought not to do something arise, then, when a question cannot be answered by appeal to the special or restricted considerations governing simple, clearly defined, and justifiable roles or practices. Here one must enlarge the frame of reference and identify and critically examine all the relevant considerations. It is this matter of a completely unrestricted frame of reference that makes ethical inquiry so difficult. The range and complexity of relevant factual and value-laden considerations often outstrip our initial capacity to comprehend and evaluate them. This is especially true of problems that arise within the medical and nursing context. The problems are more difficult now than ever before partly because the complexities of contemporary health care have required the development of health care "teams" made up of different sorts of professionals whose respective roles cannot always be precisely defined. Given the complexity of the clinical encounter and the nature of ethics (with its completely unrestricted frame of reference), no simple code—together with common sense—can relieve the thoughtful health professional of the difficult and demanding task of ethical inquiry. The reflective nurse cannot put her moral course on "automatic pilot."

4. ETHICAL INQUIRY

Even if a widely accepted code of ethics could provide unambiguous solutions to moral dilemmas in nursing, we would want to know whether these were the best or most nearly correct solutions and if this were the best code. To answer these questions, we would have to rely on conventional ethical analysis and reasoning. The same sort of analysis and reasoning must be applied directly to the dilemmas that resist a codified solution. The first step in this analysis is to identify the ethical or other value-laden issues in nursing in a particular case, and to distinguish them from purely technical or empirical concerns. Next, we use various skills of ethical analysis and reasoning in an attempt to reach a well-grounded solution. At various points in this process, we may also have to consider the nature and limits of ethical knowledge as well as the nature and justification of basic ethical principles.

A. Identification of Ethical Issues

Health care professionals who are unaware of the value-laden elements of their practice may, in the name of technical expertise, impose their (often unexamined) personal values on others without adequate justification. Once it is recognized, however, that a particular question is not solely—or even mainly—a function of medical or nursing expertise, the health care professional can then try to determine who can best answer it and what, all things considered, seems to be the best-grounded solution or range of solutions.

Thus, a decision to withhold troublesome details of a surgical procedure from a patient cannot, like a decision to intubate, be justified by a physician's *medical expertise.* If a nurse and a physician disagree over whether a patient should be intubated, surely the presumption must be that the physician, by virtue of his or her more extensive training and knowledge, is correct. But if, for example, Mary Evans and Dr. Lampson disagree over whether a couple like Mr. and Mrs. Vasquez should be told that Luis's surgery had not quite "got all" of the cancer cells in his prostate gland, the matter of whose opinion should prevail is not quite as clear as it is where intubation is the question. The question of what Mr. and Mrs. Vasquez should be told is basically an ethical one, and the decision and reason underlying it are more a matter of ethical analysis and reasoning than medical knowledge and expertise. Neither the physician, as a physician, nor the nurse, as a nurse, occupies a privileged position for making this decision. Once an issue is identified as basically an ethical or value-laden one, those who address it should employ ethical analysis and reasoning to try to reach a well-grounded, mutually satisfactory solution.

B. Ethical Analysis and Reasoning

Critical reflection and inquiry in ethics involve the complex interplay of a variety of human faculties, ranging from empathy and moral imagination on the one hand to analytic precision and careful reasoning on the other.

The following are among the more cognitive skills one employs in thinking an ethical issue through:

1. *Determining and obtaining relevant factual information.* Although genuine moral dilemmas cannot be resolved simply by an appeal to or understanding of "the facts," certain factual matters will always be relevant to ethical inquiry. If we must reach beyond the facts in attempting to resolve a moral dilemma, we must also guard against reaching without them. Thus, for example, in "Withholding troublesome details," it is important that Mary Evans be very clear about such things as the pathology report, whether her experience of other patients with similar pathology reports choosing to begin additional treatment within six months after surgery is representative of most patients, Mr. and Mrs. Vasquez's capacity to deal with the knowledge of "positive margins," and various other psychosocial and biomedical data.

Although our account of ethical analysis and reasoning begins with determining the facts, we do not want to give the impression that this can always—or even mostly—be completed at the outset. Often, we cannot determine what counts as relevant factual information until we are well into an analysis. As we clarify concepts, construct and evaluate arguments, anticipate and respond to objections, identify relevant ethical principles, and so on, certain factual considerations that we initially thought to be relevant may come to seem less so, and we may perceive a need to obtain other information that, at the outset, seemed less important. In short, what counts as a relevant fact is dynamically related to the other elements of ethical analysis and reasoning. We list the determination of factual information first because it is usually a good way to begin. But the list is not strictly serial; the skills of ethical reasoning are dynamically related, and we will often revise our understanding of an ethical issue and the relevant facts as we employ first one skill and then another.

2. *Aiming at conceptual clarity and drawing relevant distinctions.* The complexity of ethical inquiry often requires careful conceptual analysis and the recognition of important distinctions. For example, many controversies in health care involve conflicting claims of rights. These include the "right to life," the "right to die," "patients' rights," "society's rights," the "right to one's own body," the "right to health care," and numerous other "rights," all of which are often invoked to support one or another resolution to a moral dilemma. But what, exactly, is a "right"? What, we may ask, does it *mean* to say that people have a "right to life"? Does it mean that it is wrong, under any circumstances (e.g., self-defense, war, or capital punishment) to kill people? Or that killing is only wrong when it is "unjust" (and, how, exactly, do we determine whether a particular killing is "unjust")? In

addition, does the "right to life" require that people be given whatever is necessary to sustain their lives (even if so doing requires enormous expenditures and forces significant reductions in other areas such as education, housing, and treatment for illness and injuries that are not life threatening)? A satisfactory analysis of the concept of a "right" and of the various "rights" *in* and *to* health care (including the "right to life") is necessary if appeals to "rights" are to play any but a rhetorical role in the resolution of moral dilemmas in medicine and nursing. The same is true of such concepts as "health," "disease," "care," "death with dignity," "sanctity of life," "euthanasia," "benefit," and "mental illness." One of the reasons ethical debates often become frustrating and fruitless is that the participants fail to clarify adequately what they are talking about.

The result of a careful conceptual analysis is often the recognition of one or more distinctions that had not previously been explicitly recognized. Drawing an important distinction in ethical inquiry can be likened to using fine instruments in surgery. The surgeon needs very fine instruments to cut or suture one particular part of the body while leaving others untouched. Neither a woodsman's axe nor a kitchen knife is suited for surgical incision because each is too crude or blunt and will cut far more than should be cut. So too, in ethical inquiry, one needs fine tools to outline a defensible position on one particular issue without thereby being committed, less defensibly, to the same position on a different kind of issue. It is one thing, for example, to argue for allowing conscious, competent, adult Jehovah's Witnesses to refuse lifesaving blood transfusions for themselves and quite another to allow them to do so for their minor children. Our tools here are words; fine linguistic distinctions, like fine surgical instruments, make possible more precise analysis of complex questions.

As an example of conceptual analysis and drawing relevant distinctions, let us briefly examine the notion of a "medical decision." Patients and physicians often invoke the notion of a "medical decision" to justify the physician's authority to make one or another decision in the course of treatment. Many people, for example, might be inclined to support Dr. Lampson's decision to withhold the troublesome details of Mr. Vasquez's surgery because it is a "medical decision" and he, after all, *is* the doctor. On these grounds, Mary Evans would be overstepping the bounds of her authority by even suggesting that Mr. and Mrs. Vasquez be informed of the "positive margins" of Luis's resected prostate gland. But this line of argument reveals some confusion about the concept of a "medical decision."

There are two critically different senses in which something may be a "medical decision." In the first, a medical decision is one that is based directly on medical knowledge or expertise. Such decisions are a function of a physician's special training. Let us call such decisions "medical decisions in the technical sense" and identify this use of the term "medical decision" with the subscript "*t*." Examples of medical decisions$_t$ are decisions about the medical diagnosis and prognosis of a particular illness, the correct dosage of various medications, and how best to perform a certain surgical procedure in a given case.

The term "medical decision" can also be used to refer to any decision made in the medical context. Such decisions, however, are not always a function of medical knowledge or expertise, though they may be informed by them. They will often turn on questions of value, and, as noted above, the physician's technical expertise does not make him or her an expert on conflicts of value. Let us call such decisions "medical decisions in the contextual sense" and identify this use of the term "medical decisions" with the subscript "c." Decisions in health care that are largely a matter of resolving a conflict of values or of other factors that are not exclusively medical will thus be called medical decisions$_c$. These include decisions about whether a patient should be informed of the diagnosis and prognosis of a certain illness; whether the costs, inconvenience, or risks of a certain medication are outweighed by the benefits; and whether, all things considered, a patient should undergo a certain surgical procedure. Having made this distinction, we can say that not all medical decisions$_c$ are medical decisions$_t$.

The decision about withholding the details of Luis Vasquez's surgery is a medical decision in the contextual sense. The controversy turns largely on a conflict of values and not on matters of medical expertise; viz., whether or not Mr. and Mrs. Vasquez have a right to such a detailed explanation of the results of the surgery. To attempt to cut off ethical inquiry into this matter by an appeal to the decision's medical nature is to fail to appreciate the distinction between medical decisions$_t$ and medical decisions$_c$. Although this does not show that Mary Evans' desire to explain the troublesome details of Luis Vasquez's surgery to him and his wife is correct, it does show that she is not, in pursuing the question, mounting any sort of challenge to Dr. Lampson's expertise *as a physician*. She might be on considerably weaker ground, however, had Dr. Lampson been Mr. Vasquez's long-standing physician who maintains he knows him and his wife much better than she does.

3. *Constructing and evaluating arguments.* We use the word *argument* in the logician's sense, in which an argument is a set of reasons or premises, together with a claim, or conclusion, which they are intended to support. Having identified an ethical issue, we must not only conduct factual and conceptual investigations, we must also construct and evaluate arguments, or chains of reasoning, for and against various positions.

In so doing, we search out reasons for or against a certain position and critically examine the extent to which the reasons, as premises, constitute good grounds for accepting the conclusion. In the case of "Withholding troublesome details," for example, Dr. Lampson suggests an argument for his decision to withhold the details of Mr. Vasquez's surgery. The argument, when spelled out, might have three premises, one of which is assumed to be true, although it is not explicitly stated:

1. Postoperative issues are causing Mr. and Mrs. Vasquez considerable worry.
2. Telling them about the "positive margins" will cause them additional worry, which, based on Dr. Lampson's "good success rate" in similar cases, is unnecessary.
3. Patients and their families ought to be spared unnecessary worry. (This premise seems to be assumed, but is not stated.)
4. Therefore, the best course is for Mary Evans "to leave well enough alone."

If Mary Evans is still inclined to question Dr. Lampson's withholding what she regards as the troublesome details of the surgery, she will have to show exactly where and why this argument fails to support the conclusion that Mr. and Mrs. Vasquez should not be told of the "positive margins."

An argument must meet two principal conditions if its premises are to be regarded as good grounds for accepting the truth of the conclusion. The first has to do with the argument's *validity*. "Validity," as used in logic, is a technical term referring to the logical connection between an argument's premises and its conclusion. An argument is valid if the assumption that its premises are true gives us very good grounds for supposing that its conclusion is true. Validity, then, has to do not with the *actual* truth or falsity of the premises but rather with the logical connection between the premises and conclusion *if* we *suppose* that the premises are true. Thus, for example, both of the following arguments are equally valid, even though the first premise of *B* is, in fact, false:

A. 1. All doctors are human.
   2. All humans are fallible.
   3. Therefore, all doctors are fallible.
B. 1. All nurses are women.
   2. All women are fallible.
   3. Therefore, all nurses are fallible.

Although both *A* and *B* are, strictly speaking, valid arguments, *B* shows that there is more to an argument's providing good grounds for accepting its conclusion than its being valid. The premises of a good argument would not only provide support for the conclusion *if they were true*, but they must also, in fact, *be true*. A valid argument whose premises are true is called a *sound* argument. Both arguments *A* and *B* are valid, but only *A* is sound. An argument whose premises provide good grounds for accepting its conclusion will be sound as well as valid.

Let us now examine the argument we have attributed to Dr. Lampson for its validity and soundness. First, the argument seems valid. If we assume the premises are true, the conclusion will be true. But are the premises, in fact, true? Is the argument sound? It seems to us that the argument, though valid, is of questionable soundness.

Premises 1 and 3 both seem to be true: "positive margins" aside, post-operative issues *do* seem to be causing the patient and his wife considerable worry; and patients and their families ought to be spared unnecessary worry. The problem is with premise 2. Would the additional worry the Vasquez's might experience if informed about the "positive margins" really, as Dr. Lampson maintains, be "unnecessary"?

Note that premise 2 is itself a compressed argument. Spelled out, it goes something like this:

1. Dr. Lampson has had a "good success rate" in similar cases.
2. Therefore, telling Mr. and Mrs. Vasquez about the "positive margins" will cause them to worry *unnecessarily*.

This, however, is *not*, as it stands, a valid argument. First, we do not know exactly what Dr. Lampson means by a "good success rate." Is it 100%? 90%? 80%? 70%? Or is it even lower? Surely the lower the exact success rate, the stronger the reason for informing the couple about the remaining cancer cells and the less reason for characterizing the additional worry this will bring as "unnecessary." Moreover, the best judge of what counts as a "good success rate" may be the patient, not the doctor. And for the patient to make this judgment, he or she has to be adequately informed of the circumstances. Second, we need to know how many similar situations Dr. Lampson has encountered. If, for example, he has experienced only two similar situations in the past, and there were no problems, the sample is too small for his claim of a "good success rate" to be meaningful. Therefore, without further clarification, Mary Evans has no reason to accept the truth of the second premise of Dr. Lampson's argument, thus no reason to accept the truth of the conclusion.

If Mary Evans can identify these weaknesses of Dr. Lampson's argument, she can add that in her experience, other patients informed of similar pathology reports had chosen to begin additional treatment (hormone and radiation) within six months after surgery and that the same choice ought, perhaps, to be given to Luis Vasquez. Granted, this information is likely to cause Luis and his wife additional worry, but it has to be shown that it is *unnecessary*. Perhaps, when looking at the larger scheme of things, it could be argued that this worry, though regrettable, is, all things considered, unavoidable if certain other important values are to be acknowledged (such as a patient's right to make informed decisions about his or her treatment and optimizing the likelihood of a good outcome). Dr. Lampson also seems to assume that Mr. and Mrs. Vasquez would be so worried by the troublesome details of the surgery that they would be unable to make informed decisions about further treatment. Given, however, that he is not Luis Vasquez's long-standing physician, what basis does he have for making such a judgment?

Our reconstruction and evaluation of Dr. Lampson's argument have shown that it cannot, at this point, be accepted as sound. Further questions have to be answered. We have not, however, shown that his conclusion (the best course for Mary Evans is to "leave well enough alone") is false—only that the argument he appears to have in mind does not, in its present form, support his conclusion. It is still open to him to sharpen or reformulate the argument so that the premises do, in fact, provide good grounds for accept-ing his conclusion. On the other hand, those who want to show not only that his argument is weak but also that his conclusion is false must now attempt to construct a sound argument whose conclusion is something like: The troubling details of Mr. Vasquez's surgery ought to be shared with him and his wife. A more thorough examination of the sorts of arguments that might be given in this case and how Mary Evans and Dr. Lampson might discuss and examine them will be found in subsequent chapters.

We have, in this brief illustration, only scratched the surface of what is involved in constructing and evaluating arguments. Readers who want to develop their skills in this all-important activity are advised to work their way through one or more of the books listed under "Philosophical Analysis and Reasoning" in the Suggestions for Further Reading at the end of this book. Another alternative, for students, is an introductory course in logic.

4. *Developing a systematic framework.* Efforts to construct and evaluate particular arguments should draw upon and be incorporated into a devel-oping, systematic, ethical framework. The development of such a frame-work is important for two reasons. First, it provides a common ground for resolving moral disagreements. Insofar as we share a systematic framework made up of principles, rules, concepts, distinctions, standards of justifica-tion, and so on, we will then be able to use it to think through and settle certain disputes. And even in those cases—so frequent in contemporary health care—in which such a framework gives no direct guidance, it can at least provide a common background and starting point for the development of satisfactory resolutions.

Second, the development of a systematic ethical framework is of personal as well as interpersonal value. One of the qualities most of us admire in others and try to cultivate in ourselves is personal integrity. A person of integrity, in this sense, is one whose responses to various matters are not capricious or arbitrary, but principled. Such a person attempts to respond to new situations, as far as possible, in ways that are consistent with justifiable responses to past situations. The principled continuity of conduct is part of his or her identity as a person, and the degree to which he or she is able to *integrate* responses to various situations determines the extent of his or her integrity and identity as a particular person. Thus, so far as a person wants to maintain a unitary sense of identity and an accompanying sense of personal integrity and reliability, he or she will want to develop a systematic framework for analyzing and responding to ethical issues.

Given the open-ended nature of the fundamental question of morality ("What, all things considered, ought to be done?") and the complexity of our rapidly changing world (with the special difficulties created by the high stakes, personal intimacy, and enlarged range of possibilities that characterize moral dilemmas in the medical context), the development and maintenance of a personal and interpersonal ethical framework requires continual attention. As an ethical framework is repeatedly applied, tested, refined, and revised, its adequacy is gauged by the extent to which it is consistent, coherent, and comprehensive.

An ethical framework is *consistent* to the extent that its particular judgments, rules, and principles are logically compatible and do not contradict one another. An example of inconsistency in an ethical framework occurs when a nurse argues for continued, extensive treatment for certain seriously ill patients but believes that such treatment would be undesirable in similar clinical situations for herself or her relatives. Unless such a nurse can justifiably demonstrate a morally relevant difference between these particular seriously ill patients and herself or her relatives, her ethical framework is inconsistent. Other things being equal, if aggressive management is indicated for other persons, it is indicated for oneself or one's relatives; if less aggressive treatment is desirable for oneself, it is, other things being equal, desirable for other persons.[6]

An ethical framework is *coherent* insofar as its individual judgments, rules, and principles are mutually supportive. The elements of a coherent framework "hang together" so that it provides a systematic basis for addressing unprecedented dilemmas. Controversy over the use of new life-prolonging medical technology, for example, might be more readily resolved by an appeal to a set of rules and principles that are themselves related to widely accepted judgments about prolonging life in less controversial contexts.

It is often tempting to obtain both consistency and coherence by restricting a framework's domain or *comprehensiveness*. If consistency has to do with logical compatibility and coherence with mutual support, both will be easier to achieve and maintain within a restricted frame of reference. But to do so would be to retreat from one of the aims of systematic ethical inquiry: the development of a comprehensive framework that will provide guidance in a large number of contexts of moral choice. Other things being equal, then, the wider the range of situations in which a framework is able to provide systematic (i.e., consistent and coherent) guidance, the better the framework is.

Although consistency, coherence, and comprehensiveness are equally important criteria for the adequacy of an ethical framework, people sometimes overemphasize one at the expense of the others. They may, for instance, place a high value on consistency and coherence at the expense of comprehensiveness. Issues that either create conflicts among values or cannot neatly be integrated into the core of their value system are simply disregarded. It is thus that many in health care are tempted to ignore social, political, and economic considerations that would, if acknowledged, strain their framework's consistency and coherence (e.g., ignoring the social and economic costs of providing everyone the same level of care available to the President). But the gain is illusory. Since the social, political, and economic dimensions of health care create new ethical dilemmas as well as aggravate more conventional ones, they cannot be ignored. Any ethical framework that cannot or does not incorporate them is, to that extent, insufficiently comprehensive. We will have more to say about developing and revising a systematic framework in the following chapter.

5. *Anticipating and responding to objections.* No matter how careful our ethical analysis has been, it is always possible that our reasoning was defective, that we overlooked some important factor, or that new social or biomedical developments have undermined some of our basic assumptions. We must therefore be concerned not only with critically evaluating the positions of others, but also with anticipating and responding to possible objections to our own position and arguments. As John Stuart Mill argues in his celebrated essay *On Liberty*:

> He who knows only his own side of the case knows little of that. His reasons may be good, and no one may have been able to refute them. But if he is equally unable to refute the reasons on the opposite side, if he does not so much as know what they are, he has no ground for preferring either opinion.... Ninety-nine in a hundred of what are called educated men are in this condition, even of those who can argue fluently for their opinions. Their conclusion may be true, but it might be false for anything they know; they have never thrown themselves into a mental position of those who think differently from them, and considered what such persons may have to say; and, consequently, they do not, in any proper sense of the word, know the

doctrine which they themselves profess....So essential is this discipline to a real understanding of moral and human subjects that, if opponents of all-important truths do not exist, it is indispensable to imagine them and supply them with the strongest arguments which the most skillful devil's advocate can conjure up.[7]

C. Ethical Principles and Knowledge

In addition to skills in ethical analysis and reasoning, ethical inquiry often requires an understanding of the nature and justification of basic ethical principles, the status of knowledge in ethics, and the relationship among ethics, law, and religion. These very complex topics will be examined in the next chapter. What follows is simply a brief introduction to each area in order to complete our overview of ethical inquiry.

1. *Basic ethical principles.* Suppose Mary Evans and Dr. Lampson agree, after some discussion, that the question of whether to disclose the troubling details of Luis Vasquez's prostatectomy is a moral and not a purely medical matter. Suppose, too, that they agree on the facts (including that informing Mr. and Mrs. Vasquez of the positive margins will cause them additional, though perhaps not incapacitating, distress), and that they are using words in the same way. In these circumstances, it is still possible for Mary Evans and Dr. Lampson to disagree, if, for example, the principle of utility is the foundation of his ethical framework while she espouses some version of the Kantian notion of respect for personal autonomy and dignity as the basic principle of ethics.

Appealing to the utilitarian imperative to maximize the general happiness, Dr. Lampson may reason that not informing Mr. and Mrs. Vasquez is likely, on balance, to bring about more happiness than unhappiness and that therefore they should not be informed of the positive margins. If in the unlikely event there is a rise in Luis's PSA, indicating a recurrence of the cancer, in the next 18 months or so, he will start Luis on hormone treatments. Mary Evans, on the other hand, may argue that preserving a person's autonomy and right to choose is more important from a moral point of view than maximizing his or her happiness. Since withholding the troubling details of his surgery both restricts Mr. Vasquez's autonomy and violates his dignity as a self-determining person, she would argue that he ought to be made aware of the positive margins even if this makes him and his wife even more nervous and distressed than they already are. If the disagreement between Mary Evans and Dr. Lampson takes this form, there is no way to resolve it apart from examining the nature and justification of the principle of utility and the principle of respect for self-determination and attempting to determine which principle is more fundamental in cases like this where they give conflicting direction.

2. *Knowledge in ethics.* How do we determine whether one or another ethical decision or principle is better grounded than the others? Can we *know* that some position or framework is better than its rivals, or are such choices ultimately matters of personal opinion or individual taste? To answer these questions, we must say something about the extent to which ethics is a cognitive discipline. Many people believe there is no such thing as knowledge in ethics, and thus no way to know that one decision or principle is better than the others. Moral judgments and principles, they maintain, are at bottom "merely subjective" and nothing more than expressions of personal preference or taste. If this were true, our efforts to use reason, evidence, and argument to resolve moral dilemmas and disagreements would be of limited value. So it is vital to show the extent to which ethics can be regarded as a cognitive discipline and exactly what it means to have knowledge in ethics (see Chapter 2).

3. *Ethics, law, and religion.* Legal and religious considerations may be relevant in various ways to the resolution of moral dilemmas. But how are they relevant and how much weight are they to be given in various contexts? To what extent, for example, can Mary Evans or Dr. Lampson appeal to the law to support their respective positions? If something is illegal, is it also necessarily unethical? And if something is not illegal, does it follow that it is ethically permissible? Some understanding of the complex relationships between ethical and legal considerations is necessary for ethical inquiry.

So too is an understanding of the relationships between religious and ethical considerations. For we may ask to what extent, if any, are ethical claims grounded upon, and inseparable from, religious ones? And to what extent must an acceptable ethical framework allow for decisions based on appeals to religious conviction?

5. ETHICAL AUTONOMY AND INSTITUTIONAL–HIERARCHICAL CONSTRAINTS

Generally speaking, individuals are autonomous to the extent that they are self-determining or able to act in accord with a plan or course of action they have either freely chosen or at least independently endorsed. In everyday life, personal autonomy is a function of the degree to which one can be regarded as *one's own person*, capable of independent action and judgment. By regarding autonomy as a matter of degree, we suggest that people can be *more* or *less* autonomous than others as well as more autonomous in one area of their lives and less in another. Thus, for example, Anu can be regarded as more autonomous than Bonita, but less so than Claire; and she can be more autonomous as a mother than she is as a wife or teacher.

Ethical autonomy has a central place in the network of moral concepts and is closely related to the notions of personhood, self-respect, and moral responsibility. In fact, it is unlikely that a satisfactory analysis of any of these concepts can avoid referring to the others. Ethical autonomy involves being one's own person when one decides upon or judges conduct. To the extent that someone is not her own person, her will becomes the instrument of another or she may become a "cog in a machine." To be seen in this way is to fail to be respected as a person. Respect for persons, Kant pointed out, involves their being regarded as *ends-in-themselves*, not as mere means to someone else's ends. To be an end-in-oneself is to be capable of independent thought and action. Thus, the choices, commitments, and projects of an end-in-oneself are worthy of respect not because they produce good results but because they *are* the choices, commitments, and projects of a person. To have self-respect in this context is simply to respect oneself *as a person*, as a being capable of deliberation on ethical questions and one whose choices and decisions, when effected, will result in certain changes in the world. In the ethical sphere, then, self-respect includes holding oneself morally responsible for the results of one's choices and decisions. We may summarize this extremely brief account by stating that to respect oneself (and be respected) as a person, it is necessary to cultivate one's ethical autonomy and thus increase the range of things for which one is morally responsible.

A special problem, however, arises for nurses. Put bluntly, it is this: To what extent can a nurse be ethically autonomous? Consider, for example, this dated, but nonetheless influential, view of the primary role of a nurse:

> In my estimation obedience is the first law and the very cornerstone of good nursing. And here is the first stumbling block for the beginner. No matter how gifted she may be, she will never become a reliable nurse until she can obey without question. The first and most helpful criticism I ever received from a doctor was when he told me that I was supposed to be simply an intelligent machine for the purpose of carrying out his orders.[8]

Good nursing and ethical autonomy are, according to this writer, incompatible.

Although the author of this passage is reported to have been "a considerable influence on nursing in her time,"[9] that time was nearly a century ago, and her position would probably be met with disbelief or scorn if propounded to nurses today. Yet, the behavior it urges nurses to adopt may to a large extent remain even when exhortations to practice it may have become embarrassing. Nearly 50 years later, for example, a study of nurse–physician relationships revealed that nurses often complied with medical directives that they knew fell short of minimally decent standards of practice.[10] The researchers structured a situation in which a doctor directed a nurse to administer a particular dose of medication. The directive was unusual because the dosage of medication was obviously excessive; the directive was transmitted by telephone, which violated hospital policy; the voice was one with which the nurse was not familiar; and the medication was unauthorized inasmuch as it had not been placed on the ward stock list. Nonetheless, the study showed that 21 out of a sample of 22 nurses placed in this situation prepared the medication and were ready to give it to the patient when the researchers finally intervened.

This study bears on our present concerns in two ways. First, it shows that some degree of ethical autonomy is a desirable characteristic in a nurse *as a nurse*. As the authors of the study state:

> In a real-life situation corresponding to the experimental one, there would in theory be two professional intelligences, the doctor's and the nurse's, working to ensure that a given procedure be undertaken in a manner beneficial to the patient or, at the very least, not detrimental to him. The experiment strongly suggests, however, that in the real-life situation one of these intelligences is, for all practical purposes, nonfunctioning.[11]

Second, the study obviously indicates that there may be a discrepancy between a nurse's professed ethical autonomy and the actual nature of her behavior in situations where its exercise involves possible conflicts with physicians, hospitals, or others presumed to have some authority. The researchers observe that

> in nonstressful moments, when thinking about her performance, the average nurse tends to believe that considerations of her patient's welfare and of her own professional honor will outweigh considerations leading to automatic obedience to the doctor's orders at times when these two sets of factors come into conflict.[12]

The nursing context is characterized by a number of constraints that make the exercise of autonomy problematic. In 1988, the Secretary's Commission on Nursing, a 25-member public policy advisory panel established by Otis R. Bowen, Department of Health and Human Services (DHHS), reported that constraints on nursing decision making contributed to problems in nurse recruitment and retention. The commission specifically recommended the following:

> Employers of nurses, as well as the medical profession, should recognize the appropriate clinical decision-making authority of nurses in relationship to other health care professionals, foster communication and collaboration

among the health care team, and ensure that the appropriate provider delivers the necessary care. Close cooperation and mutual respect between nursing and medicine are essential.[13]

Underscoring the critical importance of clinical decision-making authority of nurses that reaches beyond effects on recruitment and retention, research in the twenty-first century indicates that workplace issues of communication and collaboration affect patient outcomes. For example, in 2007, Milisa Manojlovich and Barry DeCicco reported in a study on hospital work environments "that small but significant decreases in medication errors can be achieved when nurses and physicians communicate better."[14]

Nurses' attitudes about their professional relationships with physicians are more positive than those of almost two decades ago, according to a survey published in *Nursing2008*. The recent survey reported that 57% of nurses (compared with 43% of nurses in the 1991 survey) were generally satisfied in their professional relationships with physicians. Still, just fewer than half of nurses surveyed (43%) remained dissatisfied.[15]

Nurses who face workplace issues of communication, collaboration, and dissatisfaction with their relationships with physicians must contend not only with the conventional hierarchical structure of medical decision making in some instances but also with restrictions on behavior a hospital's bureaucratic system may impose. Thus, a hospital nurse can find herself constrained in various and occasionally conflicting ways by the hospital (which employs her), the physician (with whom she works), the patient (for whom she provides care), and the nursing profession (to which she belongs). To what extent can she be her own person—that is, be ethically autonomous—in these circumstances? The same kinds of difficulties, it should be noted, can arise for public health and visiting nurses, school and industrial nurses, and nurses working in extended care facilities. In these settings, the agency or organization for which nurses work places similar limits on their practice as does the hospital. In the following chapters, different cases will illustrate this problem of ethical autonomy, which is so basic to the consideration of ethics in nursing and so difficult to resolve.

We conclude this section with two important reminders about the notion of autonomy. First, autonomy does not mean unconditional freedom that would allow us to will or do anything. We are all aware of the formative influence of genes, culture, and social environment. Long before we were able to think for ourselves, each of us was provided with a set of emotions, beliefs, desires, principles, and so on. Nonetheless, how we use our natural, cultural, and social endowments in responding to the environment is, to varying degrees, up to us. As Gerald Dworkin has put it: "If the autonomous man cannot adopt his motivations *de novo*, he can still judge them after the fact. The autonomous individual is able to step back and formulate an attitude towards the factors that influence his behavior."[16] Autonomy, therefore, is compatible with a view of the world that includes a great deal of causal determination and constraints on our behavior.

Second, ethical autonomy involves thinking *for* oneself, not (only) *of* oneself or *by* oneself. To think only of oneself involves the object and not the manner of one's thinking. Thinking by oneself, like "thinking for oneself," does designate a manner of thinking, but in ethics this manner of thinking is unlikely to yield the best results. Given the unrestricted frame of reference and complexity of ethical inquiry, thinking *for* oneself is usually more successful if it includes at least some thinking *with* others who can call one's attention to relevant considerations that one might otherwise have overlooked or misunderstood. This is why discussion with people of various relevant backgrounds is vital to sound ethical inquiry. Thus, we may conclude, being one's own person or ethically autonomous implies neither selfishness nor isolation. One may perfectly well think *for* oneself and still think *about* and *with* others.[17]

2

Unavoidable Topics in Ethical Theory

Ethical inquiry in everyday life and in health care often proceeds without formal recourse to ethical theory. Questions may be clarified, distinctions drawn, arguments examined, and solutions found without appealing to theoretical considerations about the nature and justification of basic principles. Thus, the fact that two people have different foundations for their ethical views is sometimes irrelevant to the resolution of a particular problem.

Suppose, for example, a question arises over whether everything possible should be done to prolong the life of an elderly man in a nursing home. Suppose, too, that he has no known family and that the decision must be made by the staff. One person, Alison, might argue that the man should be treated because not to do so would be to violate a fundamental duty to preserve and prolong life. Another person, Beate, might also argue that the man should be treated, but for different reasons. Beate may argue that the man is not in severe pain and that even though his mental capacities are significantly impaired, he seems to be reasonably content. Since it is Beate's view that we ought, above all, to do what will maximize happiness, she believed that efforts to prolong the man's life should, under these circumstances, continue. So, the issue in this case can be resolved despite the fact that Alison and Beate hold different basic principles and, perhaps, different conceptions of how they are known and justified.

Yet things do not always work out this way. Sometimes different positions on a particular ethical issue are a direct function of the parties' holding different ethical principles. In this event, the issue cannot be resolved without some discussion of the nature and justification of ethical principles underlying different positions. Suppose, for example, that the facts in the case sketched above were altered so that the patient was experiencing immitigable pain and distress. In this case Beate, with her basic commitment to maximizing happiness, would have to revise her earlier judgment and say that efforts to extend the man's life should no longer be as strenuous. However, this change, in fact, would not be relevant to Alison, and her judgment that the patient's life should be prolonged would be the same. Here the resulting disagreement is rooted firmly in the difference between their basic principles. If they pursue the matter further, they will encounter questions about the nature and justification of ethical principles that have long been the subject of ethical theory.

This chapter is a bare-bones introduction to topics in theoretical ethics that cannot be avoided by anyone who seeks to develop systematic responses to ethical issues in nursing. First, we will make a brief survey of *basic* ethical principles. Second, we will identify and assess the strengths and weaknesses of comprehensive theories grounded on each of these ethical principles. Then, we will outline an increasingly popular approach called "moral pluralism" that maintains that ethical questions are too many and too varied to be satisfactorily addressed by any single principle or comprehensive theory, including theories centered on virtues like caring. Caring, though of vital importance to nursing, cannot serve as the basis of a comprehensive theory. We will then develop an account of ethical reasoning and knowledge true to the complexity of ethical questions in personal and professional life. Finally, we will address the important question of the relationships and relative priority of ethical, legal, and religious considerations in a pluralistic society.

1. BASIC ETHICAL PRINCIPLES

Persons favoring different ethical principles might well come to different conclusions about what ought to have been done by the various parties in the following case.

2.1 Plans for Suicide

During fall semester, student Beth Robinson, along with five other students under their instructor's supervision, spent a number of half days at the Community Senior Center where the College of Nursing had established a locally supported "foot clinic." The clinic was not free, but nearly; each visit costing $2.00. During a visit, senior citizens could expect to have blood pressures checked, toenails and foot problems attended to by a qualified podiatrist, and opportunities to talk about health issues with a nurse practitioner. Persons with diabetes, cardiac, and various ongoing health issues returned almost weekly.

Bill and Norma Groth came to the clinic routinely. Both, now in their mid-80s, had been volunteer workers at the center since they retired. But during the last five years, they have each developed serious health problems. Bill has cardiac problems and great difficulty in walking. Norma has declined mentally and has become increasingly dependent on Bill. She also has lost much of her sight. Although Bill has difficulty getting around, he is Norma's principal caregiver. Beth has been assigned to the couple regularly, and they have gotten to know each other rather well.

One morning, well into the semester, Bill startled Beth by talking about the horror he feels when he thinks of Norma and himself ending their lives in a nursing home "spending all their hard earned money on diapers." He said they had too many friends who had wasted money on high-priced nursing homes. Their friends had spent thousands of dollars, but had been unhappy and unable to enjoy life as they waited for what Bill characterized as "the merciful release of death." He added that he and Norma had been too old and too decrepit to buy long-term care insurance when it became available; it had simply cost too much. A year of nursing home care for both of them, he thought, would completely "eat up" what they would receive from selling their modest home and that their other savings would be gone in another year.

Beth was too surprised to make any response. Besides, she didn't think Bill was asking for one. He was simply expressing his innermost thoughts to someone he had grown to like and trust.

The next week, Bill brought up the subject again. He and Norma had thought about the high cost of nursing home care for a long time, and they both wanted to leave what money they had in savings to their children and grandchildren who, they thought, could make much better use of it. He explained to Beth that he had told their plan to his doctor and their daughter, who visited or phoned them every day: they would go into their closed garage, start the car, hold hands, and die together.

Beth discussed each of her conversations with the Groths with her clinical instructor. Beth thought that encouraging Bill to use more community support, such as meals-on-wheels, would lighten his load and help him refocus his thoughts on living rather than suicide. She had no answer, however, to the basic money issue. She knew that only after the Groths had spent their savings would they be eligible for state subsidized nursing home care. She knew of no way they could be partially subsidized and save something for their children. But she did not believe that leaving money to one's children or grandchildren justified killing oneself.

The Groths missed the next clinic, and a week later, Beth read in the local newspaper that the couple had died in their home. Neither obituary listed the cause of death, but one of their friends at the Community Senior Center later informed her that they had been asphyxiated in their garage.[1]

This case raises so many complex issues it would take an entire chapter, if not a book, to adequately sort through and address them. We will refer back to some of these issues in subsequent chapters. Our aim here is simply to illustrate how basic ethical principles occupy a central role in ethical inquiry. So, consider the following excerpt of a fictional discussion of this case by three nurses.

Livia: For me, the most fundamental ethical principle—especially for nurses and other health professionals—is to preserve and prolong human life. So, I think everyone involved—Bill and Norma Groth, their daughter, Beth, Beth's clinical instructor, and the Groths' doctor—failed in different degrees to respect this important principle. The Groths had a duty to remain alive, and Beth and any other health professional who knew of what the couple was thinking had a duty to do everything in their power to prevent them from ending their lives. Life is sacred and must be preserved *no matter what*. If a nurse doesn't believe this, she shouldn't be in health care.

Renee: But what about the pain and suffering the Groths were undergoing and their belief that ending their lives would be better for themselves and for everyone else except, perhaps, those running the nursing home?

Livia: I'm not denying that these things are important, but if you have to choose between people's being better off while alive and *life itself*, you have to go with life. Life itself is more important than making people better off.

Ursula: Boy, nothing personal, Livia, but that kind of rigid, moralistic thinking really drives me up the wall. I mean, how can you have so much confidence in an absolute rule like "Always preserve and protect life?" I can think of lots of cases where the consequences of doing that would do nothing but make everybody more miserable. And given the cost of care these days, we'd be spending nearly all our money on keeping people alive rather than keeping them healthy while alive. I really think we've got to get away from these old-fashioned dos and don'ts and start taking specific circumstances into account and being more flexible.

Livia: Then, what do you think ought to have happened in this case?

Ursula: Well, I think there are a lot of unanswered questions in this case. For example, we don't know whether Norma Groth agrees with her husband. He does all the talking. Does her mental "decline" prevent her from really participating in the discussion or decision? If so, can we know that she agreed with what Bill's thought about suicide before her mental decline? Did their daughter agree with Bill's thinking?

Moreover, the case implies that the Groths had, at least, one other grown child. What did he or she (or they) think about Bill's decision? Did the Groths have an accurate picture about what life would be in a nursing home for them—and what it would cost? What sorts of things could Beth or the Groths' doctor actually have done to prevent what happened? Once we have answers to these and, perhaps, other questions, then we can then figure out what would be best— have the best consequences—for everyone involved.

Livia: Do you really think, if your questions were answered in a certain way, the Groths would be justified in ending their lives, and Beth, their doctor, and their daughter justified in not doing everything in their power to prevent them from doing so?

Ursula: Yes, if taking everything into account, this would be the best outcome for all.

Livia: I couldn't agree with that. What do you think Renee? Which of us is right?

Renee: I don't know. Frankly, I can't go along a hundred percent with either of you. For me, the most important thing is to respect people's rights,—their right to life and, in rare circumstances, their right to end their lives. The right to end your life assumes you're fully informed of the circumstances and capable of rational deliberation and making decisions in accord with your deepest values. Granted, research has shown that most people who think about or attempt suicide are either or both not fully informed of their situation or not capable of rational deliberation (due to, for example, duress, mental illness, or poor impulse control), but still I can think of circumstances in which a patient's ending his or her life is not absolutely wrong and ought not to be interfered with. And I'm not alone in this. Some patients do it when they refuse life-preserving treatment, which is in many cases perfectly legal. In other cases, they may take more active measures. In Oregon, Washington state, and Switzerland, for example, terminally ill patients may, under certain conditions, formally request their physicians to assist them in ending their lives; and their physicians may legally comply with such requests. And I think it's okay. Granted, it's always important to do what we can to make the life-affirming decision as attractive as possible, but some people in some circumstances should have a right to make the decision for themselves.

Ursula: But, I think your right to live as you see fit, including, in certain circumstances a right to end your life, is just as old-fashioned and rigid as Livia's duty to live. As a matter of fact, it's the same thing only inside out. I can imagine a situation in which someone who exercised what you consider a right to end his or her life would make everyone else—the person's family, friends, health care professionals, and the society at large—totally miserable. And I'd say that's wrong.

Renee: I don't know, Ursula, except that here I agree partly with you and partly with Livia. I agree with you that a terminally ill patient considering physician-assisted suicide in, say, Oregon, ought to consider the consequences of his or her actually doing it on his or her friends and family. In some cases, it may be ethically wrong to *exercise* a moral and legal right. And I agree with Livia that some things are right or wrong even if they don't bring about the most happiness. And respecting people's basic right to live their lives as they see fit—including in rare circumstances ending their lives—is one of them.

In this admittedly contrived discussion, each position is based on a different basic ethical principle. Livia believes that life is sacred, and therefore her principle is that we ought always to do whatever will preserve or prolong life. Although she does not deny the importance of happiness or respecting people's rights, in cases like this, they are not as fundamental as protecting and preserving life. Ursula, on the other hand, emphasizes the principle of utility—an ethical principle emphasizing the consequences of our actions. According to the principle of utility, the right action in any circumstance is the one that will bring about the greatest net balance of happiness over unhappiness for all affected by it. Finally, Renee emphasizes the importance of people's right to autonomy or self-determination. For her, adequately informed, mentally competent adults have a right to decide for themselves not only how to lead their lives, but also, in certain cases, whether to hasten their deaths. This right occupies the same place in her thinking as the duty to preserve and prolong life does in Livia's. Although Renee does not deny the importance of happiness, maximizing it is always limited by respecting informed, rational people's right to live—and in certain circumstances die—as they see fit.

In the remainder of this section, we will elaborate each of these three principles and their justifications. We begin with the principle enjoining us to protect and preserve life. We turn then to the principle of utility and after this to the principle of autonomy (sometimes also called, for reasons that will be made clear, the principle of "respect for persons"). In the following section, we will show how each of these principles has been taken to be the foundation of a comprehensive ethical theory.

A. The Principle of the Sanctity of Life

Livia is certainly correct that a principle directing us to preserve and prolong life has long been a cornerstone of medical and nursing morality, and there is no question that it is still the reigning principle in certain contexts, such as the battlefield and the emergency room. In its strongest form, the principle is based on a doctrine called "vitalism," which holds that human life is an absolute moral value. Vitalists believe it is wrong either to hasten death or refrain from prolonging life regardless of pain, suffering, patients' wishes, or expense. No effort or costs should be spared in attempting to preserve or prolong human life.

Though there may be significant numbers of vitalists in other cultures, this doctrine is no longer as central to Western medicine and nursing as it once was. This is partly due to advances in medicine and technology that permit us to preserve and prolong life in circumstances where the burdens in terms of pain, suffering, and sometimes cost seem greatly to outweigh the benefits. Refusing to compromise vitalist doctrine in such circumstances—for example, aggressively treating anencephalic infants, the permanently comatose, and those undergoing immitigable pain and suffering in the last states of terminal illness—borders on fanaticism. It is also due to the recognition, at least in the United States, of the importance of respecting personal choice (or autonomy) and the belief that in some cases, the principle of autonomy may be more important than the principle of preserving or prolonging life. This is exemplified in situations in which informed, mentally competent patients are permitted to refuse life-prolonging treatment. The most dramatic example is, perhaps, the refusal of life-saving blood transfusions by informed, mentally competent, adult Jehovah's Witnesses *even if* after the transfusions they would be "good as new." Here, we say legally, if not also morally, that a person's right to live according to his or her deepest convictions—in this case religious convictions—is more important than (earthly) life itself. In 1990, the U.S. Supreme Court in the case of *Cruzan v. Director, Missouri Department of Health* recognized a (Constitutional) right to refuse medical treatment, even life-preserving medical treatment, on the part of informed, competent adults. The Court indicated that this right could also be exercised in the event of a loss of competence if there were clear and convincing evidence (usually in the form of a written advance directive) of the patient's wishes.

Thus, a duty to preserve and prolong life, while still very important, no longer reigns supreme in health care. It is not absolute or unconditional. It sometimes conflicts with, and must give way to other important values and principles including a duty to respect patient autonomy. Still, it may be argued, respecting a patient's right to refuse life-prolonging treatment is one thing, and respecting—or worse yet, aiding—a patient's decision to actively end his or her own life is quite another because intentionally ending one's own life, is *always* wrong.

The principal arguments for this view may be traced to St. Augustine in the fourth century. He maintained that the Biblical commandment "Thou shalt not kill" implies that it is as wrong to take one's own life as it is to take the life of another.[2] Then, in the thirteenth century, Thomas Aquinas developed a more elaborate set of arguments that remain influential to this day. Suicide, he maintained, was a sin against oneself, one's neighbors, and God. It is a sin against oneself because every living organism has a desire, built-in by nature, to prolong its life. It is a sin against one's neighbors because it prevents one from fulfilling one's social obligations. And, it is a sin against God because only God has the right to determine whether a person should live or die.[3]

Contemporary support for a duty not only to refrain from killing oneself but also to prevent others from killing themselves comes from sociological research indicating that in most cases those who attempt suicide don't really want to die. They are mentally ill, confused, ill-informed, or acting on momentary irrational impulse. Given this information, certainly health professionals are generally justified on parentalistic grounds (see Chapter 3, Section 1) in doing what they can to prevent nearly all patients, especially those whom they do not know exceptionally well, from attempting suicide. In the large majority of such cases, the patient does not really want to die. So, despite advances in medical knowledge and technology and the importance of patient autonomy and a correlative right to refuse medical treatment, there is considerable support for a principle directing us, as individuals, to refrain from committing suicide and, as citizens and especially as health professionals, to do what we can to prevent it.

B. The Principle of Utility

The principle of utility was articulated and developed in the nineteenth century by philosophers Jeremy Bentham and John Stuart Mill. It directs us to perform those actions likely to have the best consequences for all affected by them. Mill puts it this way: "The creed which accepts as the foundation of morals, utility, or the greatest happiness principle, holds that actions are right in proportion as they tend to promote happiness, wrong as they tend to produce the reverse of happiness. By happiness is intended pleasure and the absence of pain; by unhappiness, pain and the privation of pleasure." A bit later he adds that "...[T]he happiness which forms the utilitarian standard of what is right in conduct is not the agent's own happiness, but that of all concerned. As between his own happiness and that of others, utilitarianism requires him to be as strictly neutral as a disinterested and benevolent spectator."[4]

Even if Ursula, in the foregoing discussion, has never even heard of Bentham or Mill, she has a strong intuitive grasp of the principle of utility. Indeed, Bentham and Mill would argue that this is one of the principle's strengths: it is so reasonable—so well suited to human life and welfare—that reasonable people can't help but appeal to it, even if they've never formally heard of it (or, if in their more theoretical moments, they argue against it). What could be more reasonable in deciding what to do in a complex world than estimating the consequences of all possible courses of action and then performing the one that is likely to have the best overall consequence, in terms of happiness and unhappiness, for all concerned?

Ursula is tacitly appealing to the principle of utility in wanting to obtain as much information as possible about the situation and then making the decision likely to maximize overall happiness. She needs as much information as possible, which is why she asks so many questions about the situation before venturing an opinion. Depending on the results of such an investigation, the utilitarian principle could conclude *either* that the Groths were wrong to commit suicide and others were wrong to have either endorsed what they did or failed to prevent it (because the Groths' joint suicide would result in more unhappiness than happiness) *or* that the Groths were right to commit suicide and others would have acted wrongly if they'd tried to prevent it (because suicide in this instance would have resulted in more happiness than unhappiness). This flexibility—the rejection of absolute duties or rights and sensitivity to the specifics of particular situations—is, defenders of the principle of utility argue, one of its great strengths. Another is that it's based on a fundamental feature of all human beings, their capacity to experience pleasure and pain and their desire to maximize the net balance of happiness over unhappiness.

Contemporary utilitarians distinguish two ways of applying the principle. The first, called "act-utilitarianism," involves a fresh application of the principle of utility to each particular action. Ursula, in the foregoing discussion, seems to be employing act-utilitarianism. The second, called "rule-utilitarianism," applies the principle of utility not to each particular action, but rather in selecting a set of rules which, if always followed, would have the consequence of maximizing utility (or overall happiness). A difficulty with act-utilitarianism, rule-utilitarians argue, is that it is often humanly impossible to gather all of the relevant information and to consider it impartially before applying the principle of utility in particular cases. It's more practical to have at one's fingertips a set of rules which, if always followed, are likely to maximize utility. To see how establishing such a rule may be more effective than case-by-case utilitarian decision making, consider a rule to the effect that a government will never negotiate with hostage-taking terrorists. Although such a rule may, at the outset, result in the possibly preventable deaths of a certain number of hostages, in the long run, always following the rule is likely to reduce terrorist hostage-taking. For, once it becomes known by terrorists or potential terrorists that under no circumstances will the government negotiate with hostage-takers, there will be no point in taking hostages, and the practice should wither away. So, too, some have rejected physician-assisted suicide (PAS) on rule-utilitarian grounds by arguing that although PAS may be justified in a small number of particular cases, because of the likelihood of abuse, overall utility is more likely to be maximized if we have an absolute prohibition than if we make decisions on a case-by-case basis. Act-utilitarians respond to this sort of rule-utilitarian criticism by arguing that unless rule-utilitarians permit some utilitarian-based exceptions to their rules, utility will not be maximized; and if they do permit such exceptions, there is little or no difference between act- and rule-utilitarianism.

C. The Principle of Respect for Persons

What is sometimes called the principle of "respect for persons" is a variation of a principle first formulated by the eighteenth century philosopher Immanuel Kant. The second formulation of what Kant called the "Categorical Imperative" enjoins us to treat human beings as "ends in themselves," not merely as "means" to an end.[5] What distinguishes us from non-human animals and what gives us our dignity, Kant maintains, is the capacity for rational deliberation and choice. Thus, to respect human beings as *rational* beings, we must respect their capacity for informed rational choice. To do otherwise is to treat them not as *persons*, but rather as mere objects, instruments, or things. And this, Kant maintains, is the most demeaning, dehumanizing thing one can do to another human being. Think, in this connection, of slavery. To enslave another human being is to treat him or her as a mere object or instrument. It is to deny that person his or her dignity as a rational, deliberative being. Think, too, of the expression "sex object." Treating another human being merely as an instrument of one's own sexual pleasure, whether by deceit or by force, is to demean or dehumanize him or her. The principle of respect for persons, then, requires that we give as much respect to others' capacity for informed rational choice as we give to our own.

We can now better appreciate the reasoning underlying Renee's belief that in some circumstances, individuals may have a right, based on the principle of respect for persons, to elect to hasten their own deaths. Though Kant himself would disagree, preventing a mentally competent adult from acting on an informed, reasoned decision to end his or her own life in order, for example, to please God or to maximize utility is to treat him or her as a mere means to the satisfaction of these other values. It is not to respect him or her as an end-in-himself or herself, his or her capacity for informed, reasoned self-determination.

The question now becomes whether a rational, informed person could ever prefer inducing his or her own death to continued life. We cannot hope to resolve the matter here, but consider a widely publicized case similar in some respects to that of the Groths in Case 2.1. Dr. Henry Pitney Van Dusen, 77, was the former president of New York's Union Theological Seminary and a distinguished Presbyterian minister. He and his wife, Elizabeth, 80, discussed suicide with their friends and then signed a pact before together taking an overdose of sleeping pills. In it, Mrs. Van Dusen wrote:

> We have both had very full and satisfying lives....But since Pitney had his stroke five years ago, we have not been able to do any of the things we want to do...and my arthritis is much worse. There are also many helpless old people who without modern medicinal care would have died, and we feel God would have allowed them to die when their time had come. Nowadays it is difficult to die. We feel that this way we are taking will become more usual and acceptable as the years pass. We are both increasingly weak and unwell, and who would want to die in a nursing home?... "Oh Lamb of God that takes away the sins of the world, grant us thy peace."[6]

As one commentator noted, "Although they did not say so, they were probably also disturbed by the thought of the loneliness that would follow if one survived the other."[7]

Suppose the Van Dusens, as they appear to have done, had given long and serious thought to what they ultimately did. Suppose, too, that: (1) they were informed about their condition and prospects; (2) they were mentally competent; (3) they had discussed the matter with family and friends and explained their reasoning; and (4) their family and friends understood their perspective and reasoning and, with mixed feelings, felt that to respect them as persons, they must not prevent them from ending their lives. Under these conditions, was their act morally wrong? Writing in *The Christian Century*, William E. Phipps concludes,

> There may well be situations in which suicide can be a conscientious act resulting from a careful weighing of alternatives. The Van Dusens' suicide note, for example, displays serious and rational decision making by Christians. After the couple died a committee of the Presbytery of New York City wisely concluded that for some Christians, as a last resort in the gravest of situations, suicide may be an act of their Christian conscience.[8]

The principle of respect for persons is designed to protect not only "Christian conscience" but also the capacity for all informed rational beings to lead and, in rare circumstances, end their lives as they see fit.[9]

2. COMPREHENSIVE ETHICAL THEORIES

Philosophers have long sought to discover or develop comprehensive ethical theories that could provide consistent guidance on all ethical questions. Each of the three principles outlined above—Livia's principle of the sanctity of life, Ursula's principle of utility, and Renee's principle of respect for persons—has been conceived as the foundation of a single comprehensive ethical theory capable of providing consistent (or non-conflicting) answers to *all* ethical questions "without remainder." Part of the attraction—one might say the charm—of comprehensive theories is that they promise to eliminate conflicts between ethical values and principles.

Comprehensive ethical theories grounded on certain conceptions of Christianity and Islam categorically prohibit suicide. Following Thomas Aquinas, for example, orthodox Catholicism maintains that suicide violates the sixth commandment, rejects God's gift of life, violates obligations to others, and repudiates the Christian duty to endure suffering in the image of Christ. This is a key component of a comprehensive "life" ethic that also prohibits abortion, sterilization, contraception, euthanasia, almost all reproductive technologies, research on human embryos (including embryonic stem cells), and the killing of the innocent, in times of war as well as peace. Though in many ways an attractive and noble comprehensive outlook, in a morally complex world, its purity is difficult to maintain. Strictly speaking, such an ethic would, for example, prohibit abortion even in cases of rape and incest, but few opponents of abortion, including otherwise devout Catholics, are willing to go this far. There are other important values that occasionally conflict with the sanctity of human life and that we sometimes regard as more important. Sometimes, for example, considerations of utility or respect for persons conflict with a doctrinaire commitment to the sanctity of life, and it is hard to argue that the sanctity of life must always prevail. It is easy to cite or imagine cases like that of pregnancy resulting from rape or incest in which sticking to a prior rank ordering of principles is, at best, rigid or hidebound. It is one thing, then, to regard a principle of the sanctity of human life as one extremely important ethical principle among others; and quite another to regard it as an uncompromisable absolute and the foundation of a comprehensive theory. We can endorse the first, without embracing the second.

The same is true of the principle of utility. Bentham and Mill not only articulated and defended the principle of utility, but they also developed a comprehensive ethical theory called utilitaria*nism*. It is one thing, however, to say that the principle of utility is an extremely important ethical principle; and quite another to say, as do comprehensive utilitarians like Bentham and Mill, that it is, at bottom, the *only* or *most basic* ethical principle and that all other ethical principles are either derived from the principle of utility or subordinate to it. Here, too, it is easy to cite or imagine cases or situations in which this would be at best too simple and at worst absurd. Consider, for example, circumstances in which a small increase in utility would require large scale violations of the principle of the sanctity of life or the principle of respect for persons. Or consider a dangerous, life-threatening medical experiment on human subjects, the results of which are likely to provide a cure for some cancers and hence maximize utility, but which cannot be conducted unless the subjects are deceived about the hazards they are about to run. Comprehensive utilitarianism, like a comprehensive sanctity of life doctrine, suffers from *simple-mindedness*, which, as Bernard Williams puts it, means having "too few thoughts and feelings to match the world as it really is."[10]

Immanuel Kant, who most famously articulated the principle of respect for persons, thought it was not only an extremely important principle, but also the "supreme principle of morality," and he developed a comprehensive ethical theory we call "Kantian*ism*" that made this principle an absolute that, in cases of conflict with other important ethical considerations, was always to triumph. Comprehensive Kantianism, however, runs into the same difficulties as comprehensive sanctity of life and utilitarian theories. It is easy to identify real and plausibly fictional situations in which a small violation of the principle of respect for persons would come at the cost of large violations of either or both the sanctity of life or the principle of utility. Comprehensive Kantianism, then, can be as rigid or doctrinaire as either a comprehensive sanctity of life view or utilitarianism. It is one thing to say that Kant's principle of respect for persons is an extremely important ethical principle, and quite another to say that it is the *only* such principle.

As bioethicists John Arras, Bonnie Steinbock, and Alex John London have observed,

> In recent years, a number of philosophers have come to doubt that any ... [comprehensive] ... theory can plausibly claim to be *the* correct theory. It may be that moral reality is sufficiently complex that any one theory gives only partial insight. Utilitarians are certainly right that achieving human happiness is an important goal of morality, but nonconsequentialists are also right in insisting, first, that other values such as justice and autonomy are also important, and second, that these values cannot be reduced to happiness. We conclude that it is a mistake to view the various ... [comprehensive] ... theoretical alternatives as mutually exclusive claims to moral truth. Instead we should view them as important but partial contributions to a comprehensive, although necessarily fragmented, moral vision.[11]

To say this moral vision is "necessarily fragmented" is to reject what Stuart Hampshire has dubbed the "doctrine of moral harmony"—the belief that all good things and all right actions must ultimately fit together in a single harmonious scheme of morality.[12] It is to embrace instead "moral pluralism"—the belief that so long as individuals and groups enjoy a certain amount of freedom to think and act for themselves, there will be conflicts between good and important ethical values and principles that cannot neatly or easily be resolved by a single comprehensive theory consisting of a rigid, hierarchically-ordered set of values and principles, such as a comprehensive sanctity of life ethic, utilitarian*ism*, or Kantian*ism*.

3. MORAL PLURALISM

Moral pluralists[13] believe that a number of *good* and *important* ethical values and principles such as the sanctity of life and the principles of utility and respect for persons are inherently incompatible.[14] They cannot be combined *once and for all* into a single harmonious scheme of morality for all. We emphasize "good and important" to distinguish "pluralism *as such*" from "reasonable pluralism."[15] Pluralism as such includes both: (1) plural and conflicting values and principles attributable to selfishness, prejudice, ignorance, bad reasoning, and so on; *and* (2) plural and conflicting values and principles that remain even if selfishness, prejudice, ignorance, bad reasoning, and the like are eliminated. *Reasonable* pluralism is restricted to (2). Pluralism is reasonable when plural and conflicting values are not the result of selfishness, prejudice, ignorance, bad reasoning, bias, or other deficiencies. Even when we exclude obvious "bad guys" like Nazis and hitmen, ethical conflicts will remain between (and within) informed, clearthinking, well-meaning "good guys," such as the readers of this book and ourselves. From here on, when we talk of moral pluralism, we will mean *reasonable* moral pluralism.

Moral pluralism is, as political philosopher John Rawls puts it, "a permanent feature of the public culture of democracy." Everyone's adhering to the same, unified, comprehensive ethical theory—whether the sanctity of life theory, utilitarianism, Kantianism, or some other—can be maintained, as Rawls adds, "only by the oppressive use of state power."[16] If, for example, we want to live in a society in which everyone agrees and complies with orthodox Roman Catholic morality, we will have to reinstitute the Spanish Inquisition. Similarly, if we want to live in a society in which everyone agrees and complies with either comprehensive utilitarianism or Kantianism, we will have to institute a kind of utilitarian or Kantian "inquisition."

Moral pluralism has a number of sources. Isaiah Berlin points out that many good and important moral values and principles are logically incompatible.

Justice, rigorous justice, is for some people an absolute value, but it is not compatible with what may be equally ultimate values for them—mercy, compassion, as arises in concrete cases. Both liberty and equality are among the primary goals pursued by human beings, but total liberty for wolves is death to the lambs, total liberty of the powerful, the gifted, is not compatible with the rights to a decent existence of the weak and less gifted.[17]

To this list we might add occasional conflicts between the principle of preserving and prolonging life and either the principle of utility or the principle of respect for persons as well as conflicts between utility and respect for persons. These and other conflicts between good and important values and principles, Berlin persuasively argues, cannot be entirely eliminated.

Rawls identifies additional sources of reasonable disagreement.[18] First, in considering difficult issues like those addressed in this book, the relevant empirical and scientific evidence is often complex and hard to evaluate. Different, informed, and thoughtful individuals will, in some cases, draw different, yet nonetheless reasonable, conclusions from the same evidence. Second, even when we agree about relevant factual considerations, we may reasonably disagree about their weight, and thus arrive at different conclusions. On suicide, for example, Livia, Ursula, and Renee may all agree that facts about the Groths' pain and suffering are important, but Ursula will give them more weight than either Livia or Renee. Third, in many cases, our concepts will be vague and subject to different interpretations. Think here of concepts like "health," "disease," "benefit," and even "suicide." Does someone who exercises her right to refuse medical treatment by refusing hydration and nutrition in order to hasten death commit suicide? Why or why not? Fourth, the way we assess evidence and weigh moral and political values is often shaped by what Rawls calls "our total experience, our whole course of life up to now; and our total experiences must always differ." Sociologist Kristin Luker's illuminating description of the background beliefs and ways of life of pro-life and pro-choice activists on the abortion question provides an excellent illustration.[19] The upshot is that informed, thoughtful individuals, like the readers of this book, will not always agree about complex moral issues. A number of divisive conflicts will have no simple or clear resolution.

Nor, as some might suggest, are advances in knowledge likely to contribute to convergence on a single comprehensive ethical theory in the future. New knowledge brings new possibilities—possibilities that create or aggravate as many conflicts as they eliminate or reduce. Think of how better understanding of human reproduction and the development of various reproductive technologies have provided new and conflicting conceptions of motherhood and the family. Who, for example, is *the* mother of a child when: (1) Anna provides an egg that is fertilized *in vitro* with Harold's sperm; (2) the embryo is then transplanted into Bettina, who becomes pregnant and gives birth; and (3) Carrie, who is married to Carlos, takes the infant home from the hospital and with him raises the child. Different thoughtful individuals with different experiences and different world views and ways of life will take different reasonable positions. This is only one among many ethical conflicts generated by advances in knowledge and technology.

4. A COMPREHENSIVE ETHICS OF CARE?

In addition to various values and principles, our ethical frameworks consist of a number of virtues or commendable character traits that dispose us to do the right thing in certain circumstances. Honesty is an important virtue as, for example, are courage, integrity, conscientiousness, and cooperativeness. We will discuss and illustrate these and other virtues in some detail in subsequent chapters. We will also discuss conflicts among virtues—for example, between loyalty and integrity or honesty and kindness—and suggest that moral pluralism is a feature of various virtues as well as of good and important values and principles.

An especially important virtue for nurses is *caring*. As suggested by the term "nursing care," it may be the principal nursing virtue. Some, however, see caring as not only an important virtue for nurses but more importantly as the foundation of a comprehensive ethical theory unique to nursing. Rejecting standard comprehensive ethical theories based on the sanctity of life, utility, or respect for persons, they hope nonetheless to develop a comprehensive theory based on caring. Though we believe virtue plays an important role in ethics in general and that caring plays an indispensable role in nursing ethics, we are as dubious of a comprehensive ethical theory based on care (or any other virtue) as we are of comprehensive theories based on a particular principle. To adapt the title of a chapter in Helga Kuhse's book, *Caring: Nursing, Women and Ethics*, we are inclined say, "Yes" to caring—but "no" to a *comprehensive* nursing ethics of care.[20]

Kuhse distinguishes two primary senses of 'caring' in the nursing context.[21] The first is caring *about* the patient—evincing concern, compassion, or empathy for the particular patient and his or her plans and projects in a particular health-related context. This is the same general sense of care in which, for example, good teachers care about their students and good doctors care about their patients. The second sense of care has to do with caring *for* the patient—looking after or providing for the particular nursing-related needs of the patient. This has no direct counterpart in, for example, teaching or medicine. Teachers look after or provide for the educational, not the nursing-related, needs of the student, and physicians look after or provide for the uniquely medical, not the (directly) nursing-related, needs of the patient (though we hasten to add that there is considerable overlap between nursing and medical needs).

The complexity of caring, in general, and in nursing care, in particular, raises many important questions to which a large literature is devoted. What exactly is involved in caring about and caring for particular patients in particular contexts? How does the virtue to care about others develop in human beings? Can it be taught, cultivated, or reinforced by parents or teachers? Can it be subverted or even destroyed by parents or teachers? Can it be cultivated by individuals themselves? Can one resolve to become and then succeed in becoming a more caring person? Is there anything admissions offices in departments or colleges of nursing can do to distinguish applicants who are likely to be caring from those who are not? Are there things colleges or hospitals can do to either foster or undermine caring in student or practicing nurses? These and many others are important questions that have yet to be fully answered.[22]

As for ethics, it is generally accepted that a nurse cannot make good ethical decisions unless she is also caring. Caring supports good ethical decision making. But good ethical decision making in and out of nursing requires more than just being caring. Consider once again the disagreement between nurse Mary Evans and Dr. John Lampson in Case 1.1 "Withholding troublesome details." Each of them seems to care about the patient in the sense of evincing concern, compassion, or empathy for Mr. and Mrs. Vasquez. Yet, they disagree on whether the troublesome details of Mr. Vasquez's surgery should be disclosed to the couple. It is difficult to understand, then, how an appeal to the notion of caring can by itself resolve the disagreement. We can see now that the issue turns partly on a conflict between considerations based on the principle of utility and considerations based on the principle of respect for persons. Dr. Lampson seems to favor the former while Mary Evans' position seems based on the latter. The notion of caring itself (unless considerations of utility or respect for persons are somehow covertly built into it) cannot settle the matter.

Other issues, too, show that while caring is important, it is not *all*-important; it cannot serve as the basis of a comprehensive ethical theory. Consider, for example, situations in which limited resources mean that a nursing unit cannot provide optimal nursing care for all the patients for which it is responsible. How are the supervisors to determine who gets more care and who less? It is difficult to see how the concept of care can itself resolve this issue. A good nurse will care *about* and hope the staff will be able to provide optimal care *for* every one of the patients. But this is not in this instance possible. So, considerations of the sanctity of life or overall utility or respect for persons or some combination of these values and principles (and perhaps others such as justice or fairness) will have to be called into play.

There is an additional reason nurses should be wary of focusing only on a comprehensive ethics of nursing care. It is related to one of the limitations of nursing (or medical) codes of ethics identified in Chapter 1. Nurses will invariably be involved in discussing and attempting to resolve conflicts of values and principles with other health professionals, patients, and their families. If these parties are to discuss and address these conflicts together, they must speak a more or less common language. There is such a common vocabulary (or *lingua franca*) developed over the centuries by moral philosophers and "spoken" with some success by mainstream health professionals and bioethicists. It is the vocabulary employed by, for example, nurses, doctors, social workers, lawyers, clergy, philosophers, and others making up hospital ethics committees and state and national ethics commissions and in bioethics books and journals. This is the vocabulary presented in the first two chapters of this book. If nurses are to successfully address ethical issues in nursing and incorporate the nursing perspective into the interdisciplinary conversation of contemporary bioethics, they will have to become more or less "fluent" in it.

Philosopher Virginia Held has written that, "Caring, empathy, feeling with others, being sensitive to each other's feelings all may be better guides to what morality requires in actual contexts than may abstract rules of reason or rational calculation, or at least they may be necessary components of an adequate morality." While we agree that "caring, empathy, feeling with others, being sensitive to each other's feelings" are indeed "necessary components of an adequate morality," we cannot agree that "caring, empathy, feeling with others, being sensitive to each other's feelings all may be better guides to what morality requires in actual contexts than may abstract rules of reason or rational calculation."[23] This is a false dichotomy. There is no need to choose between caring, on the one hand, and the "abstract principle" of respect for persons or the "rational calculation" of utilitarian reasoning, on the other. Both are essential to good ethical reasoning and decision making. Thus, we conclude "yes" to caring and "no" to the idea of a comprehensive ethics of nursing care.

5. ETHICAL REASONING

How, then, without the benefit of a clear, consistent, comprehensive theory can moral pluralists reason about ethics? How can they come up with well-reasoned answers to the difficult questions posed by, for example, Case 1.1

"Withholding troublesome details" or Case 2.1 "Plans for suicide?" The answer, we think, is the development and constant testing and revision of a coherent *moral framework* aimed at a *reflective equilibrium*.[24]

As we grow up, each of us is socialized by our parents, our religion, our ethnic and socioeconomic groups, and the larger society into one or another general, moral framework. A working moral framework is enormously complex; more complex, in fact, than anyone currently understands. A useful, though *highly simplified*, diagram identifies three main elements. In no particular order they are: (a) judgments about particular cases; (b) general rules and principles; and (c) beliefs and theories about the nature of the world and ourselves. The elements are related as follows:

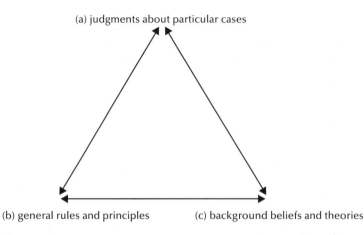

Each element consists of a set of presumptively true beliefs. Initial judgments about particular cases include beliefs like "sharing toys is right" and "hitting your sister is wrong." Rules and principles include "tell the truth" and "don't steal." Background beliefs and theories include our general understanding about persons (for example, they can experience pain) and the world (for example, fire is dangerous). The three elements are interdependent and mutually supporting. Judgments about particular cases are, if challenged, supported by showing they cohere with general rules and principles and background beliefs and theories. General rules and principles are supported by showing they cohere with highly secure judgments about particular cases and with well-grounded background beliefs and theories. Background beliefs and theories are supported by showing they cohere with highly secure particular judgments and with plausible rules and principles. We can thus think of an ethical framework in reflective equilibrium as an approximation or representation of a person's moral outlook—the background and dispositions that he or she brings to the consideration of ethical problems or questions.

Before long, however, as we encounter the larger world and acquire a capacity to think for ourselves, we become aware of various shortcomings of our inherited moral framework. Some judgments about particular cases now seem wrong. Some of us, for example, may have been raised to believe that atheists or homosexuals are somehow bad, but we meet or learn of some atheists and homosexuals (or perhaps come to realize that we ourselves are basically atheist or homosexual) and discover they aren't any worse than most of the theistic heterosexuals we know and read about. Certain rules or principles come to seem wrong. Some of us may have been raised to believe that life is sacred and ought to be preserved for as long as possible, but we find this doesn't make sense in the case of an infant born without a cerebral cortex or when an informed, competent adult refuses painful, marginally beneficial, life-prolonging medical treatment. Some background beliefs or theories seem wrong. Some of us may have been raised to believe that black people, white people, gay people, poor people, or rich people don't have the same *basic* hopes, fears, wishes, and values as we do or that there can be no morality without God, but what we read and see for ourselves makes these seem doubtful.

In such instances, we revise our inherited moral framework to achieve a better overall fit among its elements. No element is basic or sacrosanct. Each may be modified in the interest of the framework's achieving greater overall breadth and coherence. Sometimes we will revise an increasingly dubious particular judgment in the interest of coherence with more secure rules or principles or background beliefs and theories. At other times, we will revise an increasingly obsolete rule or principle (for example, "*Always* do whatever you can to preserve and prolong life") to fit with a particular moral judgment and background belief and theory. In some cases, as we will illustrate below, we will even revise a background belief or theory— our understanding of what the world is like—to square with particular judgments and rules and principles. The relations between the elements are dynamic, not static. Particular moral judgments, rules and principles, and background beliefs and theories are each subject to modification or replacement in the interest of achieving a more consistent, comprehensive, and coherent overall "fit" with the others. The three types of elements are in *equilibrium* if they are mutually supportive. The equilibrium is *reflective* if it is based on a continuous dialectical interplay among them.

Once we have restored reflective equilibrium among the elements of our inherited moral framework, we extend it to new contexts and circumstances—such as those presented in Cases 1.1 and 2.1 and the many cases in subsequent chapters. In some instances, the rules and principles in our current framework will provide straightforward guidance. In others, we can find analogies between the new situation and cases in which our judgments are secure or we can easily refine our rules and principles to handle the new situation. If, however, a novel situation cannot readily be accommodated by our current framework—if indeed the new situation reveals possible flaws or limitations in it—we may have to revise one or more of its elements. This may require modifying or replacing judgments about particular cases, general rules or principles, or background beliefs and theories. The following example shows how equilibrium may sometimes be restored by revising our factual or metaphysical understanding of the world—in this case what it means to be living or dead.

In the late 1960s, advances in medical knowledge and technology were beginning to allow physicians to maintain the lives of patients whose brains had been completely and irreversibly destroyed. In the past, such patients' hearts would have stopped within minutes, and the patients would have been declared dead; modern respirators and other technology were now, however, enabling doctors to prolong breathing and heartbeat. A rule directing doctors and nurses to preserve and prolong life, at (b) in our diagram, seemed to require that treatment be continued. But to many this was intuitively wrong, economically wasteful, or even silly. Intensive care units might soon be teeming with such patients, leaving no room for those whose prognosis was more favorable. This prospect clashed with more secure judgments about particular cases at (a) in our diagram. Two fairly obvious ways of eliminating the disequilibrium—weakening the rule directing doctors and nurses to preserve and prolong life or affirming that continued treatment for such patients is right—were rejected in favor of a third: the modification of one of our then widely held background beliefs at (c) in the diagram.

An interdisciplinary committee at Harvard Medical School proposed criteria for identifying respirator-dependent unconscious patients whose brain function has been totally and irreversibly lost.[25] It then suggested that we modify our understanding of those patients satisfying such criteria. Individuals whose brain function has been totally and irreversibly lost should not be considered alive, despite the presence of respirator-dependent breathing and heartbeat. They should instead be conceived as (brain) dead. And the rule directing doctors and nurses to preserve or prolong life does not apply to those who are dead. Thus, a new problem generated by a conflict between the application of (b) an entrenched moral principle and (a) a strong particular judgment was resolved by altering (c) particular fundamental background belief. Equilibrium was restored without either modifying a principle or accepting a counterintuitive application of it. What we decided to change was our understanding of the world.

In other cases, it will be the rule or principle that will be modified or the particular moral judgment. For example, in addressing Case 2.1 "Plans for suicide" with Ursula and Renee, Livia is forced to consider some troubling consequences of her very strong, unqualified conception of the sanctity of life. A principle directing doctors and nurses to *always* do everything in their power to preserve and prolong life conflicts with the principles of utility and respect for persons as well as with Constitutional law. So she will probably have to modify or constrain the principle in some way—perhaps, among other things, restricting the strong version to prohibiting and preventing suicide. Further discussion of the principle of utility and its unconstrained application, for example, to research on human subjects may also induce Ursula to put some distance between the principle of utility in her moral framework and comprehensive utilitarian*ism*. If she was not a moral plural- ist before considering this implication of the principle, she may eventually revise her framework to become one. And if Renee believed individuals who are rational and informed about their medical condition have a more or less absolute right to end their lives if they see fit, she may want to reconsider this in the light of what we know about the devastating effects suicide often has on friends and family members. Here, considerations of individual rights to autonomy may have to be balanced by considerations of utility.

In proceeding in this general way—going back and forth between secure judgments about particular cases, rules and principles, and background beliefs and theories, and then applying the framework to new, previously unconsidered, or problematic cases—one is using the method of *reflective equilibrium*. Although the label may be new to you, the process is probably not. Most of us who have discussed and deliberated about difficult ethical issues have engaged in this process with various degrees of sophistication even if we were not explicitly aware of it. Readers familiar with the test- ing and revision of scientific theories and hypotheses will note a similarity between this never-ending process and the method of reflective equilib- rium. In both cases, changes in the world and our growing appreciation of its complexity sometimes require modification of the frameworks we have developed for understanding and acting in it. Thus, a distinct advantage of the method of reflective equilibrium is that it incorporates and allows us to make use of the wisdom of the past while remaining responsive to a changing future.

It follows that whatever ethical framework seems to you at a certain point in time to meet the conditions of reflective equilibrium better than any other, it does so only provisionally. As convinced as we may be of the superiority of our current framework to others, we should be prepared to reopen the matter and reexamine our position on certain questions and our overall framework in the light of new circumstances or challenges to it. Once one makes a provisional commitment to a particular framework, then, one should put it to use by (1) trying to make one's position on particular ethical issues reflect it; (2) continually testing the framework under conditions of wide reflective equilibrium and, when necessary, trying to refine it so as to make it more comprehensive and consistent; and (3) remaining open to new or newly recognized implications or criticisms that may require significantly modifying the framework.

Given the fact of moral pluralism and the complexity of and rapid social and technological changes in contemporary health care, there is no avoiding a certain amount of reasonable disagreement on matters of ethics—disagreement among good people, not bad, people who are trying to do the right thing but, due to the complexity of the subject matter, cannot yet agree on what is right. Our aim in this chapter and the previous one is to identify and illustrate the cognitive skills and understanding necessary for addressing ethical issues in nursing. Continued, disciplined, mutually respectful, give-and-take discussion and reflection among thoughtful nurses, physicians, patients, and families are likely to foster well-grounded consensus.

Granted, the results of our reasoning and reflection will not always be as simple or clear as we would like. We may console ourselves, however, with an observation of Aristotle that is as true now as it was more than 2000 years ago. It is a mark of an educated person, Aristotle pointed out, to ask for as much precision from a particular discipline as the subject matter allows. To ask of the same sort of precision in ethics as, for example, in mathematics is to reveal a misunderstanding about the difference between ethics and mathematics.[26] Given the unrestricted frame of reference of ethics (What *all things considered* ought to be done in a certain situation—and why?), together with the fact of moral pluralism and our rapidly changing social and technological circumstances, the best we can hope for in many cases is to find answers to our questions that, falling short of perfection or universal agreement, are better than any practical alternatives. As in selecting medical treatments, we must often settle on an answer to a difficult ethical question not because it is perfect or flawless, but because it seems, on reflection, to be better than any practical alternative.

In this respect, there is a sense in which ethics, as a living body of practical knowledge designed to address a certain set of practical human problems, is no less objective than medicine. By "objective," we mean what Hilary Putnam calls "objectivity humanly speaking."[27] To say that something is objective *humanly speaking* is, as Putnam puts it, to say that it is "objective from the point of view of our best and most reflective practice." In medicine, for example, our best and most reflective practice for comparing the efficacy of two or more treatments is the randomized clinical trial. A particular medical treatment is objectively (though not absolutely or eternally) better than others if impeccably designed and conducted randomized clinical trials clearly reveal it to be so. That it is generally the best treatment is not a matter of a particular physician's subjective preference; it is (humanly speaking) an objective fact. Still, our knowledge is fallible. It's possible we've made a mistake or that a new treatment will be discovered that is objectively better than this one. In ethics, our best and most reflective practice is the method of reflective equilibrium. If what some individual or individuals *happen* to believe is ethical cannot, all things considered, be supported in reflective equilibrium, it is not "from the point of view of our best and most reflective practice" objective. We can thus reject the stagnant ideal of ethical absolutism without, at the same time, rejecting objectivity.

If what we have said about ethical reasoning and justification is correct, there are two important consequences for ethical dilemmas in health care. First, if, parties to a controversy rooted in disagreement over basic ethical principles (for example, Livia, Ursula, and Renee) were to: (1) acknowledge the truth of moral pluralism; (2) acknowledge the limitations of all ethical frameworks, including their own; and (3) engage jointly in the method of reflective equilibrium, they would be more likely to arrive at a well-grounded, mutually agreeable solution. As K. Danner Clouser rightly observed:

> We generally quit the discussion of values long before we have exhausted meaningful argument. We are too quick to say, "You have your values and I have mine." Further discussion can elicit much more agreement either by pursuing the *consistency* of the value in question with other values that you hold or in "unpacking" the conceptual and empirical criteria underlying the values in question. Persistent pursuit of each other's values [and principles] with "why" questions will elicit a lot of hidden assumptions and reasoning, and consequently more agreement than one would initially expect.[28]

Second, even when agreement is not reached, an extended, mutually respectful, reflective discussion will usually convince the parties that those holding opposing positions are not thoughtless, callous, or otherwise "defective" from a moral standpoint. As a result, personal acrimony will be limited, and the parties may come to realize that as thoughtful persons struggling with the limitations of the human condition and the enormous complexities involved in reasoned ethical decision making, there is more that joins than divides them. And the recognition of this, in particular cases, may provide both the motivation and the groundwork for developing mutually respectful, compromise positions that preserve the integrity of the opposing parties (see Chapter 4, Section 4).

Finally, let us reemphasize a point made at the outset of this chapter. In the vast majority of cases, the actions required by the most plausible basic ethical principles are the same. Defenders of the principle of the sanctity of life, the principle of utility, and the principle of respect for persons will all conclude, for example, that permitting an ill-informed, mentally ill, impulsive teenager to commit suicide is morally wrong. They will differ only in the exact reasons they offer when pressed for an explanation as to *why* it is wrong. Therefore, it would be a mistake to assume that all ethical disagreement is a function of a conflict in basic principles. On the contrary, most ethical disagreements are rooted in misunderstandings of what is at issue, different understandings of the facts, conceptual ambiguity and confusion, faulty reasoning, and so on. Only if our analysis reveals that a particular disagreement is rooted in a conflict of basic principles, need we address their justification and priority. And although this cannot be entirely avoided, it arises much less often than specialists in ethical theory would have us believe.

6. ETHICS, LAW, AND RELIGION

Legal and religious considerations often play a prominent role in discussions of ethical issues. But to what extent and in what manner are law and religion relevant to the resolution of moral dilemmas in nursing? We may begin our brief inquiry into this difficult question by addressing the legal and religious considerations raised by the following case.

2.2 Religious and Legal Considerations in Conflict

Jean Lyons, employed by the county health department, provided community nursing services to a rural area, including the schools. While Jean was at the high school, Kathy Jorea, a 17-year-old junior student, told her that she was pregnant but that she knew her parents, especially her mother, would never "get over it" if they found out. There was no law in their state requiring that parents be either informed of or consent to abortions for 17-year-olds. A friend had told Kathy about someone who had had an abortion in a nearby city. Kathy believed that she needed more specific information about the costs, the time it would take, and where to go.

Jean was strongly opposed to abortion on religious grounds. Appealing to the edicts of her church, she held that abortion was tantamount to murder, and had become an active member of a church-related group seeking either a Supreme Court decision or a Constitutional amendment prohibiting abortion. The thought of Kathy, healthy and obviously intelligent, destroying her baby angered and frustrated Jean. The thought also crossed her mind that the county had few public health nurses and, since she alone covered Kathy's township, no other professional nurse was readily available to help Kathy.

In deciding how to respond to Kathy's request for information, how much weight should Jean give to her religiously based belief that abortion is as grave a moral wrong as murder? And to what extent does the fact that Kathy's abortion would, at present, be legal bear on her decision?

Let us begin by examining the complex relationship between law and morality. The first thing to note is that, although legal and moral prohibitions often coincide, certain acts may be morally but not legally justified, and vice versa. In Chapter 1, for example, we assumed that a man taking his pregnant wife, whose labor has begun, to the hospital in the early hours of the morning is justified in cautiously driving through red lights. What he is morally obligated to do is nonetheless illegal. The circumstances may *excuse* him for violating the law, but they *do not suspend* the law. Similarly, abolitionists who violated the fugitive slave laws and civil rights activists, like Martin Luther King Jr. and his supporters, who violated certain laws as a last resort in protesting institutionalized racism, broke laws but did not act immorally. On the contrary, one may plausibly argue that what was immoral were laws that supported racism. In this case, one would be saying that certain acts, though legally justified, are not morally justified.

The fact that we can identify acts that are morally justified but not legal, and vice versa, is not simply an indication of a remediable imperfection in our present legal framework. There will always be acts that are morally permissible or obligatory, but not legal, and vice versa. The former will occur because the completely unrestricted framework of ethical inquiry always allows for the possibility of new or unanticipated considerations overriding the prima facie moral obligation to obey the law. And the latter will always be with us because certain immoral acts (such as one person's falsely promising another to be committed to a long-term relationship solely to manipulate his or her consent to short-term sexual relations) cannot be made illegal without resulting in either costly additions to the police force and unacceptable incursions on liberty and privacy or an erosion of respect for the law in general because the law will be unenforced. A simple appeal to an act's legal standing, therefore, is never by itself a sufficient response to questions of ethical justification. And although a strong case can be made that in a reasonably just society individuals have a prima facie obligation to obey the law, it can be overridden if necessary to fulfill a more stringent moral obligation.

How does all this bear on Jean Lyons' problem in "Religious and legal considerations in conflict?" First, Jean might correctly argue that the legality of abortion (since the Supreme Court's *Roe v. Wade* decision in 1973) is no more sufficient to show that it is morally justified than its illegality (before 1973) was sufficient to show that it was not morally justified. It is still possible, she might maintain, that abortion is morally wrong, even though legal, just as slavery in this country was morally wrong even when it was legal. So, *if* (and only if) Jean can provide strong reasons to show that abortion is tantamount to murder and hence morally wrong, regardless of present legal opinion, she may not only try to dissuade Kathy from seeking an abortion but also refuse to help her, withholding relevant information and possibly even notifying Kathy's parents of her predicament and intentions. Of course, this would include a refusal to provide certain legal nursing services and a breach of confidentiality—a serious violation of most codes of nursing ethics. Therefore, Jean's case for the immorality of abortion must be extremely strong if it is to justify such drastic measures.

Jean, we are told, is strongly opposed to abortion on religious grounds. Now, to what extent can arguments resting only on religious belief be used to justify judgments about conduct in ethical dilemmas? It is widely held that all ethical decisions are ultimately grounded upon, and inseparable from, some set of religious beliefs. If this is correct, people in a religiously pluralistic society will be unable to develop a systematic framework for resolving basic ethical disagreements. Ethical disagreements will be regarded as a function of religious differences, and ethical reasoning and discussion will be interpreted as an attempt at religious conversion.

But what does it mean to say that all ethical decisions are ultimately grounded upon, and inseparable from, religious belief? For some, this may mean simply that our ethical principles are *historically* rooted in one or another religious tradition. Even if this is true, however, it does not follow that the principles cannot be justified on their own terms, quite apart from the tradition from which they emerged. We do not, for example, say that the validity of modern chemistry depends on the validity of Renaissance alchemy, even though the former had its origins in the latter; nor does the fact that astrology was the mother of modern astronomy imply that controversies arising in the latter cannot be resolved without appeal to the former. Similarly, even if there is a historical connection between religion and basic ethical principles, we cannot conclude that the validity of an ethical principle depends upon the validity of the religious tradition from which it emerged.

But when people claim that ethics is based on religion, they may also mean that religion alone can provide the ultimate justification of our most basic ethical rules and principles. Many believe these rules and principles are correct only if they have been issued by God. If this is true, a secular framework will have no foundation, and basic ethical differences will be beyond the reach of reasoning and empirical evidence.

Nonetheless, we think that secular considerations offer at least as much support for ethics as religious considerations and that questions of public policy in a religiously pluralistic society can be resolved only by an appeal to secular reasoning. In the previous section, we suggested that the method of wide reflective equilibrium provides the most plausible approach to justifying ethical rules and principles as well as particular ethical judgments. Whatever cognitive difficulties attach to this method, they are no greater than the cognitive difficulties raised by the notion of God, or any other purely religious authority, as the ultimate source of ethical justification. Moreover, the striking similarity among the basic ethical principles held by people of widely diverse religious convictions is difficult to explain if ethical principles can be justified *only* within the context of religion. According to P. H. Nowell-Smith, this similarity

> can be explained only on the hypothesis that when men think morally they think as they do when they think technologically—that is, rationally and on the basis of experience. The human needs that morality serves, nonaggression and cooperation, are everywhere the same, and it is not surprising that intelligent beings, reflecting on their own experience, have evolved broadly similar codes for meeting them.[29]

Thus, although people may attribute certain principles like the Golden Rule to religious authority, it is likely that insofar as these principles are widely accepted and presumed to be binding on believers and nonbelievers alike, they are also grounded on reason and empirical evidence.[30]

Our reasons for suggesting that questions of public policy be discussed in secular terms are mainly pragmatic. Agreement on basic policy in religiously heterogeneous societies like ours is possible only if the reasons for accepting such policies are independent of any particular religious doctrine. For example, patients and health professionals of various religious persuasions, as well as agnostics and atheists, will be able to reach agreement on recurring ethical issues in health care only if they can appeal to secular principles and justifications. Therefore, to the extent that it is important for people of differing religious convictions to adopt common basic policies, it is important that they support their views in the "public square" with secular arguments, even if their views had their origin in, and can also be supported by, religious arguments.

To suggest that basic ethical principles can be justified by secular considerations is not, however, to imply that people's religious beliefs, principles, and practices are irrelevant to the *content* of these principles. On the contrary, they are of central importance. To the degree that religious beliefs form a part of one's identity as a person, respecting the exercise of these beliefs is part of respecting the individual *as a person*. Therefore, if a secular framework is to be acceptable to people of various religions, it should include among its basic principles the *principle of respect for persons* so as to allow considerable freedom of religious observance and practice. In

health care, this will require that health professionals respect the importance of their patients' religious beliefs when these bear on decisions about
their care. Thus, for example, religious holidays, dietary restrictions, and
attitudes toward contraception, sterilization, autopsy, and so on, will often
be important in determining a course of treatment. Similarly, clients and
various health care organizations and agencies must, when possible, respect
the religious beliefs of various health professionals.

We may now apply this brief analysis of the relationship between ethics
and religion to Jean Lyons' dilemma in "Religious and legal considerations
in conflict." The first thing to note is that Jean's opposition to abortion is
based on her identification with certain religious ideals. This means that
others, in their interactions with Jean, must, if they are to respect her as a
person, respect her views on abortion *as they apply to herself.* But unless
Jean can also provide strong, nonreligious arguments in support of her
opposition to abortion, her personal, religiously grounded opposition is
not sufficient to override her prima facie obligation to provide legal nursing
services and to preserve the patient's right to privacy. For, if Jean's views
are grounded in nothing more than her religious teachings or convictions,
any attempt to dissuade Kathy from seeking an abortion (assuming Kathy
does not share Jean's religious beliefs) would amount to an imposition of
the nurse's religious beliefs on the patient. And although people may try to
convert others to their religious beliefs, the nurse-patient encounter is certainly not the proper place for it.

There are reasonably strong, nonreligious arguments to show that abortion is a serious moral wrong.[31] The problem is, however, that there appear
to be equally strong, nonreligious arguments showing that abortion, though
always regrettable, is not usually a serious moral wrong and that it is, therefore, unjustifiable to prevent a woman who wants an abortion from obtaining one.[32] Thus, even if Jean's opposition to abortion were based on secular
considerations, we may hope that attempts to anticipate and respond to
objections to her position would have revealed to her that decent, thoughtful people—people who are neither callous nor "ethically challenged"—
can hold an opposing view. Since purely religiously based convictions are
inadmissible, secular arguments are inconclusive, and abortion is not illegal, we would state our position by saying that Jean must not interfere with
Kathy's efforts and probably ought to give her the information she wants.
But if there were another nurse who could provide this information, Jean
might be able to "conscientiously refuse" to do so (see Chapter 4, Section 5)
and refer Kathy to the other source.

3

Nurses and Clients

Moral dilemmas arising from encounters between nurses and clients generally raise one or more of the following questions. First, under what circumstances, if any, and for what reasons, if any, may a nurse treat an adult client as if he or she were a child? In other words, how can what we will call "parentalism"[1] be justified? Second, under what circumstances, if any, and for what reasons, if any, is a nurse justified in deceiving a client? Modes of deception may range from nonverbal pretense to withholding relevant information to outright lying. Third, under what circumstances, if any, and for what reasons, if any, may a nurse divulge information that has been given to her in private under the assumption that it would be held in confidence? Fourth, what is the relationship between professional obligation and personal risk? For example, when, if ever, may a nurse refrain from caring for a highly contagious seriously ill patient? And fifth, how does the nurse determine to whom she owes fundamental allegiance when she cannot satisfy the interests of all those whom she has some prima facie obligation to serve? For example, how should a nurse balance the welfare of a family with the needs of individual members?

Although for purposes of analysis we will examine each of these five kinds of questions separately, individual cases will often raise more than one of them. For example, one of the most common forms of parentalism involves deceiving patients in one way or another so that they will consent to procedures that the doctor or nurse believes to be "in their best interest" or "for their own good." The following case raises not only questions of parentalism and deception but also questions about who ought to be regarded as the principal subject of nursing care and concern.

3.1 Helpful Lies?

Public health nurse Linda Stone first met Arlene Knox when she was referred to the County Public Health Department by an emergency room nurse who

(*Continued*)

was concerned that Arlene's bouts of intoxication might be harmful to her unborn child. Linda soon learned that Arlene had previously been addicted to heroin, but when her boyfriend threatened to leave her, she had stopped taking the drug. Shortly thereafter, Arlene had become pregnant. Over a period of several months, Arlene repeatedly told Linda that she was no longer drinking, but Linda, aware of Arlene's past need for drugs and suspicious that she had not actually stopped drinking, continually worked to educate her about the danger of alcohol to the baby.

After delivery, Arlene's doctor told her the baby had fetal alcohol syndrome. When Linda made a home visit a few days later, Arlene, still crying and distraught, asked Linda to reassure her that she had not harmed the baby, that he did not have fetal alcohol syndrome. Linda assumed that Arlene had not seen her or the baby's medical records, which she had a right to do, nor would she ever ask to see them, especially since she was already home.

Linda suggested they both look at the baby, and she was surprised by his good health and vigor. He had no obvious signs of the syndrome. She immediately suspected that the physician had lied to Arlene in an attempt to shock her into awareness of the seriousness of her drinking. Linda did not contradict the doctor, but told Arlene to ask him again. Linda also calmed Arlene by pointing out the baby's strengths and by reassuring her that she would help her learn ways to stimulate his development over the next year.

Later Linda phoned the physician and learned that she was right in suspecting a ruse; any problem the baby might have from alcohol would probably be small. The doctor said he would tell Arlene the case was slight when he next saw her, but he had no intention of changing his story since it seemed to make her realize what could have happened and, as a result, seemed to have strengthened her resolve to stop drinking.

Linda knew that lying and shocking Arlene was no substitute for helping her deal with problems underlying her drinking. However, Linda also thought that perhaps she should also lie to Arlene; she definitely did not want to see Arlene drink excessively during another pregnancy and damage a child. Telling the truth might lead Arlene to believe she had no need to worry about the amount of alcohol she could consume during another pregnancy. Linda thought that she would begin to help Arlene with some of her underlying problems whether or not she contradicted the physician's story. After several days of deliberation, Linda finally decided to go along with the deception since, she reasoned, it seemed to be in Arlene's best interest.[2]

Insofar as Linda seems ultimately to justify her complicity in deceiving Arlene by appealing to what she believes to be Arlene's best interest, the justification is parentalistic. But there may be nonparentalistic factors in Linda's mind as well. If her concern for the welfare of Arlene's baby and the children resulting from possible future pregnancies was the principal basis of her decision, the justification would no longer be parentalistic. She would not be deceiving Arlene mainly for her own good but for that of her future children. Here, of course, questions arise as to whom Linda owes fundamental allegiance: Arlene, the new baby, or possible future babies? Finally, the deception in this case, as in most others, does not involve a straightforward decision to tell a bold lie. It is more a question of withholding the truth. Of course, the situation is complicated by the fact that the physician initiated the deception, and a decision to unmask it could be costly to Linda's working relationship with him.

This brief discussion indicates just how complex cases of this kind can become. To attempt to analyze them, the rest of this chapter will be divided, somewhat artificially, into sections on parentalism, deception, confidentiality, personal risks and professional obligations, and conflicting claims. Discussion of the complications from the involvement of a physician will be deferred until the following chapter. The reader is reminded again, however, that in everyday life these considerations frequently overlap.

1. PARENTALISM

In its most general sense, parentalism means that an adult is being treated as if he or she were a child by persons acting as if they had the authority and concern of a parent.[3] Just as a parent may force an unwilling child to go to bed at a certain hour or take bitter medicine, so too, it is argued, a nurse may sometimes force an unwilling patient to get rest or receive treatment. Like the parent, the nurse will claim to be acting *on the behalf*, although *not at the behest*, of the patient; for, like the child, the patient is presumed unable to appreciate the connection between the nurse's behavior and his or her own welfare.[4]

When a parent forces or manipulates a child into doing something for his or her own good, the assumption is that the child lacks the capacity to understand, endorse, and act in accord with the parent's benevolent aims. When a child is, in fact, able to understand and appreciate the parent's reasoning, but nonetheless disagrees with it, parental force or manipulation may no longer be justified. Thus, it is one thing for a parent to force a four-year-old to brush his or her teeth; it is quite another for a parent to prevent a 14-year-old from going to any but "G"-rated movies. Parents are justified in coercing or manipulating children into doing things "for their own good" when (1) it is reasonably clear that the result will be in the child's best interests; (2) the child is unable to understand or resists rational appeals to the connection between the act in question and his or her own (long-term) interests; and (3) it is reasonable to assume that, in the absence of special "brainwashing" or indoctrination, the child will endorse or ratify the parents' behavior at a later date when he or she can understand and appreciate the parents' aims and reasoning. It is because forcing four-year-olds to brush their teeth clearly meets all of these conditions, while preventing 14-year-olds from going to any "PG" movies does not, that we are inclined to think the former more justifiable than the later.

Insofar as parentalistic coercion or manipulation of an adult involves a refusal to accept at face value the choices, wishes, or action of an individual who is presumed to be autonomous and self-determining, it bears an even heavier burden of justification. Parentalistic behavior, regardless of benevolent motives or the magnitude of the benefit to be secured or the harm to be avoided, overrides the right of an adult to be respected as a person. (See Chapter 2, Section 1.) To be a person, as the term is used here, is to regard oneself as having the ability and right to formulate various projects and make various commitments, and then to attempt to fulfill them. A human being is identified as a particular person by the values and life plan that guide his or her conduct. To respect another as a person, then, is to take full account of his or her values and life plan and to give them as much consideration in determining the effects of one's conduct as one wants given to one's own values and life plan. Conversely, to disregard or give only perfunctory consideration to the values and life plans of others is to disrespect them as persons. It is to regard them as mere objects or things rather than one's equals as persons, *even if one's aim is to benefit them or protect them from harm.* In Kant's terms, it is to treat them as mere means to an end, and not as ends-in-themselves.[5] And nothing is more demeaning to a person, more damaging to self-respect, than to be so treated. To care for a sick individual as a person, then, is to place his or her values and plans, so far as possible, in the center of the picture and to attempt to preserve his or her sense of capacity for reflective choice.[6]

Nonetheless, as the following case illustrates, there may be times when an adult's capacity for reflective choice is seriously impaired.

3.2 Parentalistic Control

Professor Roger Neff was angry. His anger was directed at Nina Patton, a nurse's aide who had just dashed into his room at the sound of the shrill beeping of an alarm attached by a small cord to the back of the professor's shirt, which had sounded as he was attempting to get out of bed. After disarming the bed alarm, Nina told Professor Neff that since he had finished his nap, she would help him into a wheelchair. Then she would wheel him out to the multipurpose room where he could read, watch TV, or participate in the afternoon activities program. As she attached the wheelchair alarm cord

(Continued)

to his shirt, Professor Neff pursed his lips and firmly said, "No, I won't go."
Nina rang for help from Kirsten Li, charge nurse.

Professor Neff, age 77, had enjoyed a successful career as a research biologist and university dean. Although he had become somewhat forgetful during the past few years, he had gone to his university office several times a week and had lived alone in his home until he suffered a stroke. Following hospitalization and a few weeks in a rehabilitation unit, he had recently moved to the nursing home, where he continued to receive physical therapy. On his second day at the nursing home, Professor Neff had fallen while attempting to walk unattended and had badly bruised his face and arm. Recognizing that additional falls might result in serious injuries, the nursing staff had instigated the alarm system and required that he not sit in his room unattended.

Professor Neff protested vigorously that he was being deprived of his dignity, that he felt as if he were on a leash, that he was on "display" in the public room, that he was perfectly competent to be left alone in his private room and responsible for his own safety. In response, Kirsten repeatedly told him that the alarm and his being where the staff could see him were "standard procedures" for patients in his condition, and that he had no choice in the matter as long as he remained in the nursing home and his condition remained unchanged.

Underlying her decision was the fact that, as is not uncommon in such cases, Professor Neff's mental capacities seemed to swing back and forth, so that sometimes he was undoubtedly competent to move about at liberty, but at other times he became confused and lost some motor control. It had been, in fact, during such a confused period that he had suffered his earlier fall. Another important consideration was that the nursing staff did not have time to be in his private room continually to keep watch over him. Thus, as Kirsten had explained to Professor Neff's son, the control measures were "for his own good," even though contrary to his wishes. All things considered, she maintained, it was best for him to be attached to the alarm and not be left alone in his room, except for sleep, even during periods of mental clarity, to insure that he would not, when unattended, lapse into mental confusion and hurt himself seriously. Professor Neff's son agreed with Kirsten and fully supported the nursing staff's decision.[7]

If we assume that Kirsten's appeal to Professor Neff's best interests is not a rationalization for a more basic concern with the nursing home's legal liability, the convenience of the nursing staff, or an authoritarian desire to exercise complete control over all patients, her reasons for keeping him in restraints are purely parentalistic. She believes that Professor Neff's capacity to decide for himself on this question has been seriously impaired and that because he runs a significant risk of harm from being left alone without supervision, he must, for his own good, wear the alarm and sit where he can be observed even if he resists and protests. The question now is whether this parentalistic intervention is justifiable.

Parentalistic behavior requires justification because it refuses to accept at face value the choices, wishes, or actions of an individual who is presumed to be autonomous and self-determining. Thus, in justifying a particular parentalistic intervention, one must show that the presumption of autonomy or self-determination no longer holds—that the choices, wishes, or actions of the individual are not genuinely autonomous or authentically self-determined.[8] Even John Stuart Mill, whose defense of individual liberty is often considered to be antiparentalistic in the extreme,[9] allowed that we may interfere with a person's acting on his or her expressed desires when we can be certain that they are not his actual desires:

> If either a public officer or anyone else saw a person attempting to cross a bridge which had been ascertained to be unsafe, and there were not time to warn him of this danger, they might seize him and turn him back without any real infringement of his liberty; *for liberty consists of doing what one desires, and he does not desire to fall into the river.*[10]

Similarly, we might conclude that Professor Neff does not desire to injure himself while walking around unattended. Thus, insofar as he is prevented from doing so, the nursing staff no more violates his right as a person to do what he (genuinely) wants to do than the intervener in Mill's example violates the rights of the person crossing the bridge.

In both Mill's example and the case of Professor Neff, the defense of the intervention rests on two conditions: (1) the ignorance or impaired capacity for rational reflection, decision, or action of the agent and (2) the magnitude and probability of harm that would result without parentalistic intervention. Although some would argue that only the limited autonomy of the first of these conditions is *necessary* to justify parentalistic interference, and others would maintain that the prospective harm of the second is by itself *sufficient* to justify such interference, we believe that both are necessary.[11] If a person meets condition (1) but does not thereby run an increased risk of significant harm, one cannot say that the "lesser evil" (the deprivation of liberty or choice) is justified by appeal to the avoidance of a "greater evil" (harm to the person whose liberty or choice is restricted); hence, the intervention is not clearly in the person's best interests. And if a person meets the harm condition (2) but is mentally competent and fully aware of the magnitude and probability of harm that may result from his or her action, interference cannot be justified on parentalistic grounds unless one is willing to say that autonomous people should not be free to drive racing cars, smoke cigarettes, or refuse certain forms of medical treatment.

Although a parent may be justified in making a child do things judged to *benefit* the child as well as to protect him or her from harm, we believe that generally a health care professional can override an adult client's right to self-determination *only to prevent harm*. Although the difference between preventing harm and providing a benefit is not always clear, often it is both clear and useful. The main difference between the promotion of benefit and the prevention of harm, for our purposes, is that it is much easier to obtain agreement on what constitutes a harm than on what constitutes a benefit. People may, for example, differ widely about whether public funds should be used to promote the arts, athletics, ethnic festivals, libraries, or parks, but there is usually significant agreement among the same people that such funds should be used to prevent foreign invasions, crime, and disease. The latter (invasions, crime, and disease) are regarded as harms of great magnitude by most any set of values, while whether one or another of the former (promotion of arts, athletics, etc.) is regarded as vital benefit will vary widely from one set of values to another. Thus, unless one has a more or less explicit prior consent for interventions conceived mainly as providing a benefit rather than preventing a harm, the *presumed* benefit (which may simply reduce to the imposition of one's own values on a vulnerable patient) cannot override the *certain infringement of a person's right to self-determination*.

Underlying this emphasis on harm as opposed to benefit is an assumption that parentalistic behavior is justifiable only if the subject of the intervention in some sense consents to it. For example, a parent's forcing the child to brush his or her teeth is justified, in part, by the reasonable assumption that the child at a later date, when the parent's aims and reasoning can be understood and appreciated, will endorse or ratify the parent's behavior. As Gerald Dworkin puts it, "Parental paternalism may be thought of as a wager by the parent on the subsequent recognition of the wisdom of the restrictions. There is an emphasis on what could be called future-oriented consent—on what the child will come to welcome, rather than on what he does welcome."[12] Similarly, just as Professor Neff, the stroke victim in Case 3.2, does not want to injure himself, and the person about to walk over the bridge in Mill's example does not want to fall into the river, those who parentalistically interfere should be reasonably sure that their interventions will later be ratified by the subjects of the interference.[13] Thus, we may now add a future consent condition to the two we have already provided for the justification of an act of parentalism. An act of parentalism will now be said to be justified if and only if:

1. the subject is, under the circumstances, irretrievably ignorant of relevant information, or his or her capacity for rational reflection, decision, or action is significantly impaired (the *autonomy* condition);

2. the subject is likely to be significantly harmed unless interfered with (the *harm* condition); and
3. it is reasonable to assume that the subject will, at a later time, with greater knowledge or the recovery of his or her capacity for rational reflection, ratify the decision to interfere by consenting to it (the *ratification* condition).[14]

Discussions of the justification of parentalism often distinguish two forms: "strong" and "weak." Strong parentalism emphasizes doing what is ostensibly for the patient's own good or welfare regardless of his or her capacity to consent. Weak parentalism, on the other hand, involves acting to benefit a person or limit harm when, due to irretrievable ignorance or mental impairment, the patient is substantially unable to make the decision for him- or herself. Our emphasis on the autonomy and ratification conditions indicates that we are endorsing a "weak" and not a "strong" form of parentalism. Our restriction of condition (2) to harm, and excluding benefit or welfare, indicates that ours is also among the weaker versions of "weak" parentalism. Our main reason for rejecting strong versions of parentalism is that they are usually too quick to override the patient's autonomy in the name of a conception of the good that cannot be shown by cogent argument to be superior to the patient's own conception of the good. On the other hand, the form of weak parentalism outlined here can, in many instances, be justified in the context of health care.

Let us now become more thoroughly acquainted with our three conditions for justifiable (weak) parentalism by applying them to three more cases.

3.3 Postexposure Rabies Treatment

Mindi Yaeger, single mother of three elementary school children, phoned the Health Department to report that she had found a dead bat in her home inside a bedroom window fan at about 6:00 p.m. the previous evening. She said that the bedroom was one of three 2nd floor bedrooms that the family used every night. Mia Torres, the county Communicable Disease nurse, told Mindi that if the bat was rabid, family members would need postexposure rabies treatment, a series of injections. Mindi said that she hadn't told her children about the dead bat because she hadn't wanted to upset them. The nurse told Mindi how to make arrangements with Animal Control so they could pick up the bat.

Mia was concerned because six bats had tested positive for rabies during the past month in the urban area where Mindi lived. The following day Mia called the state laboratory for test results, but they did not have the specimen. Tracking events backwards, Mia learned that Animal Control had gone to

(Continued)

get the specimen, but since no adult was home, they could not get it. Mia immediately phoned Mindi to reschedule the pick up. Mindi, however, had left the bat outside in a can for two days in summer heat, and the lab found it too decomposed for testing.

If the bat had tested positive, the family would have been considered exposed. With the bat's status unknown, anyone who slept in the bedroom with the bat, or even in another room on the same floor as the bedroom with the bat, would be considered exposed. To prevent the fatal disease, County Health Department policies require that anyone exposed to rabies undergo treatment, an injection of immune globulin and Postexposure Prophylaxis (PEP), which is a series of five injections over a month. In Mia's county the cost of PEP for a family of four is over $4,000. But if a family has no insurance or doesn't qualify for Medicaid, the county uses a sliding scale for payment going as low as $24. The County Health Department oversees treatment for any person exposed to rabies and finds ways for bills to be paid.

The following day, Mindi gave a revised account of the situation. Rather than repeating that the bat had been found in one of the three 2nd floor bedrooms the family used, as she had initially reported, she now said she didn't know if the children had actually slept in the upstairs bedrooms or had remained downstairs near the family TV all night. In addition, she was unsure whether the bat had been there during the night. Since she hadn't found the bat until early evening, she thought it probably hadn't been in the house while they slept. She also said no one had slept in the bedroom during the day. Since there was no positive exposure based upon either test results or her revised history—that is, her denial that family members had slept in the bedroom with the bat—she didn't believe the family needed treatment. She didn't like the idea of preventative shots. Mindi's reluctance to participate in a disease prevention program was not new. In the past, she had allowed her children to be immunized only to the extent required by law to attend public school.

Mia called the county Medical Director, who agreed with her that the family still ought to have treatment even though, given the mother's stories, they probably had not been exposed. Mia talked at length with Mindi, and stressed that even though the chance Mindi or her children had been exposed was slight, the disease was fatal. Simply because of that fact, Mia told Mindi, the entire family should take the rabies treatment. Mindi did not immediately agree, but Mia persisted and they all received the PEP.[15]

At an internal review of the case in the Health Department later in the summer, Mia acknowledged that she had stretched her authority. Had Mindi not changed her story, Mia could have simply required the family to follow Health Department policies and take the PEP. She justified her actions because, in her own words, "Rabies is a *fatal* disease. I don't know why some people just don't get it."

Mia's parentalistic intervention in this case meets the first condition because there is evidence that Mindi's capacity for rational reflection, decision, or action was significantly impaired. When Mindi initiated contact with the Health Department and described the situation as one in which the family had been exposed, she apparently recognized the seriousness of the situation. But after learning about the extent of the treatment, she changed her story; she may have decided that the trouble and bother of organizing her family to get the injections outweighed the risk of rabies. Or she may have allowed her opposition to immunizations to influence her judgment. On the other hand, as a nurse Mia believed anyone capable of rational reflection would agree that the risk of contracting a preventable fatal disease outweighed the burden of a series of injections for the family.

Mia's intervention meets the second condition because she believed that the family could possibly be significantly harmed by not having the PEP. Mia thought that the family could well have been exposed since six rabid bats had been found in the area recently, and a bat had been found dead in the family's bedroom fan. Importantly, as well, her emphasis that rabies is a *fatal* disease underscored her recognition that great harm could occur. The case points to two factors in simple probability judgments: (1) the *likelihood* that harm will occur and (2) the *magnitude* of the harm if it were to occur. A low likelihood of a low-level harm may sometimes be overlooked. But a high likelihood of a low-level harm or a low likelihood of a high-level harm is more serious. For example, the low likelihood that a person will be critically injured in an automobile accident is such a serious concern that we equip automobiles with expensive safety-related devices. Mia's concern was that, although the likelihood of anyone in Mindi's family having been bitten by the bat may be low, the magnitude of the harm if someone has been bitten and does not receive the PEP is very great.

Finally, Mia's parentalistic intervention meets the third condition. Mia could likely cause Mindi to change her assessment of the situation. Mia knew that Mindi understood the seriousness of finding a dead bat in her home because she had contacted the Health Department. Mia could reasonably assume that Mindi, when given opportunities to thoroughly discuss the fatal nature of rabies and the effectiveness of postexposure treatment, would likely value the treatment program more positively. Mia could also address financial worries Mindi might face since their county routinely found ways to pay for PEP. Finally, Mia and other nurses could provide supportive nursing care to Mindi and her children by minimizing fear, anxiety, and pain during the treatment program. Given the likelihood that Mindi might change her views about the burden of injections and the positive benefit of preventing rabies in one or more persons in her family, Mia could reasonably assume that Mindi would later consent to her interference and hence ratify it.

The question of justified parentalism also arises in the following case.

3.4 Breaking the Smoking Habit

Twenty-three-year-old Fred Winston had attempted suicide by shooting himself in the head. Permanent brain damage left him largely helpless and his body deformed by muscular contractions. He required assistance for almost every activity. He was usually incontinent, although this was attributed more to lack of concern than to physical incapacity. In addition, his speech was barely audible, and the combination of brain damage and emotional difficulties resulted in stammering, repetitious speech patterns.

Fred failed to eat well, and his primary pleasures seemed to be watching television and smoking cigarettes. He lived in a "no smoking" nursing home, but a small number of staff and residents, including Fred, smoked frequently out-of-doors in a covered walkway that joined the large facility's two wings. After his initial period of transition to the nursing home, those responsible for his nursing care decided to try to limit his smoking "for his own good." Thus, he was often falsely informed that his cigarettes were all gone, or that there were only one or two left and he ought to save them for later, or that no one was available to supervise him while he smoked (a safety requirement necessary because of his limited fine motor control). The nursing staff reasoned that since he did not appear to care about what was in his own best interest, they would have to take measures to limit his smoking, even if he protested.

When he sensed what was happening, Fred protested as strongly as his limitations would allow. In response to the nurses' explanation that what they were doing was for his own good, he insisted that since there was little hope that his condition would improve, he was entitled to whatever gave him pleasure at the present moment. Given his condition, he maintained, smoking was "for his own good." But inasmuch as his physical debilities and difficulties with speech limited his capacity to resist or vociferously protest the nurses' behavior, their will prevailed.[16]

Before determining whether the nursing staff's conduct meets our three conditions for justifiable parentalism, we may want to ask whether their actions are, at bottom, parentalistically motivated. Parentalistic reasons for forcing or manipulating people to do certain things often function as rather high-minded rationalizations for conduct that is actually motivated by anger or a concern for one's own advantage or convenience. In such cases, parentalistic reasoning, which we may characterize as primarily other-regarding, simply acts to conceal reasoning that is basically self-regarding, though we may be reluctant to admit this—even to ourselves. In Case 3.4, for example, it would not be surprising if the nursing staff's behavior were motivated by an underlying, unarticulated anger with Fred. After all, patients like Fred are not likely to make the nurses' already difficult job any easier. He requires a great deal of care and shows a lack of respect and consideration for the nurses by his apparently willful incontinence. His failure to eat well is also likely to frustrate the nurses and, like most people, they are probably threatened to some degree by Fred's self-destructive repudiation of society and all they hold dear, regardless of what drove him to attempt suicide. Thus, it is important in this case for the nursing staff to determine whether their conduct is actually, or only apparently, parentalistic.

Even if their plan to help Fred cut down on his smoking is intended for his own good, and not simply a rationalized expression of anger, it does not meet the conditions we have set out for justified parentalism. It does not meet the autonomy condition because, as far as we can tell from the case description, Fred is neither ignorant of the dangers of smoking nor is his capacity to reason about his decision less impaired than that of other smokers. (It should be noted that other patients in the same nursing home, subject to safety rules, are allowed to smoke in the designated out-of-doors covered walkway as they wished.) The staff's parentalistic behavior fails to meet the second condition not because cigarette smoking is not harmful but rather because it has not been regarded by the society as a whole to be *so* harmful that adults, after being duly warned, are not free to decide for themselves whether the benefits outweigh the risks. Consistency demands, then, that we regard the probability and magnitude of harm to Fred from smoking at this point no greater than that to him before his attempted suicide or to other people in or out of the nursing home. Finally, the nurses cannot reasonably assume that Fred will, at some later date, ratify their decision by consenting to it. As he himself suggests, given his limitations, the pleasure derived from smoking has taken on a greater significance than it had before his suicide attempt. As his limitations are apparently permanent, it is unlikely that he will ever be able to replace the pleasures of smoking with anything else.

If the nurses' conduct is not an instance of justified parentalism, it must be regarded as an attempt to take advantage of Fred's dependence and vulnerability to impose their values on him. Surely if he were strong enough to smoke without supervision or to protest vociferously, the nursing staff would be forced to change their treatment of him. Insofar as their force prevails, so too does their will. This, of course, is not the first time that professional dominance has violated the rights of patients to be treated as persons. But here as elsewhere, a precedent for the violation of someone's personhood ought never to be confused with an ethical justification for it.

The emphasis in nursing on health promotion and teaching constantly raises questions about justifiable parentalism. How far may a nurse go in trying to alter a client's way of living in the name of better health? Can one be parentalistic when the situation is very complex and the likelihood of harm cannot be reliably gauged? And if so, what form should the parentalistic interference take? Are exaggerated threats and lies acceptable if nothing else appears likely to be effective? Consider, in this connection, the following all-too-typical case.

3.5 Promoting a Healthier Lifestyle

Aisha Cleaves, clinic nurse, faces the task of interpreting Paul Spencer's current health risk appraisal form to him. The appraisal, a computer printout sheet, indicates the risks he faces from various health problems, given his age and physical condition. In Aisha's professional judgment, Paul's health risk appraisal shows that he should reduce his smoking and intake of food and alcohol, exercise more, and take his medicine with greater regularity. Although Paul, who is 50 years old, reports that he watches his diet, has cut down on his smoking, and regularly takes his medicine, he has nevertheless gained 15 pounds during the past year; he came into the clinic with a blood pressure of 190/100 and a laboratory report of his lipid profile that placed him in risk group 3X. Aisha knows that during hospitalizations and clinic visits, other nurses have tried to persuade Paul to change his lifestyle, but he has become irritated by such efforts and what he has termed "preachy nurses." He has indicated that he wants no further discussion of his personal behavior. Aisha, however, is strongly inclined to make another effort to get him to change his ways, for his own good.

Since previous discussions to this end seem to have been unsuccessful, what should Aisha do? Should she simply hand Paul the assessment with no further comment? Should she try to overcome his reluctance to change by using subtle or open threats, or even lies, about the likelihood of a painful and early death? Or is there a more plausible course of action that lies between these two extremes?[17]

We leave it to the reader, at this point, to answer these questions for him- or herself. The answers, we believe, are not obvious. A good way to begin is to determine whether parentalism might be justified in this case; and, if so, whether threats or deception about the likelihood of a painful and early death can in this case be parentalistically justified. Other relevant considerations include the possibility that further efforts to alter the client's lifestyle might only increase his antagonism to medicine and nursing and thus be counterproductive, and whether or not the nurse can reasonably expect the high value she, quite understandably, places on health to be shared by the patient. In addition, we assume that Aisha, if she respects him as a person and refrains from being parentalistic, could indicate that she continues to care about him and his health by asking whether he has questions and ensuring that he has information about the clinic should he choose to return.

2. DECEPTION

The foregoing case raises questions about the use of deception in trying to regulate a client's conduct. Deception is a form of manipulation, and manipulation, like coercion and rational persuasion, is a way of inducing others to do what one wants them to do. Before the forms and possible justifications of deception in the context of nursing are directly examined, it will be useful to compare and contrast manipulation with coercion and rational persuasion as ways of inducing clients to comply with various medical and nursing directives.

Rational persuasion consists of appealing to another person's rational capacities in order to influence his or her behavior. Reasons and information are provided for or against various courses of action with a view toward changing the other person's beliefs or conduct in some specific way. Ideally, rational persuasion is conceived as a dialogue in which the persons attempting to do the persuading recognize that those to whom they direct their arguments are their equals as persons. As Lawrence Stern has pointed out, "There is in general, no point in reasoning unless the other person is capable of seeing reason, getting the point. If he can do that he can also correct *me* if I am mistaken. We are co-members of the rational community."[18] Thus, for a nurse to obtain a client's compliance with one or another directive or procedure by rational persuasion or client education is to recognize and respect his or her personhood. It is, for this reason, ethically preferable to manipulation or coercion in this interpersonal context as well as others. Despite her professional status, then, the nurse must be prepared to engage in genuine dialogue with the client, which means that the client must be allowed the same opportunity to alter the nurse's views that the nurse has to alter the client's views.

Manipulation, on the other hand, puts a premium on the results of one's intervention and less emphasis on the means. It is a mode of altering another's beliefs or behavior by subverting or bypassing his or her rational capacities. As Stern indicates, manipulation includes "such things as deceit, the deliberate by-passing of conscious processes, and various conditioning techniques (real or science fiction) which place belief or action beyond rational criticism."[19] Etymologically, the terms *management*, as in the phrase "patient management," and *manipulation* both have to do with *handling* things (*hand* is *mano* in Italian and Spanish and *main* in French). Raymond Williams, in his study of language and cultural transformation, has pointed out that "the word *manage* seems to have come into English directly from *mannegiare*, It.—to handle and especially to handle or train horses."[20] Horses are not handled or managed as if they were persons; one needn't pay attention to their capacity for rational reflection or personhood because they haven't any. To treat a person in the same manner bears a heavy burden of justification. Manipulation of persons with the aim of achieving a certain result places an overriding value on that result. The benefits of the result, in the view of the manipulator, are more important than the moral and emotional costs to the manipulated individuals from disregarding their personhood and treating them as if, say, they were horses. On the face of it, then, nurses should be reluctant to resort to manipulating their clients unless there are strong ethical grounds for doing so.

There is an interesting contrast between manipulation and *coercion*, understood here as one person's bending another to his or her will by force or the threat of harm. As Stern has pointed out:

> Coercion is not dialogue. But in a sense it is closer to dialogue than is manipulation. Generally speaking, when successful, coercion achieves only unwilling compliance with the wishes of the person who uses it. There is no change of belief on the part of the coerced person; nor does he lose his capacity to do otherwise should opportunity offer. He gives in but is not convinced; and he remains an independent center of action. By contrast, manipulation brings about willing compliance or psychological incapacity to do otherwise. Coercion leaves open the possibility of dialogue; manipulation forecloses it.[21]

This suggests that coercing clients to comply with nursing directives or procedures, though needing justification and falling short of the ideal of compliance grounded on rational persuasion, is in some ways preferable to manipulating them.

Instances of rational persuasion, manipulation, and coercion can be found in the case studies we have already set out in this chapter. Linda Stone's initial response to Arlene Knox's drinking problem in Case 3.1 is an attempt to educate her about the danger of alcohol to her baby and thus rationally persuade her to stop her heavy drinking. Later, however, she also supports the doctor's decision to rely on manipulation in order to curb the drinking problem. In Case 3.2, Kirsten Li decides to use coercion to restrict Professor Neff's freedom of movement in the nursing home. She might, however, have been able to take advantage of his lucid periods to persuade him rationally, that, all things considered, being attached to the alarm system and seated in a public area whenever unattended was in his best interest. Case 3.3 provides an interesting example of nondeceptive manipulation. Here Mia

Torres uses her status as the county Communicable Disease nurse and her persistence to manipulate Mindi Yaeger's agreement for the postexposure rabies treatment. Finally, in Case 3.4 the nursing staff first tries to manipulate Fred Winston into cutting down on his smoking, and when this effort fails, they fall back on force or coercion.

Deception is the most common form of manipulation but, as Mia's use of her nursing position and her interpersonal skills in "persisting" in Case 3.3 illustrates, it is not the only form. The clearest, most widely recognized form of deception is lying. To lie is to intentionally say what one believes to be false with the aim of having others come to believe that it is true. There are, however, a number of ways to deceive people apart from lying.[22] One may, for example, deceive people simply by one's nonverbal behavior. Pretending to be busy when you want to avoid an inveterate bore or faking left before cutting right while playing basketball are just two of many examples of nonverbal deception.

Verbal deception can also take other forms. Saying something that deliberately creates a false impression but, because it is literally true, is not a bald lie is nonetheless an act of deception. An example from a widely used logic text[23] provides a particularly apt illustration of this distinction. Aboard a certain ship, the first mate was repeatedly drunk. The captain was rightly very angry at this serious offense, and every such day despite the mate's pleas, entered into the ship's log: "The mate was drunk today." One day when the captain was ill and couldn't keep the log, the mate himself kept the log. Smarting and eager for revenge, he wrote: "The captain was sober today." Now this joke trades on the distinction between saying what is literally true on the one hand and conveying a true impression on the other. When the mate writes "The captain was sober today," what he says is literally true, but in the context it creates a false impression—namely, that the captain was drunk *every other day*. Thus, we must not allow a fastidious preoccupation with lying to blind us to the important distinction between saying what is literally true and conveying a true impression.

Other modes of verbal deception turn on negative as opposed to positive verbal acts, such as intentionally refraining or forbearing from doing something.[24] Negative acts of deception include deliberately refraining from correcting an existing mistaken belief or allowing someone to acquire a mistaken belief. Imagine a situation in which a patient who has just been diagnosed with a mildly leaky heart valve is strongly urged by a cardiologist to undergo an immediate angiogram. The patient then looks at the physician and says, "I have no choice, do I?" The patient doesn't seem to expect an answer, and the physician gives him none. The patient then says, "Okay, doctor, set it up." But the consent in this case is not truly informed. The physician should have responded, "Yes, you *do* have a choice, but I strongly recommend that you choose to undergo the angiogram." By withholding this crucial bit of information, the cardiologist has manipulated the patient into consenting to the angiogram in a manner that is no less deceptive than if he had told an outright lie.[25]

To summarize this brief account of the various forms of deception, we may say that deception is a form of manipulation that is aimed at controlling people's behavior by inculcating, or allowing them to retain, false beliefs. As a form of manipulation, it subverts people's rational capacities and restricts their autonomy. Insofar as a person acts on the basis of false beliefs that have been deliberately conveyed or uncorrected by others, his or her freedom and dignity as a person have been compromised. Indeed, it is the possibility of participating in deception by refraining from correcting Mr. and Mrs. Vasquez's beliefs in Case 1.1, "Withholding troublesome details," that troubles nurse Mary Evans.

Both the principle of utility and the principle of respect for persons outlined in Chapter 2 contain strong presumptions against deception. Although the grounds will differ with each principle, the result is the same: deception requires justification, and the burden of proof rests on those who wish to initiate or maintain deceptive acts.

It is widely held that the principle of utility allows much more leeway for deception than does the principle of respect for persons. Indeed, we have echoed this bit of conventional wisdom in our use of examples in the two preceding chapters. But the issue is not so clear. Although on short-run utilitarian grounds it may appear that deception would produce a greater net balance of happiness than would truthfulness in many cases, a more long-run utilitarian outlook may indicate otherwise. As Sissela Bok has emphasized, those who engage in deception

> often fail to consider the many ways in which deception can spread and give rise to practices very damaging to human communities. These practices clearly do not affect only isolated individuals. The veneer of social trust is often thin. As lies spread—by imitation, or in retaliation, or to forestall suspected deception—trust is damaged. Yet trust is a social good to be protected just as much as the air we breathe or the water we drink. When it is damaged, the community as a whole suffers; and when it is destroyed, societies falter and collapse.[26]

Thus, insofar as the consequences of each act of deception may have a corrosive effect on the sort of trust that is necessary for the preservation of essential, but fragile, social bonds, there is a strong utilitarian presumption against deception.

The principle of respect for persons grounds the presumption against deception on a person's right to autonomy or self-determination. Since deception, as a type of manipulation, subverts or bypasses one's capacity to exercise rational deliberation and choice, it undermines one's personhood. As Alan Donagan puts it, the duty to be truthful rests

> Simply on the fact that the respect due to another as a rational creature forbids misinforming him, not only for evil ends, but even for good ones. In duping another by lying to him, you deprive him of the opportunity of exercising his judgment on the best evidence available to him. It is true that the activities of a lying busybody may sometimes bring about a desirable result; but they do it by refusing to those whom they manipulate the respect due to them.[27]

It is important to note, however, that this sort of case for truthfulness leaves open the possibility of deceiving young children, those with severe mental disabilities or impairment, and others with a significantly diminished capacity for rational deliberation and choice. But even when one is justified in deceiving such persons, one must consider their capacity or potential for rational deliberation.

Given this presumption against deception common to the principles of utility and respect for persons, it comes as something of a surprise to learn that codes of medical and nursing ethics have traditionally been mute on the subject of truthfulness. Bok points out that, through the years, the oaths, codes, and writings of physicians have made little or no mention of being truthful.[28]

Whatever the reasons for this omission, the contemporary shift of emphasis in health care from the parentalistic dominance of professionals to the individual rights of clients is beginning to change professional codes. For example, a concern for truthfulness is reflected in the International Council of Nursing Code of Ethics for Nurses that states, "The nurse ensures that the individual receives sufficient information on which to base consent for care and related treatment."[29] The Patient Care Partnership, a document replacing the American Hospital Association's Patients' Bill of Rights,[30] also recognizes the patient's right "to consent to or refuse a treatment." To make informed decisions with one's doctor according to that document, the patient needs to understand

> the benefits and risks of each treatment. Whether your treatment is experimental or part of a research study. What you can reasonably expect from your treatment and any long-term effects it might have on your quality of life. What you and your family will need to do after you leave the hospital. The financial consequences of using uncovered services or out-of-network providers.

This emphasis on honestly informing the patient is echoed in the most recent version of the American Nurses Association (ANA) Code for Nurses with Interpretive Statements, Provision 1.4 "The right to self-determination," which states that patients have the moral right "to accept, refuse, or terminate treatment without deceit."[31] This emphasis on truthfulness places a clear burden of proof on any health care professional who decides to engage in any form of deception.

Yet this burden of proof can sometimes be met. The question is: Under what conditions and for what reasons is it permissible or obligatory to deceive a client? In what follows we will try, through a consideration of cases, to address this question.

3.6 Placebos

Sandra Seamans, staff nurse, is caring for Dorothy Langley, whose doctor has ordered placebos to wean her off pain medications that she has persistently requested since being hospitalized after a car accident. The day nurses have already given Mrs. Langley two placebo doses, each of which seemed to relieve her pain for several hours. Sandra does not want to give a placebo. She is worried about what she will say if Mrs. Langley should ask what medication she is giving her. She has thought about warding off such questions with, "Oh, the same thing you got last time" to avoid lying; Sandra does not believe in lying to patients. Yet she acknowledges, "You can't tell the patient it's a placebo because that ruins the whole effect. I know placebos are given to help the patient—to ease off medication. But it is still going behind the patient's back, and I don't feel comfortable with it."

Before determining under what conditions Sandra could be considered to be participating in a justifiable act of deception, let us briefly call attention to the way in which this case illustrates the distinction between telling the literal truth and conveying a true impression.

First, since the effectiveness of the placebo requires Mrs. Langley to believe that she is receiving biochemically active medication, she is deceived even if she is never actually told a lie. Second, even if Sandra should respond to a question from Mrs. Langley about her medication by saying what is literally true ("It's the same thing that you got earlier") she nonetheless conveys a false impression. Sandra would be compounding deception with self-deception if she were to believe that there is a significant ethical difference between saying "It's a pain medication" and "It's the same thing you got last time."

We turn now to the question of justification. It is, in general, much more difficult to justify administering placebos than is commonly supposed. Too often, for example, the administration of placebos reinforces the patient's mistaken belief that there is a "pill for every ill." As a result, patients often fail to understand the inevitability of certain aches and discomforts, the limitations of medical understanding and techniques, the healing power of time, the importance to health of certain patterns of living, and so on.[32] In addition, the cavalier administration of placebos involves needless expense. But most important is the corrosive effect of placebos on the trust which is an essential element in the relationships between patients and health care professionals. As Bok points out:

> The practice of giving placebos is wasteful of a very precious good: the trust on which so much in the medical relationship depends. The trust of those patients who find out they have been duped is lost, sometimes irretrievably. They may then lose confidence in physicians and even in bona fide medication which they may need in the future.[33]

Finally, it is important to distinguish the placebo *effect* from the administration of placebos. The former is a way of characterizing healing that is attributable to the interaction between patient and professional, though not to any specific medication. The placebo effect adds greatly to the professional's effectiveness and requires no deception. It must be noted, however, that an indiscriminate reliance on placebos, which do require deception, will in the long run severely impair the capacity of nurses and physicians to take therapeutic advantage of the placebo effect.[34]

It follows, then that placebos should be used with great reluctance and only when nondeceptive means to the desired end have been exhausted. For the sake of analysis, we will assume that various nondeceptive attempts to reduce Mrs. Langley's dependence on pain medications have been eliminated on grounds other than convenience or expedience. Thus, we assume that Mrs. Langley has been unresponsive to attempts to educate her about the danger of addiction and to persuade her rationally to go without the pain medication. Further, we assume that she is indeed running a significant risk of addiction, that in her present mental state further efforts at persuasion will be fruitless, and that her apprehension about the drug's being cut off will significantly magnify her pain and distress. If these assumptions do not hold, then we believe that the resort to placebo has been premature. But if they do hold, there is a fairly strong parentalistic justification for employing a placebo.

Recall the three conditions set out in Section 1 for justifiable parentalism. If, as we have assumed, Mrs. Langley has been unresponsive to education and rational persuasion about the dangers of addiction, we can infer that her capacity for rational reflection has been impaired (either by the drug or by her inordinate fear of the temporary pain and distress of being weaned from it); thus, the first condition will have been met. The second condition will be met if significant harm is likely to result if she is not given the placebo; and it appears that it will. And the third condition will be satisfied because it is reasonable to assume that when Mrs. Langley is successfully weaned from the pain medication and later informed about the way in which it was done, she will ratify or endorse the deception by retroactively consenting to it.

The following deception, although seemingly innocent, is much more difficult to justify.

3.7 Immunization Clinic

Lykendra Smith and two other public health nurses offer an immunization clinic once each month in a conveniently located church. Lykendra and her colleagues try to dispel children's fears of medical personnel by wearing pleasant, attractive clothing rather than white uniforms and by being friendly and cheerful.

One busy afternoon when the clinic was unusually crowded, David Winn, a four-year-old, was becoming apprehensive while waiting to get his MMR (Measles, Mumps, Rubella) immunization. When his turn came, David reluctantly walked with Lykendra and his mother to an area behind a screen usually used to separate Sunday school classes. As Lykendra picked up the syringe, David started to cry softly. Lykendra noticed his distress and feared that he was building up to a long, loud scream that would upset children who were still waiting. So, she smiled and reassuringly said, "Don't worry, you won't feel a thing." Then, as quickly as she could, she gave the injection. Although he did not cry out, David winced and emitted a little gasp as the needle entered his arm.

It is ironic that, after trying to allay the children's fears through special attention to clothing and friendliness, Lykendra's panicky lie to David is likely to compound his subsequent fear of doctors and nurses with mistrust. Trust is perhaps the most important element in the nurse–client relationship, and once lost it is exceedingly difficult to regain. If what David felt was not as bad as he had anticipated, it was nonetheless worse than Lykendra said it would be. The next time a nurse attempts truthfully to mitigate his fears, it would not be surprising if his response were suspicious.

To conclude this brief discussion of deception in nursing, we want to emphasize that the presumption on behalf of being truthful does not imply that clients have an obligation to learn about their illness or treatment. Although people generally have a right to such information, they may, if they wish, choose not to exercise it. Just as a right to freedom of speech does not imply an obligation to speak, so too the right to be informed about one's illness and treatment does not imply an obligation to be so informed. Clients may indicate that they would rather not know all they are entitled to know.

3.8 How Much to Tell?

The nurses in a particular chemotherapy unit always try to sit down and talk with patients before they begin chemotherapy. Depending on the person's ability to understand and accept information about the effects of chemotherapy, the information they provide is more or less detailed.

However, Juan Zaragoza, a 49-year-old carpenter, was extremely anxious about receiving chemotherapy. He tried to keep his mind and conversation on other things and would only say half jokingly that he was sure the chemotherapy was going to turn him into a "sniveling idiot."

After consulting with another nurse, Diane Fetterson, a staff nurse, decided that Juan did not want detailed information about certain effects and possible complications. Therefore, before his chemotherapy began, Diane explained briefly that he might become nauseated; might lose some of his hair; might not feel like eating; and would need to drink many fluids. She did not tell him, however, everything she might have told other patients. She withheld more detailed information that she thought would be needlessly distressing to Juan in his present state and which he, himself, had indirectly indicated that he did not want. As Diane put it, she was sure he did not want to know all the "gory side effects that could occur."

Although Diane withheld certain information, we would not characterize her conduct as deceptive. Insofar as we assume that Juan had chosen not to exercise his right to know more about the side effects of chemotherapy, Diane was under no obligation to tell him more. To have done so in this case would have been to confuse a right to be informed with an obligation to be informed.

As nurses and doctors rightfully move away from a norm of parentalistic deception, they must be careful not to embrace a norm of parentalistic honesty. If patients clearly indicate that they do not want to know more about their illness or treatment, it is not up to the health care professional to make stronger persons of them or to bring them up to some ideal of lucid awareness. Here, as elsewhere, genuine respect for persons requires sensitivity to genuine personal differences.

3. CONFIDENTIALITY

An obligation to preserve the client's privacy and hold certain information in strict confidence has long been a part of nursing and medical ethics. As Provision 3.2 of the ANA Code for Nurses states: "Associated with the right to privacy, the nurse has a duty to maintain confidentiality of all patient information."[35] As with deception, the principles of utility and respect for persons imply a strong presumption against disclosing information about a client that has been obtained under the supposition that it will be held in confidence.

The principle of utility will base this presumption on the negative long-term effects of arbitrary disclosure of information given in confidence. Such a line of reasoning can also be found in Provision 3.2 of the ANA Code for Nurses: "The patient's well-being could be jeopardized and the fundamental trust between patient and nurse destroyed by unnecessary access to data or by the inappropriate disclosure of identifiable patient information."[36] After all, if clients were afraid that certain embarrassing or incriminating information about themselves would be arbitrarily or maliciously disseminated by health care professionals, they would be disinclined to share such information, often to the detriment of their health.

The principle of respect for persons will emphasize the patient's right to privacy and the confidential nature of communications and records pertaining to his or her care. To casually share information about a patient's condition or treatment is to fail to respect him or her as a person.

Nonetheless, as with deception, there are cases in which the presumption against disclosing information obtained in the clinical encounter can be overridden. Health care professionals are required by law to report cases of venereal disease, gunshot wounds, and child abuse even though they learn of them within the clinical encounter with its presumption of confidentiality. Reporting such information to government agencies, though not uncontroversial, is frequently defended because it is designed to protect the public interest. In addition, it can be argued that such acts of disclosure do not involve a breach of confidentiality because, insofar as the relevant laws are public and knowable in advance, the health care provider does not obtain the information in question under the supposition that it will be held in confidence. More troublesome, however, are ethical dilemmas about confidentiality that do not involve a prior suspension of the principle of confidentiality. Consider, for example, the following case.

3.9 "I Don't Want Anybody to Know"

Sandy Wilson, 14 years old, had just completed a six-month checkup for a fractured ankle. The fracture had healed completely without complications, but her hemoglobin level was in the low-normal range. As a precautionary measure, she was sent to Maria Gomez, a nurse practitioner, for diet counseling. Before long, Sandy confided that she thought she was pregnant and that she did not want anyone else to know, especially her mother. Upon brief questioning, it became evident to Maria that Sandy had no clear idea of what she was going to do about the suspected pregnancy. Before Maria could

> begin to help her think the situation through, however, Mrs. Wilson came in. Mrs. Wilson said that Sandy had been nauseated and very tired lately, and she asked Maria if she had any idea of what would be causing it. As Maria prepared to respond, Sandy remained silent and glared at her.[37]

Although there is a presumption that nurses should maintain confidence, there is also a presumption against deception. Maria's dilemma in this case is due to a conflict between these presumptions.

A decision to override the presumption against deception for the sake of confidentiality could be based upon the importance of maintaining trust in the nurse–client relationship. Maria is well aware that a young pregnant girl's trust in her, as a nurse, must be preserved. Moreover, since the law in their state does not require Maria to tell parents about a 14-year-old's sexual activities, there is no legal ground for suspending confidentiality.

On the other hand, arguments can be made for truthfully answering Mrs. Wilson's questions. Although the presumption for maintaining confidentiality is strong, Provision 3.2 of the ANA Code for Nurses states that information of a confidential nature must be judiciously, not absolutely, protected.

> The rights, well-being, and safety of the individual patient should be the primary factors in arriving at any professional judgment concerning the disposition of confidential information received from or about the patient, whether oral, written or electronic. The standard of nursing practice and the nurse's responsibility to provide quality care require that relevant data be shared with those members of the health care team who have a need to know.... Duties of confidentiality, however, are not absolute and may need to be modified in order to protect the patient, other innocent parties...[38]

This statement provides a basis for arguing that "professional judgment" in Case 3.9 dictates that the nurse should share information with the mother since it relates directly to Sandy's "well-being and safety." Teenage pregnancies pose a high risk to both mother and baby. If Sandy decides (or has already decided) not to have an abortion, obtaining good prenatal care is important, and Sandy's mother may be instrumental in helping her get it. If Sandy does want an abortion, her mother could help her by arranging the abortion and, perhaps, by giving emotional support.

Another reason for being truthful with Mrs. Wilson is to refrain from reinforcing Sandy's avoidance of her problems. If Maria were to support Sandy's deception, she would undercut her own professional efforts to help Sandy develop effective ways of coping with difficult problems.

Given the limited information available to Maria, choosing between maintaining confidence and avoiding deception is very difficult. We hope that Maria would try to soften the dilemma by asking if Mrs. Wilson would leave the room for a short while so that she could talk to Sandy alone. Maria would then have time to assess Sandy's perception of family relationships. Maria could also indicate why she would like Sandy to release her from confidence so that Maria could deal more openly with Mrs. Wilson. If Sandy agreed, they could decide when and how best to tell Mrs. Wilson about the situation.

If Sandy does not release her, however, Maria would have to determine whether Mrs. Wilson's having knowledge of the suspected pregnancy would in any way jeopardize Sandy's well-being. If the knowledge would not place Sandy in jeopardy, either physically or psychologically, we believe that Maria has several reasons for telling Mrs. Wilson. First, Maria could justify breaking confidence on parentalistic grounds if Sandy seems not to appreciate the situation or is unable to deal with it, the pregnancy puts her at risk, and in the future a good chance exists that she will look back and agree that involving her mother was the right course of action. Maria could also justify breaking confidence on the grounds that, if Sandy does not choose abortion, the unborn baby's claims to health care override Sandy's claims to confidentiality. Finally, Maria could justify breaking confidence on the grounds that Mrs. Wilson's rights as a parent override Sandy's right to secrecy. The mother's responsibility for her daughter requires that she be informed of current or potential problems. To do less would be to hinder her exercise of parental responsibility.

Dilemmas concerning confidentiality figure prominently in debates over testing for acquired immune deficiency syndrome (AIDS) and other blood borne diseases such as hepatitis C (HVC). Many AIDS patients and those infected with the human immunodeficiency virus (HIV) are understandably reluctant to have others learn of their condition. Numerous persons have acquired the virus through either homosexual relationships or intravenous drug use. Each is associated with social stigma. Consequently, individuals with AIDS or those who have tested positive for the HIV virus are at increased risk of losing their jobs, housing, life and health insurance benefits, and possibly the support of friends and family. Both testing and treatment for AIDS must therefore be protected by the highest standards of confidentiality. If, for example, those at risk for AIDS cannot be assured that information about their medical condition will be held in the strictest confidence, they will very likely avoid being tested or seeking treatment. The consequences will be detrimental not only to their health but possibly also to that of the larger public. Consider the following case.

3.10 Confidential Information: Test Results

Anita Lopez, a nurse who has spent the past year working in various hospitals for several nursing pools, and who now works as a staff nurse on a diabetic unit, wonders if she should inform the community college clinical nursing instructor who uses the unit as a clinical placement for students that David Whitefield, a recently admitted patient, has tested HCV and HIV positive at another hospital. When she spoke with David about the matter, he acknowledged being her former patient but denied being infected with hepatitis C and HIV.

Anita is troubled. She believes that students who are inexperienced in giving injections face a risk of accidental needle sticks. Any patient is potentially a source of infection, but Anita believes David is a known source. She does not think that students ought to be placed in a situation where they may be in harm's way if it can be avoided. Should Anita tell the clinical nursing instructor that David is HCV and HIV positive? Can she do so without violating confidentiality?[39]

Before considering the question of whether or not she should tell the nursing instructor that David has tested positive for HCV and HIV, Anita should try to persuade him to be more forthright about his condition. She may, on the one hand, have legitimate concerns about his well-being in light of recent findings about drug therapy. If David is in fact HCV- and HIV-positive, his squarely facing up to his condition and seeking appropriate medical care may improve the efficacy of subsequent treatment. For his own sake, she may maintain, it is important that he confirm the results of the earlier test and make his caregivers fully aware of his medical history. This will assure that he and his caregivers have an opportunity to identify possible treatments. If, on the other hand, David appears to be in the grip of denial or genuinely unconcerned about combating the diseases, Anita can appeal to his concern for others. Is he aware, she might ask him, of the risks run by the student caregivers? If, in fact, he is HCV- and HIV-positive, shouldn't they be so informed so as to reduce their risk of contracting the virus? If out of concern for his own well-being or that of others, David agrees to be more forthcoming about his medical history, Anita will not have to consider the possibility of violating confidentiality.

Suppose now that Anita's efforts have been unsuccessful—David refuses to acknowledge his having previously tested HCV- and HIV-positive. Should she inform the nursing instructor of his medical history? Would so doing be a justifiable breach of confidentiality? The strongest argument for Anita's revealing what she knows about David's medical condition turns on her concern for the welfare of the students. Yet this is likely to be outweighed, first, by legal considerations and, second, by the utilitarian importance of strictly adhering to the rule of confidentiality.

Federal privacy rules and some states prohibit disclosing this information. Although such disclosure's being illegal does not make it immoral, the burden of proof is in this case quite heavy. Underlying the legal prohibition is a rule-utilitarian argument to the effect that overall good with respect to combating AIDS and other blood borne diseases will best be furthered by invariably following a rule against disclosure. Only if those who suspect they may have contracted the diseases agree to be tested will the disease's possibility be contained. And such individuals will, for reasons indicated above, submit to testing only if they are assured that test results will be kept protected by the highest standards of confidentiality. Thus the long-run consequences of Anita's preserving David's confidentiality are likely to be much better, in terms of overall social welfare, than if, for the sake of securing more protection for the students, she were to reveal his previous test results.

Moreover, it may be possible for her to alert the nursing instructor without violating David's confidentiality. Suppose, without naming any particular individual, Anita were to tell the nursing manager and the nursing instructor that she had good reason to believe that one of their patients had, on a previous occasion and at a previous hospital, tested positive for HCV and HIV. While refusing to identify this patient by name or anything else, she would strongly urge that the nursing students adhere to the standard precautions for minimizing the chance of infection when caring for all of their patients. In addition, knowing that research has shown that needle sticks are underreported by nurses,[40] she could request that both the nurse manager and the nursing instructor inform all students, as well as all nurses, that they must report all needle sticks no matter how insignificant, slight, or embarrassing, and that supportive postexposure prophylaxis treatment for HIV is in place for them.[41]

Students might at this point object that good care plans require a full knowledge of a patient's condition. Unless a nurse is fully aware of a patient's medical condition and history, she cannot provide adequate nursing care. Therefore, nurses must know about David's previous HCV and HIV tests if they are to provide adequate nursing care. In response we may argue that good nursing care centers on assessed clinical manifestations as well as laboratory and diagnostic study findings. In David's case, nurses are able to provide high-quality care without having to have the information he is reluctant to disclose. Apart from the students' taking greater care to protect themselves from infection and following protocols to report needle sticks, little, if anything, about David's nursing care would be altered by this additional information. It is thus possible for Anita to alert the nursing instructor to urge students to take precautions to minimize chances of becoming infected and to teach the importance of taking care of one's self by reporting all needle stick injuries without violating the principle of confidentiality.

4. PERSONAL RISKS AND PROFESSIONAL OBLIGATIONS

The following case raises another ethical dilemma in nursing practice associated with infectious disease: When, if ever, may a nurse refrain from caring for an infectious patient?

3.11 Refusal to Care for SARS Patients

During the 2003 SARS outbreak, in one Canadian hospital insufficient numbers of nurses volunteered to care for SARS patients. Therefore, Crystal Mahorn, a nurse manager, assigned Mary Duncan-Keilman, a registered nurse, to the special SARS unit. Crystal specifically chose Mary because she was a long-term employee, had excellent skills, and some emergency room experience.

When Mary learned of her assignment, she immediately informed Crystal that being exposed to such a deadly disease violated her rights. She refused to place herself at risk by caring for patients with SARS. Mary explained to Crystal that should she have to run the risk of caring for SARS patients, she would instead leave her position "flat out," without giving notice. Mary also said that she believed that her life and the lives of her husband and children were worth more than keeping her job.

Crystal believes Mary's threat to leave her position if Crystal does not find another nurse for the assignment. If this situation happened in the United States, would Mary have a professional obligation to care for SARS patients? If a pandemic of avian influenza in humans occurred in the United States,[42] would Mary have a professional obligation to care for those patients?[43]

What roles should nursing tradition, estimates of personal risk, and fear play in determining a nurse's professional obligation to care for infectious patients with possibly lethal illnesses?

As a profession, nursing traditionally holds that nurses are obligated to care for all persons. Provision 1 of the ANA Code for Nurses underscores this commitment: "The nurse, in all professional relationships, practices with compassion and respect for the inherent dignity, worth, and uniqueness of every individual, unrestricted by considerations of social or economic status, personal attributes, or the nature of health problems."[44]

The history of nurses' commitment to care for infectious patients is underscored by Florence Nightingale's scorn of medical attendants who "take greater care of themselves than of the patient" and by her praise of "true nursing" and the "true nurse":

> Perhaps the best illustration of the utter absurdity of this [cowardly] view of duty in attending on "infectious" diseases is afforded by what was very recently the practice, if it is not so even now, in some of the European lazarets—in which the plague-patient used to be condemned to the horrors of filth, overcrowding, and want of ventilation, while the medical attendant was ordered to examine the patient's tongue through an opera-glass and to toss him a lancet to open his abscesses with!

> True nursing ignores infection except to prevent it. Cleanliness and fresh air from open windows, with unremitting attention to the patient, are the only defense a true nurse either asks or needs.[45]

The nursing profession's *Suggested Code* of 1926 continued to support the ideal that nurses serve others even in face of danger to themselves. The code claimed that "the most precious possession of this profession is the ideal of service, extending even to the sacrifice of life itself... "[46]

More than 60 years later, nurses did not routinely support the ideal of serving others in the face of risk to their own well-being. Although nursing has a long history of service to others, including care of infectious patients, in 1988 nearly half of nurses surveyed in two studies believed that they had the right to refuse to care for an AIDS patient.[47] Nurses' concern for their own well-being may indicate a shift in estimating personal risks inherent in nursing. Many contemporary nurses entered the profession believing that providing nursing care included virtually no health risk to themselves. Since the middle of the twentieth century, widespread use of antibiotics and immunizations has offered a shield of protection. Antibiotics and immunization, however, do not completely protect health care workers against all infections. A twenty-first century nurse must use techniques and take precautions to control the spread of infection in her or his practice.

In 2006, to help nurses analyze the issue of personal risk versus responsibility to care for patients, the American Nurses Association recognized that the issue might arise from the nature of certain health problems, dangerous patient behaviors, and catastrophic events:

> ...it is the nature of health problems such as acquired immunodeficiency syndrome (AIDS), cytomegalovirus (CMV), hepatitis B or C, human immunodeficiency virus (HIV), severe acute respiratory syndrome (SARS), the threat of bioterrorism agents, including bubonic or pneumonic plague, smallpox, and viral hemorrhagic fever, and other newly diagnosed infectious diseases, which may raise questions for the nurse regarding personal risk and responsibility for care of the patient. Violent and combative behaviors of patients also pose dangers to the nurse and catastrophic events can require nurses to evaluate

their personal risk and responsibility for patients in unique and unimaginable situations.[48]

The American Nurses Association concluded, as it had 20 years previously, that a nurse is obligated to care for patients if:

1. The patient is at significant risk of harm, loss, or damage if the nurse does not assist.

2. The nurse's intervention or care is directly relevant to preventing harm.

3. The nurse's care will probably prevent harm, loss, or damage to the patient.

4. The benefit the patient will gain outweighs any harm the nurse might incur and does not present more than minimal risk to the health care provider.[49]

In discussing these criteria, the statement concluded that "in certain situations the risks of harm may outweigh a nurse's moral obligation or duty to care for a given patient," and that, "Accepting personal risk exceeding the limits of duty is not morally obligatory; it is a moral option."

In the twenty-first century evaluating potential personal risks in caring for patients with AIDS/HIV is not as difficult for nurses as it was in the early 1980s when little was known about the disease.[50] Research indicates that caring for such patients does not present more than a *very low risk*, if that phrase means an extremely low probability of contracting an HIV infection. Not only is the actual probability of nurses' contracting HIV infection from patients very low, but risks involved with delivering health care to such patients can also be well managed with correct infection-control measures.[51]

Evaluating potential personal risks in caring for patients with newly diagnosed, potentially fatal diseases lacking known treatments is, however, more challenging and requires health care workers to obtain as up-to-date correct information about the diseases as possible. The high risk of caring for SARS patients during the outbreak in 2003 was alarming. The doctor who diagnosed SARS died from it.[52] Worldwide, 1,775 health care workers (20% of all cases) contracted the disease.[53] As correct, up-to-date information about SARS became known, caregivers reduced their personal risk through the rigorous use of personal protective equipment and innovative procedures. In Asia, for example, one hospital instituted an "isolation-buddy" system in which one nurse completely covered with protective equipment attended a patient while a "buddy" nurse observed the caregiver from outside the patient's room. When the caregiver made any movement that compromised his or her personal protection, the "buddy" quickly acted to alert the caregiver to leave the room. The "buddy" system of continuous and undivided support helped to reduce risk of contamination through quick response to breaks in technique. It also lent needed support to the caregivers.[54]

If a nurse gave her life in providing nursing care in a high-risk situation, one could reasonably assume that many Americans would view such a nurse as a hero, as they did the firefighters, police officers, and rescue workers who died on 9/11. But a nurse is not required to take life-threatening risks. Like the lifeguard in the following example, a nurse is not obligated to give his or her life.

> If a swimmer in an isolated but supervised beach starts to drown 50 meters from the shore, the lifeguard may reasonably be expected to attempt a rescue. This, after all, is the lifeguard's duty as a qualified professional. If, however, the person is drowning 2 miles out and is surrounded by a school of hungry, man-eating sharks, then one cannot expect the solitary lifeguard to dive among the sharks to save the swimmer, even if that means the swimmer will certainly die and even if the lifeguard has a small chance of saving him or her (at great personal risk).[55]

If, however, the lifeguard has been prepared with a high-speed shark proof boat and qualified helpers, one would expect the team to launch an attempt to save the drowning person. Preparations that reduce the lifeguard's personal risks would change expectations about his or her obligations to attempt a rescue 2 miles out in shark infested waters even if the lifeguard team has a small chance of saving the person.

Nurses, too, can reduce their own personal risks in nursing care situations that carry higher than average personal risk. Such preparation requires them to address important questions: What is the likely occurrence of man-made or natural catastrophes or epidemics such as bioterrorism or an influenza pandemic? Who is responsible for instituting measures to reduce personal risks in unknown, potential situations? Are plans in place to keep nurses and patients safe if there is such an occurrence? What is the degree of preparedness within various settings in the health care system? Are adequate supplies such as protective equipment available locally or regionally? Are sufficient numbers of nurses competent in the use of such equipment? And finally, the very personal question of how much risk is too much risk.[56]

High personal risk that carries a high likelihood of a nurse's debilitating illness or death is not acceptable. The loss of a nurse would not only be felt by her relatives and friends, but by the population as a whole since the community would no longer benefit from her care. High risk can be lowered, however, through the competent use of protective equipment, informed policies, and nursing skills, to a risk level nearer to that found routinely in nursing practice. For example, nurses during the SARS outbreak reduced high personal risk through well-informed actions to tolerable levels for themselves. But if lack of institutional preparedness, insufficient protective equipment, and low competency in using special protection left a nurse little or no way to reduce personal risk to a reasonable level, the nurse would not be obligated to give care.

One nurse may judge a level of risk as reasonable for herself, and in the same nursing care situation another nurse may judge the risk as too high for herself. Age, personal health, family obligations, ability to handle stress, religious or spiritual beliefs, fatigue, education, experience, as well as level of confidence in one's own nursing skills, influence a nurse's judgment about personal risk. Fear, too, may play an important role.

A few decades ago, not only fear of HIV as a contagious fatal disease may have influenced a nurse's refusal to provide care to HIV and AIDS patients; prejudices may also have been influential, such as those stemming from attitudes about venereal disease, homosexuality, and drug abuse. Today, xenophobia and fears of terrorism may play a similar role. Prejudices stemming from attitudes about people and diseases that cross international borders, as well as fears of unknown risks of infection and injury from chemical and biological agents secretly used as weapons, may influence a nurse's refusal to provide care to patients with potentially fatal diseases.

If only one or two nurses judge a particular situation as presenting too high personal risk and other nurses are available to provide care, patients could rely on those other nurses. But if all nurses and caregivers in a particular situation decide personal risk is too high and no one is willing to provide nursing care, patients would be left to fend for themselves. In discussing a discovery that doctors, caregivers, relatives—everyone—had abandoned a hospital in Africa and left 30 patients dying of Ebola, Daniel Sokol argued that the doctors could justifiably abandon their patients. His argument depended on an assessment of high risk of infection for the doctor, of futile treatment with "no, or trivially small, benefits" for patients, and a belief that patients would not force a doctor to care for them since patients "have a duty to care for healthcare workers."[57]

Sokol's discussion of the abandonment of patients dying of Ebola points to a need for extensive examination specifically of whether nurses could justifiably abandon patients in similar situations. Basic to nursing, care and comfort, even if cure is impossible, are not "trivially, small benefits." If the American public is to support nurses and other caregivers in their decisions about providing care in particular epidemics and catastrophes in which not everyone can be saved and caregivers face great personal danger, much public education and reasoned discussion concerning risks, responsibilities, and benefits may be necessary.[58]

When patients die during epidemics and catastrophes, questions about decisions made during the crisis may arise. For example, in a New Orleans hospital during the chaos of Katrina in 2006, a doctor and two nurses, in an attempt to alleviate suffering, gave morphine and sedatives to very ill, fearful patients housed on a long-term acute care unit that no longer had adequate staff or resources to adequately care for them. The patients died before evacuation. The caregivers were initially arrested for murder, and only after approximately a year were all three cleared of criminal charges.[59]

To return to Mary Duncan-Keilman's refusal to care for SARS patients in Case 3.11, the case does not mention whether the hospital was prepared for catastrophes and epidemics with special self-protective equipment and procedures. If such equipment and procedures were not in place, Mary ought to be excused from her professional obligation to provide nursing care for the SARS patients. If, on the other hand, the hospital had institutionally prepared for such events and provided nurses and other caregivers sufficient self-protective equipment and training, Mary may have already participated in readiness training and catastrophic/epidemic preparation. If Mary has not been trained, she can be expected to learn quickly. A long-term employee with excellent nursing skills and emergency room experience, she ought to be able to learn promptly how to use self-protective equipment and how to apply all special procedures relating to the hospital's plan to care for SARS patients. If Mary is prepared to use self-protective equipment and to follow all special procedures, her professional obligation to care for SARS patients is clear: First, according to nursing tradition and the ANA Code of Nurses, "The nurse, in all professional relationships, practices...unrestricted by...the nature of health problems." Second, the ANA's criteria for analyzing personal risk and responsibilities supports Mary's obligation to care for SARS patients (if she is provided with self-protective equipment and training) in the statement, "A nurse is obligated to care for patients if...the benefit the patient will gain...does not present more than minimal risk to the health care provider." And third, since Mary accepted employment as an RN in the hospital and had emergency room experience, she implicitly promised to provide service to all patients who needed such care.

Mary seems to believe that she would be in mortal danger if she were to care for SARS patients. Since risks of infection can be managed, Mary's refusal to care for SARS patients may be related to ignorance about information concerning SARS infection and its control. Her refusal may also be related to her fear of and attitudes about biological terrorism or to xenophobia. Such fears and attitudes, however severe or however supported by her husband or others, do not override professional obligations inherent in her employment on a unit that provides nursing service to SARS patients. (A discussion of nurse manager Crystal Mahorn's response to Mary Duncan-Keilman's refusal to care for SARS patients is included in Chapter 5.)

In a pandemic of avian influenza in humans, questions about professional obligations to care for patients would require, as in the discussion of Mary's refusal to care for SARS patients, an analysis of the availability of up-to-date techniques and procedures to control the spread of infection. Problems concerning institutional and community preparation, lack of protective equipment, and insufficient training in the use of special equipment could result in a dire situation for nurses assigned to care for infectious patients during a pandemic. As the ANA concluded, "in certain situations the risks of harm may outweigh a nurse's moral obligation or duty to care for a given patient." A nurse's duty to care for patients is not absolute.

5. CONFLICTING CLAIMS

In Case 3.9, "I don't want anybody to know," the nurse had to balance her obligations among three parties: the young teenager, her mother, and the potential child. Whose needs or claims are to be given priority when a nurse cannot respond to all of those to whom she has a prima facie obligation? Consider, for example, the following case.

3.12 Who Is the Client?

Louise Russell, staff public health nurse serving the inner city, made a home visit to Kathryn Simmons and her young baby. During the visit, Kathryn told Louise that she thought she might be pregnant again. Not one to seek medical care until absolutely necessary, Kathryn had not planned to see her doctor. Louise immediately reminded Kathryn that her doctor had increased her epilepsy medication just after her baby's birth, and that she would probably need to get the prescription changed to safeguard the unborn baby's development. After a short discussion about the importance of checking her medication if she were pregnant, Kathryn phoned for a doctor's appointment. When Louise left Kathryn that day, she was pleased that Kathryn had assumed responsibility for herself and her unborn child rather than letting Louise take control and call the doctor for her.

A week later Louise wondered if Kathryn had actually seen the doctor. Although Kathryn had made the phone call in her presence, she was not convinced that she would follow through. She wondered if she should call Kathryn and check if she had, but she knew that Kathryn would immediately understand the unspoken message that Louise did not entirely trust her. Or, Louise thought, she could call the doctor and find out if Kathryn had kept

(Continued)

the appointment, which would also be an admission that Louise did not trust her client. In the past, Louise had struggled with the question of whether she trusted clients to act on information she gave them, but in this situation she had to consider the unborn baby, too. She didn't know how to balance her respect for Kathryn as a person against her responsibility as a nurse to protect the health of the unborn child.

Louise's dilemma is clearly drawn: if she treats Kathryn as a responsible adult, harm may come to the fetus; if she intervenes on behalf of the fetus, she will not be treating Kathryn as a fully responsible adult. Although the case raises a number of different issues, our primary concern is this: Whose interest, Kathryn's or the unborn child's, ought to be given priority when Louise cannot, on the face of it, satisfy both?

In cases like this, we would suggest applying the principle that the client who runs the greatest risk of significant harm should be the primary concern. Thus, Louise should insure that Kathryn keeps her appointment because the risk of significant harm to the unborn baby if she does not keep it is higher than the risk of significant harm to Kathryn if she is upset by Louise's intervention. An important consideration in making this judgment is that it would be much easier for Louise to repair Kathryn's wounded self-esteem than it would be to reverse the harm that might befall the fetus in the event that Kathryn neglects to have her medication changed.

The principle we have appealed to does not imply either that Kathryn has no right to be regarded as a responsible adult or that a fetus's or child's rights always outweigh those of a parent or adult. First, both Kathryn and the unborn baby have a right to Louise's respect and concern. In this case, however, the fact that the unborn baby runs a greater risk of significant harm than does Kathryn gives Louise strong grounds for overriding Kathryn's right. To say that Kathryn has a right that Louise has reluctantly overridden in the name of the unborn baby's more stringent right implies that Louise ought to do what she can to justify her act to Kathryn and indicate in other ways her respect for her as a person. Second, there may be occasions when the foregoing principle will indicate that it is a child's, and not an adult's, right to respect and concern that must be overridden. Thus, for example, if Louise makes a routine home visit to assess the development of a premature infant and discovers the mother has a badly infected cut on her leg requiring immediate treatment, her first concern should be for the mother.

Although we think it is fairly clear that Louise ought to insure that Kathryn has visited the doctor, it is not so clear whether she should do this by simply calling Kathryn or by calling the doctor. On the one hand, it may seem better to call the doctor. If the doctor indicates that Kathryn has kept the appointment, Kathryn may never learn of Louise's doubts, and the doctor's confirmation that Kathryn has kept the appointment is, perhaps, stronger evidence than Kathryn's saying that she has done so. On the other hand, making the initial call to the doctor shows less trust in Kathryn than does calling her directly; if she has in fact not visited the doctor and learns that Louise has been checking up on her "behind her back," the perceived insult and breach of trust will seem greater and the relationship between her and Louise will be more difficult to repair. We leave it to the reader to determine which of these alternatives is preferable and why. A more difficult case of competing client claims is the following:

3.13 Advocate for Parents and Children

As the community health nurse assigned to the city's northwest corner, Sharon Brinker believes that she is responsible to all the people on her case load. Recently, she was called into court to testify in a child abuse and neglect case involving Larry and Carolyn Trice and their three children (David, seven years old; Linda, five; and Sandra, four). Sharon found it difficult to think in terms of individual clients because she usually looks at a family as a whole. Yet the court considers a child's welfare and safety separately from a parent's wishes for the family to remain together. One option before the court is to place the Trice children in a local institution that offers therapy to whole families; children are returned to parents who successfully participate in treatment programs. Other options require more lasting separation. The judge will base his or her decision in part on the recommendations of expert witnesses—doctors, nurses, psychologists, and social workers.

Sharon first met the Trices six months ago when David was unable to stay awake in school. She thinks she has made good progress with Carolyn in that she has gained her trust and goodwill. David has been doing better since Sharon suggested that Carolyn could leave food out for him to eat before school. But many problems remain, including some relating to David's asthma. Carolyn cannot or will not keep medical appointments for David, enforce rules for the children, or keep the children on any kind of simple routine of meals or scheduled bedtimes. Larry, who works seasonally at pouring cement, usually takes little interest in the children's daily activities.

Recently, Linda has been caught stealing repeatedly from local stores on her way to and from kindergarten, with the result that Larry or Carolyn or both beat her badly enough to result in the court hearing. Sharon feels responsible for the children. She thinks that Linda especially needs her protection; if she steals again, she will probably be beaten. But Sharon also believes that the children need their parents. She thinks she must be the parents' advocate as well as the children's. She has built a positive relationship with Carolyn and thinks that, though she cannot meet all of Carolyn's many needs, Carolyn's trust in her as a professional and friend should be protected.

(Continued)

Sharon's problem is to determine what she could say to the court that would best preserve Carolyn's trust, protect the children, and preserve the integrity of the family.

Those, like Sharon, who consider the family or a similar social group as the unit of nursing or medical care occasionally find themselves in the following dilemma: If they do what appears best for the family as a whole, they may violate the rights or neglect basic needs of individual members; yet if they focus on the rights or needs of particular members, the result may be the weakening or disintegration of the family. Those who advocate regarding the family as the unit of care believe that what is best for the individuals and what is best for the family are generally the same or at least are not in conflict. But sometimes, as in this case, familial and individual interests do not appear to coincide. Thus, if Sharon is concerned primarily with preserving the mother's trust and the integrity of the family, she may be putting the children at significant risk. On the other hand, if her primary concern is the control of David's asthma, regularly scheduled meals and bedtimes for all the children, and an alternative to beatings as a way of dealing with Linda's stealing, her testimony in court may help weaken the integrity of the family.

This is an extremely difficult issue, and it is impossible to take a position that is beyond question or controversy. Nonetheless, we are inclined to agree with Goldstein, Freud, and Solnit that a policy of minimum coercive intervention by the state is most in accord with individual freedom, human dignity, and the intricate developmental processes of children: "So long as a child is a member of a functioning family, his paramount interest lies in the preservation of his family."[60] But where the dynamics of particular family interactions place the child at risk of serious bodily injury inflicted by the parents or the parents have repeatedly failed to prevent the child from suffering serious injury, there are grounds for intervention. One restriction on state intervention in such cases, however, is that the state must also be able to provide a better situation for the child. "If the state cannot or will not provide something better, even if it did not know this at the time the action was initiated, the least detrimental alternative would be to let the *status quo* persist, however unsatisfactory that might be."[61]

The questions in Case 3.13 are the following: (1) How severe will the long-run negative consequences of the lack of regularity in their home life be to all the Trice children? (2) What are the special risks to David because of his asthma and to Linda because of her stealing and the subsequent beatings? If, on the basis of her knowledge of the situation, Sharon believes that one or more of these alternatives poses a significant risk of lasting harm to the children *and* if the state is able to provide something better, she should advise the court to intervene. If, on the other hand, both of these conditions are not met, she should not advise the court to intervene. Furthermore, if intervention is advisable, the less extreme alternative—placing the children in an institution that offers family therapy and the possibility of family reintegration—is, at least initially, preferable to options requiring more lasting separation.

4

Recurring Ethical Issues in Interprofessional Relationships

1. CONFLICTS BETWEEN NURSE AND OTHER HEALTH CARE PROVIDERS

Conflicts arise when either the nurse or another health care provider disagrees with the other's professional practice. In some situations the nurse believes that the health care provider's orders or actions may result in poor care or be unsafe; in other instances the health provider believes the same about the nurse's activities; in still other instances each disagrees with the other about questions of ethics or values. The following is an example of a conflict resulting from a nurse's independent assessment of a need for immediate medical care.

4.1 The Doctor Won't Come

After working eight years as a nurse in an emergency room in a medium-sized city and in an inner-city hospital pediatric unit, Jackie Nardi presently is charge staff nurse two afternoons a week on a 16-bed pediatric unit in a community hospital.

Six-year-old Laurie Thoma was a new diabetic who, in Jackie's judgment, was close to respiratory arrest. Jackie first phoned the resident on call, who happened to be new to the hospital. When he arrived, he was not only younger than Jackie but seemed to be uncertain of himself. Jackie gave him some suggestions regarding immediate medical care for Laurie, but according to her, he "just threw it down the tubes because I'm the nurse and he's the doctor." Then he left, saying he'd return after dinner

Meanwhile, Jackie still believed it was a life-threatening situation for the child and called the pediatrician, Dr. Bauerlein, who was working in the hospital emergency room. When he learned that the resident had been there moments earlier, he refused to come. Jackie was frustrated: "I could

---

see Laurie's condition worsening. I could see a lot of things that needed to be done, but I couldn't do anything about it because I can't write orders." She thought Laurie needed more than her observations and decisions, so she started calling Dr. Bauerlein every five minutes. She also called her supervisor and convinced her that Dr. Bauerlein had to come immediately. Finally, the supervisor went to the emergency room and brought him over. He was angry at Jackie for her persistent calls, but he ordered, basically, the medical care Jackie had suggested earlier to the resident.

Although Jackie never regretted getting emergency help for Laurie, she dislikes the way Dr. Bauerlein now treats her. At times when a resident or another nurse, especially her supervisor, is within hearing distance, he asks Jackie medical questions relating to his various patients—questions he knows she cannot, without a medical education and pediatric background like his, answer correctly.

This case raises a number of questions: What should a nurse's responsibility be in making medical decisions (in the technical sense)? What should a nurse do when her well-grounded recommendations are ignored? What, if anything, should a nurse do when she disagrees with a physician's actions or lack of action? On the face of it, the easiest solution for Jackie, of course, would have been simply to wait for the doctor and follow his orders; but the result, if her assessment of Laurie's precarious situation was correct, might have been Laurie's death. Jackie's awareness of the medical situation placed her in an acute conflict between complying with Dr. Bauerlein's wishes to be left alone and meeting Laurie's need, as Jackie saw it, for emergency medical care.

Several factors contribute to tension in this and similar situations. Among them are the historical legacy of nurse–physician relationships, the expanding scope of nursing practice, the socioeconomic and educational distance between nursing and medical professionals, and the ideology of professionalism in nursing. Since these factors often impede or distort efforts to engage in ethical inquiry, it is important to have some understanding of them.

A. Historical Legacy

During the earliest period of nursing history, nursing and medicine developed independently and had little contact until recognition of the medical value of bedside nursing brought them together in the late nineteenth century. With the development of the modern hospital came the introduction of the trained nurse, and patterns of relationships in hospitals developed that affect current nurse–physician relationships.[1] Physicians developed the medical staff, but as a part of that staff, they were not employed by, subordinate to, or responsible to the hospital administration. Physicians could and did, however, issue orders directly to nurses. The nursing staff's position was quite different from that of the medical staff. Nurses were employed by, subordinate to, and directly responsible to the administration. Thus, nursing developed under the dual command of physicians and hospital administrators. The two lines of authority severely limited and complicated the decision-making role of a hospital nurse.[2]

The Nightingale plan for nursing schools, which included instruction in both scientific principles and practical experience, appeared in the United States in 1873. Unfortunately for American nursing, the schools had no endowment or financial backing, and hospitals quickly seized the opportunity to gain inexpensive student nurse labor. Nursing education was essentially an apprenticeship, and, as late as the 1930s, student nurses received little formal instruction in some hospitals.[3]

Under the dominance of male doctors and administrators, schools of nursing grew, and they were not noted for encouraging nurses to think critically and for themselves. Students entered nursing schools already expecting that women would defer to men, and, therefore, that nurses would defer to doctors. Adding to the traditional subordination of nurses to physicians, nursing school faculties often culled out overly questioning and rebellious students.[4] The students' socialization and education taught them to be deferential. Many diploma schools included the study of textbooks such as L. J. Morison's *Steppingstones in Professional Growth*, published in a revised edition in 1965, which tells the student to cultivate loyalty, prudence, willingness, and cooperation since the physician has the right to expect such qualities. Further, the nurse must follow orders and uphold the physician's professional reputation.[5] Expected by society and trained by the nursing school to act as subordinates, most nurses behaved accordingly.

Yet tradition and nursing education alone cannot be blamed for the dominance of physicians and the deference of nurses. In the late 1970s, Beatrice and Philip Kalisch argued that a physician who sees himself as an independent, omnipotent man with mystical healing powers relates to coworkers as he does to patients and therefore insists that nurses and other health care providers serve him in his "so-called captain of the ship role."[6]

The relegation of nursing to the subordinate position in the nurse–physician relationship limited collaboration between the two professions. Empirical studies showed that physicians were at the center of the decision-making process and that nurses carried out those decisions.[7] In 1968, psychiatrist Leonard Stein described nurse–physician relationships in terms of a doctor–nurse game in which a nurse must appear to be passive. In this game any suggestion a nurse makes to a doctor must be masked in such a way as to seem as if it were his idea, and a doctor may not openly seek advice from a nurse.[8] The historical legacy of nurse–physician relationships, while affecting specific nurses and doctors in various ways, gives decision-making power to a doctor and requires passivity (or biting one's lip) of a nurse. If a nurse and physician deviate from this pattern, the exchange of information and recommendations must occur in such a way that the doctor still appears to lead, the nurse to follow.

A study published in 1985 reports, among other things, that the "doctor–nurse game" described by Stein nearly 20 years earlier was still being played. A resident interviewed for the study commented:

> I have seen nurses, who really knew a lot more than an intern, kind of gently guide him [the intern] into making the right decision....They make some very good decisions and make some very helpful suggestions sometimes....It is like trying to guide the ship without actually taking hold of the wheel....There are nurses who are good at that.[9]

A nurse in the same study claimed:

> You have to be careful whenever you talk to them [physicians] that you are not telling them what to do. You have to talk to them in such a way that you are asking their opinion and work in what you want to say without being overbearing or threatening...make them think that the idea is partially in their mind too.[10]

In 1990, Stein claimed most nurses had stopped playing the doctor–nurse game.[11] But the legacy of the traditional pattern of dominance and deference has continued. In a 2005 study involving physicians' and nurses' perceptions of collaboration and communication, researchers found a positive effect on those perceptions following three interventions: "institution of daily multidisciplinary rounds, addition of nurse practitioners, and appointment of a hospitalist medical director." Researchers concluded, however, that "physicians reported improved collaboration with nurses, but nurses did not report improved collaboration with physicians."

> The difference between physicians and nurses in their reports of a collaborative effort is striking. Physicians may define or view collaboration in a different light than do nurses. We did not specifically define collaboration for the survey, but it was distinct from communication on the survey. Perhaps the physicians thought that collaboration implied cooperation and follow-through with respect to following orders rather than mutual participation in decision making. Although communication is a necessary component, it alone is not sufficient to allow collaboration. Possibly, communication styles differ between nurses and house staff, so that physicians perceive collaboration whereas nurses feel they (i.e., the nurses) are being ordered to do something. A second possibility is that nurses did not feel comfortable "challenging" physicians by giving a different point of view. Or, possibly the input the nurses gave

was not valued or acted upon, and thus the interaction was not perceived by nurses as collaboration.[12]

Until the relationship between doctors and nurses can be fully restructured so as to be more collaborative and morally egalitarian, nurses may still have to choose, on occasion between optimally serving their clients and playing the classic doctor–nurse game.[13] In Case 4.1, Jackie was the obvious loser with both doctors, the resident and Dr. Bauerlein. The new resident rejected Jackie's recommendations because, as she said, he was the doctor and she the nurse—a statement indicating that she was well aware of the usual rules of the doctor–nurse game. Jackie forgot or ignored important rules by aggressively and publicly seeking out Dr. Bauerlein. The doctor, however, from the evidence of his later attempts to belittle or embarrass her, clearly remembered the game and placed importance on the rule that he must, as the doctor, be treated as the leader who needed no obvious assistance from her. If they continue their relationship in this historically spawned, stereotypical manner, the game effectively limits their communication, and Jackie has little chance of involving Dr. Bauerlein in an investigation of their overlapping roles and responsibilities as colleagues. In addition, had the resident and Jackie not been involved in the doctor–nurse game, the situation probably would never have developed into a problem. If Jackie and the resident had been able to exchange information freely and examine each other's ideas about Laurie's treatment, the resident would have been quick to recognize the validity of Jackie's suggestions.

B. The Expanding Scope of Nursing Practice

In some clinical situations, as in Case 4.1, a nurse believes she can correctly diagnose and treat a particular problem in an emergency, but according to the scope of her nurse's license, she is not allowed legally to act upon her knowledge. In another kind of situation, it is not the nurse but the physician who wants the nurse to perform activities that are legally prohibited in their state, such as making rounds and prescribing postoperative medications. Thus, to carry out tasks that are outside the scope of a particular nurse's licensed practice sometimes requires the nurse to break the law. However, the line between medicine and nursing is blurred and in some complex medical procedures and institutional organizations, it is difficult for a doctor and nurse to differentiate tasks that are strictly medical from those that are legitimately within the realm of nursing.[14]

The expansion of knowledge, together with the technological and social changes that have occurred rapidly in the last 50 years, has necessitated redefinitions of the scope of nursing practice and has contributed to tensions in interprofessional relationships. Such changes include the use of life-maintenance machines, automatic clinical laboratory equipment, computers, complex medical interventions, artificial replacements of human parts, human organ transplants, and resulting specialization within the health care professions.[15] Among the many social changes affecting the scope of nursing practice are increased social mobility; increased pluralism with respect to religion, culture, race, and age among patient populations seeking care; increased concern for good health among certain groups as evidenced by interest in physical fitness and health foods; increased demands for alternative care plans for childbirth and alternative health care providers in addition to physicians; and increased enrollment in managed care organizations. Given these technological and social changes, certain nurses, through in-service education, college or university courses, independent study, or experience, may know more about some aspects of a particular treatment or apparatus or machine than do other health care providers, including physicians, with whom they work. For example, an experienced and knowledgeable nurse working full-time in an intensive care unit may know more about certain treatments in that unit than a physician working there only briefly during his educational program. In addition, nurses, who usually spend more time with patients than do physicians, often know considerably more about their patients' strengths, weaknesses, desires, and needs than do some physicians, who may see patients only during short visits. Furthermore, some nurses, in viewing nursing as a "caring" more than a "curing" profession, see health education needs as important and as requiring more professional time and effort than that allotted in some medical treatment programs that focus on specific disease processes. In response to pressures to clarify the expanding role of nursing, nearly all states have attempted to redefine the scope of nursing.

In 1955 the American Nurses Association (ANA) approved a model definition of nursing practice that prohibited nurses from performing any medical act. Yet nursing education had already been strengthened to the extent that nurses were making diagnostic and therapeutic decisions in providing nursing care; disclaimers that they were not to do so were already out of date when various states incorporated the model definition into their practice acts. During the 1950s and 1960s, nursing functions continued to expand into the overlapping areas of medical and nursing practice. Pressure from both within and without the nursing profession mounted, and legal changes came rapidly in the seventies. In 1981, the ANA included "diagnosis...in the promotion and maintenance of health" in its model definition of nursing practice for new state legislation. By 1984, 23 states used the words "diagnosis," or "nursing diagnosis" or some other term for diagnosis in their nursing practice acts.[16] By the turn of the century, 33 of the 51 state nursing practice acts included the word "diagnosis." States varied, however, in usage of the term.[17]

Changes in state nursing practice acts also reflect the expanding roles of advanced practice nurses. According to the American College of Nurse Practitioners:

> Nurse practitioners (NPs) are registered nurses who are prepared, through advanced education and clinical training, to provide a wide range of preventive and acute health care services to individuals of all ages. NPs complete graduate-level education preparation that leads to a master's degree. NPs take health histories and provide complete physical examinations; diagnose and treat many common acute and chronic problems; interpret laboratory results and X-rays; prescribe and manage medications and other therapies; provide health teaching and supportive counseling with an emphasis on prevention of illness and health maintenance; and refer patients to other health professionals as needed. NPs are authorized to practice across the nation and have prescriptive privileges, of varying degrees, in 49 states.[18]

In 2004, the Health Resources and Services Administration Sample Survey reported 141,209 nurse practitioners in the United States, a four-year increase of more than 27%. Growth continues. In 2006 the number of nurse practitioners was estimated to be at least 145,000.[19]

Nurses, depending upon their state of residence, may or may not practice under a nursing practice act that allows them to carry out nursing diagnosis and treatment and/or medical diagnosis and treatment. They may live in a state that requires special certification or agency protocols, rules, and procedures before they engage in diagnosis and treatment. In some states, diagnosis and treatment functions must be delegated to nurses. In others, nurses may be absolutely prohibited from diagnosing and prescribing treatments. Finally, in some states, regulations and broad definitions only vaguely differentiate nursing diagnosis and treatment from medical diagnosis and treatment.

Given this variety and changes in legal definitions of the scope of nursing practice, it is understandable that nurses and other health care providers may disagree or be confused as to the legality of nurses' performing diagnostic and treatment procedures. As discussed in Chapter 1, before engaging in ethical inquiry, the nurse needs to have the facts about a given situation clearly in mind, and the scope of nursing practice as defined in a state's practice act is one such fact. Unless nurses keep themselves informed and educate other health care workers in their community concerning their scope of practice and current revisions of their state practice acts, nurses and other health care providers are likely to view the nurse's functions from conflicting and perhaps erroneous points of view. Nevertheless, ethical inquiry into conflicts between a nurse and another health provider may be impeded by disagreements about the nurse's rightful functions, even though both the nurse and the other provider may be aware of their state practice acts and related rules and regulations. This is especially true if the acts or rules are open to broad interpretation or if the other provider and the nurse disagree about the scope of nursing thus described.[20]

To return again to Case 4.1, both Jackie's recognition of legal constraints on her practice as a nurse and her perception of the scope of nursing practice, which differed from that of Dr. Bauerlein, influenced their relationship. Although Jackie is currently a registered nurse with eight years' experience, she did not have the required additional education for certification as a nurse practitioner. Legally, according to her state's nurse practice act, she could not treat Laurie medically. When both persons authorized by law to provide medical help for Laurie chose not to act, Jackie enlisted the help of her nurse supervisor, but she also kept calling persistently herself. Jackie clearly demonstrated that, since she recognized she could not treat Laurie herself, she had to get help from a doctor. Thus, the conflict between Jackie and Dr. Bauerlein was affected not only by the historical legacy of the health professions in the form of the doctor–nurse game and her failure in that game, but also by the scope of her duties as determined by her state's current nurse practice act.

We are not suggesting that the public should have no legal protection from unqualified health care providers. Nurses such as Jackie must recognize the general value of practice acts and observe their constraints. Nonetheless, at times the nurse must override a practice act, as she might any law, in the name of a more stringent moral obligation. Note that no matter what the practice act stated about a nurse's making a diagnosis, Jackie disregarded that issue when she observed Laurie and decided that the child was in a life-threatening situation. Dr. Bauerlein's later attempts to discredit Jackie's ability to think for herself indicate that he thought nurses should not diagnose. Quite simply, Dr. Bauerlein and Jackie did not agree about the scope of Jackie's nursing practice.

Jackie, believing that her responsibility to get immediate help for Laurie fell within the scope of her nursing practice, did not obey Dr. Bauerlein and stop calling him; rather she persisted until he came to the unit. Certainly, the nursing practice act did not forbid her from aggressively seeking his services. The tradition that the nurse should obey the doctor automatically is in conflict with the conception of a nurse who thinks for herself when she has strong grounds for evaluating a particular diagnosis and course of treatment. Yet time-worn attitudes linger in both professions. They are seen in a physician who expects a nurse's unconditional obedience and in parallel form in a nurse who hesitates to disagree with a physician even when she has good reason to do so. The following case presents a nurse in difficulty for acting independently.

4.2 A Referral

Helen Adam, a dietary aide at a local community hospital in a small midwestern town, asked Elsa Ferruolo, a nurse practitioner in gerontology who was also employed at the hospital, if Elsa knew of an "arthritis clinic" that her aunt might contact. Elsa told Helen that one of the clinics at the state university hospital 60 miles away might focus upon arthritic patients. At Helen's request, Elsa phoned and learned that the hospital did not offer an arthritis clinic, but she obtained the phone number and names of several physicians in the rheumatology department in internal medicine at the university hospital. Elsa gave the phone number and names to Helen.

A few days later, Elsa's supervisor informed her that her "unprofessional behavior" in referring a hospitalized patient, Mrs. Janice Turner, to a specialist at the university hospital was under investigation. When Mrs. Turner had told Dr. Harold Greenfield, her family doctor, that Elsa had referred her, he had immediately lodged a formal complaint against Elsa with the hospital administration. Dr. Greenfield was outraged that a nurse would interfere with his physician–patient relationship and implicitly criticize his professional care of Mrs. Turner by referring her to a physician at the university.

Elsa was shocked and confused when she learned that the hospital administration had taken such action before Dr. Greenfield or any administrator had even spoken to her. Elsa thought that she enjoyed a good relationship with Dr. Greenfield, with whom she had worked for several years, and with Mrs. Turner, who had been a patient Elsa had worked with just a few days past. She had not known that Helen Adam's aunt was Mrs. Turner until the supervisor told her of the relationship.

After Elsa finished explaining that she believed she had done nothing wrong since she had been unaware of Helen's relation to Mrs. Turner, her supervisor told her that the entire situation would be thoroughly investigated. Later, when Elsa told Dr. Greenfield she had not known that Mrs. Turner was the person who was seeking the information she had given Helen, he was noncommittal. In their daily work they exchanged necessary minimal information about ongoing care of his patients, but they did not discuss his allegations again.

The investigation became the hot topic of hospital gossip for the next few weeks, and Elsa found herself increasingly anxious about her future. She worried that if she lost her position or decided to quit, she might be forced to commute to another town for a good job. After five weeks, her supervisor told Elsa the administration was not taking any disciplinary action against her. Although relieved, her frustration and anger lingered. The damage had been done. She recognized that she had a very slim chance of stamping out community gossip that she was an unprofessional nurse. She worried that the gossip would influence her working relationships with other physicians and staff. And she questioned whether she would ever be able to collaborate fully with Dr. Greenfield in their care of patients. She also questioned whether being a nurse practitioner had anything to do with Dr. Greenfield's angry response. Had Elsa been wrong in giving the names of the university physicians to Helen?[21]

When Helen asked for Elsa's help, Elsa knew that she could provide the requested information quickly and easily. She viewed Helen as a fellow hospital employee and believed that helping Helen was appropriate. Being unaware that Mrs. Turner was Dr. Greenfield's patient, she acted independently and gave the information to Helen. Elsa asked herself only one question: Should I satisfy Helen's request? As a nurse practitioner she was legally entitled to do so. An underlying question that she did not explicitly identify was, since I am an independent care provider, that is, a nurse practitioner, would my actions infringe on another independent care provider, that is, the aunt's current physician, whoever that might be? Providing a specialist's name to a relative of a person seeking help may seem a small matter. It was no small matter to Dr. Greenfield, however, who claimed that Elsa had implicitly criticized his care and interfered with his physician–patient relationship. Whether Dr. Greenfield viewed Elsa as a staff nurse or as a nurse practitioner, his response indicates that he did not view her as a professional equal. He did not contact Elsa to discuss the issue with her before making his complaint to the administration. Rather, in immediately seeking an administrative sanction before making any attempt to talk with her, he reflects a view of Elsa as a subordinate hospital employee rather than a collegial health provider. Unfortunately, the nursing administration also seemed to do little or nothing to minimize gossip or bring about a timely resolution. In making the issue such a long public legalistic affair, both the administration and Dr. Greenfield underscored that while Elsa might be a nurse practitioner, she was still a nurse-employee, necessarily obedient to physicians and administrators, and subject to discipline. By focusing on the first question of whether she should act independently and give the information to Helen, Elsa ignored inquiry into the underlying ethical issue of infringing on another provider's practice, however slight that infringement might be.

Before continuing the discussion of obedience, two remaining major factors need to be examined since a combination of factors simultaneously contributes to tension in many interprofessional conflicts.

C. Socioeconomic and Educational Distance Between Nursing and Other Medical Professionals

Despite a recent downward trend in physicians' real incomes, medicine is one of the best-paid professions.[22] Nurses and other health care professionals are not as highly paid,[23] although nurse practitioners, as a group, have seen a significant upward trend in income over the past decade.[24] The differing incomes of medicine, nursing, and other health care provider groups have allowed physicians to remain in a much higher socioeconomic class than most nurses and other providers. With disparity of income come differences in values and lifestyles; thus, various health care providers tend to live in different neighborhoods and socialize in different groups. Of course, people do not have to be best friends to work congenially and effectively together, but they must be able to share important information.

In the past, empirical studies showed that nurses and physicians were not generally sharing colleagues; rather, they worked side by side with severely limited communication and minimal interaction.[25] Changes in the work place, however, are occurring. In a 2006 nationwide survey of 4036 currently working nurses associated with critical care, more than half of the nurses rated as positive the quality of communication and collaboration among nurses and physicians in their work units.[26]

In Case 4.2, Elsa's problem might have been resolved more quickly with better communication among the administration, Dr. Greenfield, and Elsa herself. Elsa's problem in overcoming a communication gap between herself and Dr. Greenfield is not different from problems experienced by other nurses, some much younger, less experienced, and less well educated than Elsa. Nurses, generally, have less formal education than do physicians. Nursing education for registered nurses requires two, three, or four years of study in a nursing school; for some nurses, nursing education includes an additional one or two years in a master's level graduate program, and for a still smaller number of nurses, the educational program includes several more years in a doctoral program. Medical education for doctors of medicine and osteopathy usually includes three to four years of college study, three to four years of medical school, and one to three or more years in a residency program. In simple numbers, educational programs for most nurses last two to four years while educational programs for most doctors extend from nine to thirteen years, although professionals in both groups engage in lifelong education. Needless to say, medicine remains a more prestigious and powerful profession than nursing.

D. The Ideology of Professionalism in Nursing

In the late twentieth century, nurses intensified their efforts to gain a higher level of professionalism, but the process was slow and stressful.[27] Although some nurses felt threatened, other nurses gained support and courage from positions nursing leaders took concerning various professional nursing issues, such as the goal that baccalaureate nursing education be the minimum preparation for the professional nurse as outlined by the American Nurses Association in 1965. The ANA position linked professionalism to baccalaureate preparation at a time when more than 88% of the 582,000 employed registered nurses were diploma graduates.[28] Since that time, nursing education has continued to shift from diploma programs operated by hospitals to two-year associate degree programs in community colleges and four-year baccalaureate degree programs. Twenty years after setting the goal, the ANA reported that 68.1% of an estimated 1,887,697 employed registered nurses still had less than a baccalaureate education, and pressure within the nursing profession for individual nurses to return to college for baccalaureate and master's degrees in nursing remained strong.[29] In 2004, after nearly 40 years, the ANA reported further progress toward the goal in that 51.2% of an estimated 2.4 million employed registered nurses had less than a baccalaureate education.[30]

Reflecting this drive for more education, recognition, and higher professional status, many in nursing have tried to enrich nursing's conception of itself. Advocates for increasing public support of the nursing profession stress the need for nurses to shape the image of nursing through a variety of means such as publicizing their skills, knowledge, and expertise, and challenging the media when nurses are portrayed as less than professionally competent or in a historically demeaning fashion.[31] Many nurses agree with Carol Garant's view that,

> "real" nurses do not necessarily wear white uniforms and caps, carry lamps or long stemmed roses at graduation, give bedpans, bed baths, injections, and enemas or "push" pills. "Real" nurses also engage in research, deliver babies, teach health, do group and individual psychotherapy, work with drug addicts, administer anesthesia, own their own mental health centers, and "hang out shingles" in private practice. "Real" nurses also diagnose patients and clients—no longer do they *presume* patients to be dead or are their clients *thought* to be pregnant. "Real" nurses use their brains as well as their hands and feet.[32]

Garant's "real" nurse relates directly to the advanced practice or the nurse practitioner model of practice, which is now firmly established.

The expanded role of nursing, in providing nurse practitioners with both a wider range of activities and an acknowledged role in decision making, offers meaningful incentives to other nurses to acquire new skills and a means for upward mobility in clinical nursing practice. Thus, while the nurse practitioner model of practice may change the economic distance between medicine and nursing only slightly, it reduces some of the social and educational distance between the two professions, both through the nurse's clinical experiences and formal education and through her exhibition of clinical skills that demand recognition.

But while particular physicians may respect an individual nurse's expertise and judgment, the struggle for control of nursing continues. It can be seen at the national level, for example in the split between the American Medical Association (AMA) and the Scope of Practice Partnership (SOPP) that various physician organizations have formed and the ANA and numerous health care provider organizations over the AMA's Resolution 814, "Limited Licensure Health Care Provider Training and Certification Standards."[33]

Supporting an up-to-date conception of nursing, as described above, however, are social changes related to the women's movement. While most nurses isolated themselves from the women's movement during the 1970s, and while some feminists have, at times, rejected nursing because of its stereotypical handmaiden image, nursing has gained from the movement.[34] In analyzing the use of sexist language, feminists have helped underscore the increasing awareness of nurses that the professional image of a thoughtful, independent, well-educated, responsible nurse is incompatible with the image implied by references to staff nurses as "the girls" or "the kids" or by male requests prefaced by "Hey, honey."

The struggle for recognition and respect continues. Conflicts between nurses and other health care professionals arise, at times, when a nurse tries to gain and use increased skills and education. Conflicts also can arise when a nurse responds to situations from a view of herself and her practice that is not understood or agreed upon by others. To return to Case 4.2 "A referral," Elsa made herself vulnerable to criticism by not thinking that an unnamed person (the aunt) might be the patient of an unnamed physician (Dr. Greenfield) who might take offense to her independent action. Elsa's response to Helen's request for information for her aunt exposed an underlying issue: the physician did not respect Elsa as a professional colleague with whom he could discuss a serious conflict before asking the hospital to take disciplinary action. Elsa's view that she had a good working relationship with Dr. Greenfield proved questionable. The hospital administrators' views of Elsa as an independent thinking professional and valuable health care provider could be doubted, also, since they worsened the situation through their long delay in resolving the complaint.

In summary, interprofessional conflicts are affected by the historical legacy of the health care professions, the expanding scope of nursing
practice, the socioeconomic and educational distance between nurses and
other health professionals, and the ideology of professionalism in nursing.
Although these are not all the factors involved in such relationships (and
they overlap in many respects), they are major sources of tensions. These
tensions at times not only contribute to conflicts among nurses and other
health care providers but block ethical inquiry into them.

2. NURSE AUTONOMY

The question, "Is a nurse free to act upon her own judgment?" arose in
both cases previously described in this chapter and is a central concern in
the following cases. As suggested in Chapter 3, free action as well as rational deliberation and moral reflection are necessary if a person is to be ethically autonomous. Yet, for nurses in certain situations, free action remains
problematic, as in the following case.

4.3 Disagreement with a Feeding Order

Cheryl Pulec worked during her last two years in school as a nursing assistant on a gynecology floor in a large university medical center and has had
six months' experience in a neonatal intensive care unit as a registered nurse.
When the unit is busy, she cares for two babies, but she has cared for only
one baby, Ahmed Nasser, since his admission a week ago.

Last night, one of the residents wrote orders to start feeding Ahmed and
then left the unit. When Cheryl read them, she thought they were "crazy
orders" since they included "giving sterile water over 24 hours." She had
never seen such a beginning feeding order, and she was concerned about
possible fluid and electrolyte problems. She told another resident in the unit
her grounds for objecting and that she felt uneasy about beginning Ahmed's
feeding according to that plan. Nevertheless, he told her to proceed according to the written orders.

Even though directed by two doctors to start the feedings, Cheryl thought
that since she still disagreed with the feeding plan, she would not begin it.
She liked her staff nurse position and tried to do a good job, which included,
of course, carrying out medical orders and working well with the doctors;
but she thought Ahmed's well-being was more important than the possible
repercussions she might suffer for her efforts to get the orders changed and
her refusal to carry them out. Therefore, she considered whether she should
approach a third resident and repeat her reasons for not wanting to carry out
the feeding order.

Cheryl's reasons for acting in this situation are based on her obligations to Ahmed as a health care provider, to the hospital as an employee, and to the physicians as a coworker. When she became a registered nurse, she assumed an obligation to provide safe, effective, and morally responsible care to her clients. Therefore, she has a duty to do her best for Ahmed Nasser. She is well within her legal obligations, as defined by the state nursing practice act and her contract with the hospital, to question any medical order and to refrain from implementing it if, in her judgment, the order is unsafe. Nevertheless, since nurses have traditionally obeyed physicians, she recognizes that the physicians expect her to carry out the orders as a part of the traditional nursing role. Finally, Cheryl believes she must act so as to maintain her self-respect as an autonomous, thoughtful, reliable person.

Cheryl has time to make a thoughtful decision, since the risk to Ahmed is very slight if she delays the feedings briefly. The question is, will Ahmed be harmed by the feedings in any significant or lasting way? Given Cheryl's limited experience—she has been employed in the neonatal intensive care unit for only six months—her opposition to the feedings perhaps should not be given the weight of the two resident physicians' decision in favor of the sterile water feedings since they have had more education and clinical experience than she. Her apparent lack of experience, however, is offset by her scientific education regarding fluids and electrolytes, her study of other babies during her employment, and her acute awareness of Ahmed's needs since he has been the only baby in her care during the past week. It is possible that the first physician wrote the order while thinking not specifically of Ahmed but of babies generally, and that the second physician, not recognizing a gross error in the feeding order, elected to let the order stand. Given the second physician's decision not to act, and given that Cheryl based her decision on her brief nursing experience and on the negative evidence that the order was wrong because she had never seen any like it, she could conclude that the feeding order might be within the limits of acceptable medical practice, even if it were not ideal. Therefore, she might proceed without causing Ahmed undue harm. But even though the feedings are probably not unsafe, Cheryl is convinced that they are not best for Ahmed since they may upset his fluid and electrolyte balance.

Cheryl's obligations to Ahmed and the physicians are in conflict. She cannot obey the orders and thus act as a loyal subordinate to the physicians in the traditional sense and simultaneously meet Ahmed's needs as she has defined them. But a nurse's primary obligations, in the end, are to clients, not physicians. The reason a nurse works with a physician and his medical treatment plan is to help provide a client with the best possible health care.[35] Whatever the strength of the historical legacy and the dominating status of medicine, whenever a nurse faces a choice between obligation to a physician and obligation to a client, she must recognize that her obligation to a client is primary. In Cheryl's case, her obligation to the physicians is clearly secondary to, and based upon, her obligation to the baby; the choice of overriding the obligation to the physicians carries only a relatively small risk. While Cheryl may lose her reputation as a congenial worker, Ahmed has much to gain if, in fact, a different feeding order would be better for him.

Cheryl's situation, like other situations in which a nurse considers alternatives to what a physician has ordered, rests at some point on a wide "spectrum of urgency," that is, on a continuum of cases in which the available time to make decisions varies. The spectrum begins at one end with problems that may be solved at a leisurely pace, allowing time for reflection, collection of further data, debate, and discussion, and ends at the other end with urgent questions that demand quick solutions and immediate actions. The low-urgency end of the spectrum includes such situations as those in which a physician and nurse disagree about the correct answer to a question that a young pregnant woman asks in trying to decide if she should choose a home delivery attended by a midwife or a hospital delivery attended by a physician. In such a situation, the physician, nurse, and client have several months to study and to debate all aspects of the situation. The high-urgency end of the spectrum includes emergency situations in which a physician and a nurse disagree about an order for actions that must be carried out immediately. For example, a nurse and a physician may choose to allocate care differently for three accident victims admitted simultaneously to an emergency room.

The "spectrum of urgency" can be used as a guideline for nurses who question a physician's orders in situations involving practices that fall within the range of generally acceptable medical care. In situations in which urgency is low, when ample time is available for reasonable reflection and discussion, a rule-utilitarian argument (see Chapter 2, Section 1) that nurses obey doctors as the best course of action to insure the best overall outcome for clients is much less strong than in emergency situations. To return to Case 4.3, if Cheryl agrees with the utilitarian goal of the greatest happiness for the largest number of patients, a goal supported by many hospitals in numerous policies, she might agree that she should be obedient and follow all physicians' orders that appear to fall within the broad range of acceptable practice, including the feeding order that a second physician supported. She could conclude that all nurses should follow all such physicians' orders because most of the time the orders would be correct; the greatest number of persons would thus be effectively served.

Two problems with this argument, however, immediately come to light. First, physicians' orders, like all human judgments, are sometimes wrong.

If a nurse blindly followed all of them, harm to the patient could result, as the research study described in Chapter 1, Section 5, illustrated. Thus, insofar as a nurse has an obligation to follow a doctor's orders, it is only a prima facie obligation and may be overridden in certain circumstances by other factors. A nurse must be careful not to confuse a well-grounded prima facie obligation with blind faith. Second, nurses who operate under such a regime may become automatons, unable to make the responsible decisions that are necessary for high-quality nursing care. Thus, while in the short run the result might seem to be the greatest happiness for the greatest number of patients, over the long run, the harm to some patients and the poor quality of care delivered by automatons would significantly compromise overall happiness. The idea that nurses should obey physicians, when examined in low-urgency cases, appears to have little to be said for it apart from appeals to tradition.

The nearer a case is to the other end of the spectrum, the greater the need for a nurse to follow a physician's orders without debate. In general, a physician's medical expertise should be greater than a nurse's medical expertise since a nursing education, by its very nature, focuses upon nursing rather than medicine. In most emergency situations, the greatest number of satisfactory outcomes for clients will occur if a nurse refrains from blocking acceptable orders and cooperates in delivering quick, efficient help, although she might judge that a particular course is not the one that she believes would be best. The main goal in a crisis is to provide adequate help quickly, and this goal would obviously be blocked by lengthy debate and discussion. In a cool moment after the crisis has passed, the nurse should engage the physician in a discussion regarding the feasibility and worth of alternative actions that may have been more appropriate. A nurse, especially an experienced nurse, may be more knowledgeable than a physician about a specific client, situation, or procedure. Through calm, rational discussion the nurse and the physician might learn from each other and agree how best to manage similar crises in the future.

Although a nurse generally presumes that a physician is right in an emergency situation, there are nonetheless limits to what can reasonably be presumed. When the medical care a physician orders clearly constitutes unacceptable practice, a nurse is obligated to disobey orders. For example, consider a situation in which an emergency room nurse and a resident physician disagreed about whether the use of a local anesthetic was acceptable practice in the case of a five-year-old girl who had suffered a huge vaginal laceration. After the doctor had ordered the nurse to pry the terrified and wildly struggling girl's legs apart while he repeatedly tried but failed to inject a local anesthetic, the nurse, believing that such treatment was unacceptable because of the child's fear and pain and the size of the laceration, refused to continue assisting the physician. She demanded that another resident physician be called, which resulted in the child being taken to surgery and given a general anesthetic.[36] Given the psychic trauma caused to the girl by repeated attempts to repair the laceration, further efforts in the emergency room clearly fell outside the bounds of acceptable practice.

In summary, if an order for action is clearly outside acceptable medical practice, a nurse should not obey it even in an emergency and should seek safe care for the client from another source as did the emergency room nurse in the previous example. If a physician's order is within the wide range of acceptable practice and time is pressing, the nurse should obey that order, even if she would prefer another course of action, and she should discuss the matter with the physician later.[37] At the lower levels of the spectrum of urgency—and most medical care allows some time for consideration— the nurse should calmly and rationally discuss with the physician those orders that she questions, including orders that fall within the wide range of acceptable medical practice, in order to provide the best possible care for each client. Given these guidelines, Cheryl, the nurse in the feeding order case, should discuss the situation with her nurse manager to see if she missed something a more experienced nurse should know. Then she should call the first resident to explain her reasons for not following the feeding order in the hope that he will cancel the order and write a new one. The first resident ought to learn that his order is being questioned; in addition, Cheryl's asking a third resident could confuse the situation.[38]

In the following case, a nurse who is striving to be ethically autonomous in her practice confronts the complexities of autonomy in nursing, including the question of free action.

4.4 Is It Right for Us?

Ann Fiske, registered nurse, has enjoyed the first seven months on a medical unit, her first nursing position. But since being assigned to Mr. James Bering, 71-year-old retired widower suffering from a rapidly growing, highly malignant sarcoma of the peritoneum, Ann is finding her responsibilities unsettling. Mr. Bering's days and nights are filled with intractable pain, and despite her care and that of others, he suffers much from insomnia and discomfort. Further, his various medications often cloud his mind. During the past two days, Mr. Bering has talked briefly with Ann of his approaching death.

Today, after Mr. Bering's attending physician, Dr. Rhodes, checked Mr. Bering and spoke with Mr. Bering's two children, he ordered drugs to terminally sedate Mr. Bering. The drugs would make him unconscious. The withdrawal of nutrition and hydration would then spare the family a lingering

(Continued)

death. Although the likelihood of an earlier death for Mr. Bering was not in itself troubling to Ann, she doubted whether Mr. Bering or his family had explicitly consented to this course of action.

Since Ann knew that Dr. Rhodes was a highly respected physician with years of experience, she hesitated a moment before asking him whether Mr. Bering had given his consent. When she did ask, Dr. Rhodes quietly explained that he had not discussed the issue with Mr. Bering because to do so would be needlessly cruel. Nor, he said, would he saddle his relatives with "the burden of making this decision." In fact, he added, "I never ask families to make decisions that would leave them feeling guilty." Then he said firmly, "I've made hundreds of these difficult decisions—sometimes it's a little less potassium, sometimes too much oxygen, sometimes morphine—and you, if you're a good nurse, should know better than to say anything. If you're not going to be a good nurse, I'd better call your supervisor."

Recognizing both that Dr. Rhodes expected all nurses to follow his orders unquestioningly, and that he was one of her supervisor's favorite physicians, Ann thought that if she balked at his orders she would face problems not only with him but with her supervisor. Ann did not want to make trouble for herself, but she was concerned about Mr. Bering. She asked herself, Is it right for us to administer treatment designed not only to relieve his pain and distress, but also to hasten his death without his or his family's explicit permission?[39]

Ann and Dr. Rhodes disagree on questions of ethics and values. The conflict centers on the ethical choice between: (1) simply administering the terminal sedation drugs, which will result in freedom from pain and anxiety, unconsciousness, and an inability to continue taking fluids and food naturally, leading to perhaps an earlier death; and (2) trying to determine whether, when informed of the consequences, Mr. Bering (or if he is not competent, his family) wants the terminal sedation drugs.[40] Underlying the first alternative are the utilitarian values of reducing pain, suffering, and guilt; underlying the second are the respect for persons values of self-determination and informed consent.

Inasmuch as this issue turns on a conflict of values, when Ann questions Dr. Rhodes' decision, she does not challenge his specialized medical knowledge and expertise. Nothing in Dr. Rhodes' training certified him as an "expert" on ethical matters, if indeed there are any such experts. Furthermore, in asking for his reasons and even subjecting them to critical examination, Ann is not venturing into matters beyond her competence.

If Ann discusses the matter further with Dr. Rhodes, it will be to her advantage if her position is based on rational deliberation and moral reflection rather than simply intuition or "gut feeling." Dr. Rhodes has already given reasons for preferring his course of action. If she is to maintain her position, Ann must be able to provide stronger reasons why the doctor should obtain informed consent before she proceeds to administer the drugs.

The main consideration to which Ann could appeal is the respect that is owed to Mr. Bering as a person. Mr. Bering has a right to accept or refuse various forms of medical treatment. This right is based on the right to self-determination, which is itself based on the respect that is owed persons as choosing beings. Mr. Bering, so far as we can tell, has not chosen to die sooner rather than later. He knows that death is imminent, but he has not consented that it be hastened. To administer the terminal sedation and thus end his intake of fluids and food is, of course, likely to hasten his death. To do so without his explicit informed consent is to deny his freedom and dignity as a choosing being, as a person.

On the surface, this argument for Ann's position is at least as strong as Dr. Rhodes' argument for administering the terminal sedation without further discussion with the patient or his family. If Ann is to be thorough in her deliberations, however, she must be able to anticipate and respond to the objections Dr. Rhodes might make against her reasoning. First, he might emphasize that although the principle of informed consent is fine in theory, it is often inapplicable in practice. Self-determination and informed consent presuppose that the patient (or, if not the patient, the patient's family) is capable of rational deliberation in such situations; but this, Dr. Rhodes may argue, is not often the case—and is certainly not the case with Mr. Bering or his family. Mr. Bering, Dr. Rhodes might claim, is not mentally competent to make this decision himself, and his family would be plagued by guilt if it were to be thrust upon them.

The question of patient autonomy is a complex conceptual-empirical matter.[41] If Ann is to neutralize this objection, she must be able to show that Mr. Bering or his family is capable of understanding and deciding this matter, or at least that Dr. Rhodes has not yet demonstrated their incapability. Since patient autonomy must be presumed, the burden is on him to show why they are incapable.

A second possible objection to Ann's line of reasoning is that administering the terminal sedation will maximize happiness. Appealing to the principle of utility, Dr. Rhodes could point out that not only would Mr. Bering's suffering be diminished but his family would be spared the agonies of decision making and of witnessing Mr. Bering's pain and distress. Furthermore, since obtaining informed consent takes valuable time, if Dr. Rhodes and Ann did not seek it, they would have more time to provide the high-quality medical and nursing care that they are able to give.

As is often the case, however, these utilitarian considerations may be neutralized by others. In the long run, for example, it is likely that if the practice of possibly hastening the deaths of suffering persons without their explicit consent were to become more widely practiced and more widely known, the result would be loss of trust throughout the health care system. Any suffering person with a terminal illness might wonder whether this or that treatment would hasten his or her death. Such loss of trust might create anxieties and a fear of medicine that would actually reduce the net balance of happiness.

Thus, as matters stand, Ann's doubts appear to be well grounded. The question remains, however, whether Ann in her role as a nurse can be ethically autonomous, which requires that she be free to act upon the results of her reasoning and moral reflection.

Let us suppose that Dr. Rhodes either refuses to discuss the matter with Ann any further, or that after discussing it he stands by his initial decision. Let us also assume that he has little specific evidence that Mr. Bering and his family are in no condition to decide the matter themselves and that Ann has good reason to believe that at least one of them is perfectly capable of doing so. If, then, Ann were to administer the terminal sedation drugs, she would be acting contrary not only to what she regards as Mr. Bering's rights but also to her own deeply held moral convictions. She would be compromising her integrity as a person. What, then, should she do?

An adage in ethics that "ought implies can" is pertinent to Ann's dilemma. It is usually taken to mean that if we say someone morally ought to do something, it must be true that he or she can do it. If a person cannot do something, it makes no sense or is morally unjust to say that he or she morally should do it. Thus, if a person cannot swim we cannot say that he or she ought to have gone into deep water to rescue a drowning swimmer. If a physician is prevented at gunpoint by a terrorist from treating a wounded hostage, we cannot say that he ought nevertheless to have treated the hostage. Thus, in determining what Ann ought to do in the case before us, we must try to clarify what she actually can do.

Deciding what she can do, however, is difficult because Ann's freedom of action is in doubt. On the one hand, perhaps Ann is being coerced into following Dr. Rhodes' orders. If, for example, she resists giving the drugs, Dr. Rhodes may find a number of ways to make her job very unpleasant. He may also complain about her to her nursing supervisor, who may have considerable power over her. Because she is relatively new in this unit, and this is her first position, Ann may fear losing her job. If there were no other hospital in town, and Ann were the sole support of her ailing mother, the risk of losing her job would indeed be serious. Thus, in light of such de facto conditions, we might conclude that Ann is not entirely free to act in accord with her ethical views.

On the other hand, perhaps Ann finds herself in more favorable circumstances. Experienced and with a strong record, she believes that being harassed by Dr. Rhodes, or being reprimanded or disciplined by her nursing supervisor is a small price to pay for protecting Mr. Bering's rights and for acting in accord with her deepest ethical convictions. Suppose, too, that she is not committed to living in the area where she is currently employed or that she could readily find another nursing position if her job became too unpleasant. If this were Ann's situation, we might conclude that she is not being coerced by circumstance into following Dr. Rhodes' orders. As a result, she is free to act in accord with her considered moral views, and therefore she ought to do so.

The main question, then, is this: Is Ann free to act in accord with the results of her rational deliberation and moral reflection or is she coerced into administering the drugs? If we conclude that she is not free to act in accord with the results of her rational deliberation and moral reflection, then she is neither fully autonomous nor fully responsible for administering the drugs. If, however, we conclude that, despite the circumstances, she is free to act in accord with her considered ethical judgments, then she is both autonomous and responsible for what she does.

We have no simple solution to the problem of free action in nursing. On the one hand, we admire nurses who risk punitive responses from physicians and others for the sake of patients' rights and their own moral integrity. We think such nurses should generally be commended and supported. On the other hand, we recognize that many nurses face situations in which it would be extremely difficult to withstand the threat of punitive responses. Moreover, we do not believe that nurses should have to be heroines or make harsh personal sacrifices to do what they have good reason to believe is morally right or to preserve their moral integrity. So the nurse in this case may simply have to make the best of a very bad situation. But such situations may be avoidable. In Section 3, we suggest some systematic changes in the nurse–physician relationship that can reduce both the incidence and the severity of such predicaments.

The next case, a widely discussed historical case from the 1970s, provides an additional illustration of the complexities of free action. Here, a nurse's independent actions resulted in an unfortunate nurse–physician conflict.

4.5 Giving Information to Clients

Mrs. Tuma, a junior-college nursing instructor, requested that she be assigned to care for Mrs. W., a 59-year-old woman acutely ill with myelogenous leukemia, so that one of her nursing students could learn about chemotherapy. When the physician told Mrs. W. that she was dying and that the only hope for prolonging her life was chemotherapy, he described the

(Continued)

painful and disfiguring side effects of the treatment as well as the possibility of doing nothing. Although Mrs. W. had some degree of mental impairment caused by her condition, the physician believed that she was rational when he obtained both her and her family's consent for chemotherapy.

As Mrs. Tuma prepared the first chemotherapy dose, her student reported that she had found Mrs. W. crying. When Mrs. Tuma tried to comfort Mrs. W., Mrs. W. explained that she had fought leukemia for 12 years with God's help, by faithfully practicing the Mormon religion, by eating natural foods, and by avoiding drugs and stimulants. At this point Mrs. Tuma responded by discussing natural remedies for cancer with Mrs. W. She also determined, however, that Mrs. W. still consented to the chemotherapy and consequently initiated the chemotherapy intravenously as ordered. But Mrs. W. pleaded with Mrs. Tuma to return in the evening to discuss various natural treatments with her son and daughter-in-law.

When the daughter-in-law learned of the scheduled evening meeting with Mrs. Tuma, she phoned the doctor, who told her to attend the meeting and get the nurse's name. Early in the evening, the doctor phoned an order to suspend the chemotherapy because of Mrs. W.'s changed attitude. After Mrs. Tuma's discussion with the family, which included chemotherapy and its side effects, alternatives provided by natural foods and herbs, the unavailability of Laetrile in the United States, and Mrs. W.'s problem of obtaining blood transfusions if she were to terminate chemotherapy, all agreed that Mrs. W.'s best course was to continue with chemotherapy.

Later in the evening the physician ordered the chemotherapy to be resumed. The next day he demanded that the college remove Mrs. Tuma from her position, which the college authorities consequently did. He also complained to the hospital, which notified the State Board of Nurses, which, in turn, initiated a petition for the suspension or revocation of Mrs. Tuma's license. The Hearing Officer for the Board of Nurse Examiners determined that Mrs. Tuma had interfered with the physician–patient relationship, an act that constituted unprofessional conduct, and the Board suspended her license for six months. Mrs. W. died two weeks after the chemotherapy was started.[42]

An examination of this case reveals arguments that both support and criticize Mrs. Tuma's actions. A nurse, *as a person*, has the right to function autonomously as does every other person. Every person—client, physician, or nurse—can demand that he or she be recognized as a person worthy of dignity and respect with the right to act autonomously and to make justifiable claims on others for these general rights. However, the physician did not lodge a complaint against her as a person. Rather, in her discussions with Mrs. W., Mrs. Tuma had acted *as a nurse*. As Sister Teresa Stanley pointed out in her discussion of this case, no ethical dilemma would have resulted had a neighbor discussed the same information with Mrs. W.[43]

Yet Mrs. W.'s questions about alternative treatments made a claim upon Mrs. Tuma for information; Mrs. Tuma agreed since she believed that she, as a nurse, should meet Mrs. W.'s needs. Both Mrs. Tuma and Mrs. W. perceived Mrs. Tuma's role as that of a well-informed care provider, someone who knew about and could explain alternative cancer treatments. Further, the professional nursing role, as Mrs. Tuma understood it, allowed her to insure that a client's consent to therapy was fully informed.[44] As Sally Gadow has persuasively argued, "Patients can be assisted in reaching decisions which express their complex totality as individuals only by nurses who themselves act out of the same explicit self-unity, allowing no dimension of themselves to be exempt from the professional relation."[45] Acceptance of this notion, with its requirements for recognition of a nurse *as a person*, necessitates that a nurse be allowed to be ethically autonomous in her nursing role, that is, that her actions be free from coercion or manipulation, be the result of rational choice, and be in accord with her own values and principles.

Clearly, however, Mrs. Tuma had placed herself in a risky situation. Even though she included in her definition of the nursing role that nurses function autonomously, she recognized from the outset that not all persons, including the physician, shared that viewpoint.[46] In her state, the nursing role did not confer upon nurses the privilege of autonomous action in a situation such as that involving Mrs. W. The Hearing Officer for the Board of Nurse Examiners disallowed as evidence the American Nurses Association Code for Nurses because the Board had not adopted it, as well as any testimony or definitions by the ANA. He determined that Mrs. Tuma had interfered with the physician–patient relationship, which constituted unprofessional conduct. Thus, the Board judged that Mrs. Tuma did not have the privilege of functioning autonomously in her role as a nurse in this situation since her actions interfered with the physician–patient relationship.[47] To the Board, the nurse–client relationship apparently played a secondary role.[48]

A nurse in a situation similar to that of Mrs. Tuma could respond in a number of different ways. She could assume the traditional deferential role and do nothing autonomously. Or she could play an expert doctor–nurse game, pretend that she knew nothing when the client asked, and later, if possible, indirectly get the doctor to discuss alternative cancer treatments with the client. Or she could work as if she had a collaborative relationship with the physician and view his presentation of only two choices (chemotherapy with its terrible side effects or no treatment) as morally unacceptable while at the same time recognizing that such a presentation of choices fell well within the cope of acceptable medical practice. She could, for example, contact the physician and try to persuade him that the patient and her family had a right to a discussion of alternative treatments. If he

did not want to participate in such a discussion she could offer to do it herself. If he not only refused to participate himself but also told her that she
was not to discuss this matter with the patient, she could, as an act of conscientious refusal, decide to meet with the patient and her family anyway
(see Section 5). If the physician filed a complaint, a State Board of Nurses
still might react as it did in Mrs. Tuma's case. But such a nurse would now
be perceived as having acted collaboratively as a professional who notified
colleagues of her intentions and shared her reasoning with them.

3. COLLABORATION

Collaboration implicitly assumes that nurses, in their nursing roles, like
other health care providers, in their provider roles, are morally autonomous
or self-determining.[49] Collaboration is crucially important if nurses are to
meet their social obligation to provide high-quality nursing care because,
as nurses, they are often in the middle of indeterminate and complex health
care situations. The following case summarizes such a situation, one in
which nurses and other health providers disagree as to whether they should
continue aggressive treatment.

4.6 Stopping Treatment

Susan Cory is a 29-year-old critical care nurse who enjoys the nursing challenges of a medical intensive care unit in a large medical center. Her reputation among fellow health care providers is that of a caring and exceptionally
competent nurse. At present, however, she is at odds with most persons
working in the ICU over whether aggressive treatment should be continued
for Marsha Hocking, a severely brain-damaged, young, single woman her
own age, a victim of viral encephalitis. Marsha's parents, completely over-
whelmed by the situation, are relying completely on the judgment of their
daughter's care providers. Susan and the medical, respiratory, and nursing
staffs agree as to the medical details of the case, that is, the extent of brain
damage and Marsha's very poor prognosis.

After careful deliberation, Susan concluded that aggressive treatment in
Marsha's case should be reduced sharply because no hope remained for her
recovery. Susan based her decision on her belief that no one would want to be
kept alive in Marsha's condition. Therefore, to continue treating her would
be morally wrong. Without aggressive treatment, which includes artificial
ventilation, Marsha would die quickly.

Susan has asked the other providers to think about her recommendation.
Some nurses and respiratory therapists agree with Susan. Others agree with
most of the physicians, including the one in charge of Marsha's case; they

---

believe that now is not the time to give up. They point to a variety of reasons for continuing aggressive treatment—Marsha's age, the sudden onset of the disease, her previously excellent condition, and their personal beliefs about the value of life. Throughout the discussion, which has continued for two weeks, Susan has not requested of the ICU nurse manager that she be excused from the case, an infrequent request but one that has been honored in the ICU for other nurses.[50]

In complex cases like this, an authoritarian conception of the physician–other health provider relationship is best replaced by a collaborative conception. In collaborating to meet the health-related needs of patients while respecting their rights, physicians and other providers, as well as patients and families, share knowledge, discuss differences, and work together with mutual respect.[51]

This is not to deny, however, that authoritarian structures are sometimes needed and morally justifiable. In our discussion of the spectrum of urgency, we indicated that emergency situations often require such structures. In addition, as John Ladd has suggested, specialized contexts such as the operating room are highly suited to the exercise and recognition of medical authority.

In an operating room, the authority of the surgeon might be likened to the authority of the conductor of an orchestra: the surgeon is the chief performer and the one who "orchestrates" the proceeding. Let us grant that the aim of the procedure is to save the patient's life, i.e., a morally worthy goal. But here, as with the orchestra, we are dealing with a precisely defined, limited enterprise involving goals that we may assume are shared by all the parties involved, or, to be more nearly accurate, we should say that they ought to be shared by all of them.[52]

As Ladd goes on to point out, goals in most other health care contexts are not this simply defined. And where the goals of patients, physicians, nurses, and other providers do not clearly converge, both the need and the justification for authoritarian structures are considerably weakened.

When authoritarian relationships between physicians and other providers cannot be justified by the situation, we agree with Ladd's suggestion that "we try to find more 'democratic' procedures, procedures involving mutual counseling, consultation, and collaboration. Mutual accommodation and persuasion should take the place of one person['s] issuing commands to others below."[53]

If more collaborative relationships can be established, several positive results can be expected: (1) an increased likelihood that the parties will reach a well-grounded and mutually satisfactory decision; (2) an appreciation of the ethical dilemmas nurses face in being "caught in the middle"; and (3) lower medical care costs because of reduced "burnout" among nurses.

Collaboration can result in increased willingness among all parties to reach a mutually satisfactory decision. Persons who deliberate in a spirit of mutual respect share not only their ethical positions but also bits of information about a situation that all parties may not have fully known or appreciated. No matter how carefully one analyzes an ethical dilemma, it is always possible to have overlooked an important argument or fact.

If they initially disagree, nurses and other providers (and patients and families) who carefully try to hear each other out and to see matters from one another's perspective often find themselves shifting from their original positions and meeting each other halfway. In many cases, for example, one not only comes to appreciate the strength of an opposing position but also comes to recognize that one's own motives include self-interest as well as ethical considerations. Thus, it is not unlikely that Susan Cory's concern for the patient's autonomy and for efficient use of resources is heightened by her frustration with the very difficult nursing problems the patient presents. Similarly, the desire of some of the nurses and respiratory therapists and most of the physicians to continue treatment may result in part from their desire to practice and refine certain skills. As Samuel Gorovitz has pointed out, "Skills that have been acquired at substantial personal cost are skills that people like to use.... There is an intrinsic payoff in satisfaction. State-of-the-art medicine is very sophisticated and people who can do it often find it a very beautiful thing to be doing."[54] If such possible motivations are identified and discussed, there may be less self-righteousness and more willingness to reach a mutually satisfactory accommodation.

Collaboration can lead to an appreciation among all parties of the ethical dilemmas nurses face because they are "caught in the middle." A nurse is in an especially difficult position in our health care delivery system. She is expected to be a trustworthy team member who works within a hierarchical system structured from the top down, a hierarchy in which a physician is usually in command. Yet a nurse is expected to work in that health care system as if it were structured from the base up so as to meet assessed needs of the client and the client's family.[55]

Suppose the facts in Case 4.6 are altered and Susan Cory is "caught in the middle between family and physician." Suppose, for example, that mutually respectful discussion among the physicians, Susan, and other nurses does not occur. Suppose, too, that Susan has built a close and trusting relationship with the patient's mother, a frail, nervous woman with a serious heart ailment who has asked Susan for information about her daughter's condition. Let us also suppose that the physician in charge of the medical treatment plan does not wish the mother to have this information, and that he expects and trusts Susan to put the mother's questions off, or failing this, to lie to her. Finally, imagine that Susan believes that the mother has a right to the information and has strong grounds for believing she will not be harmed by it.

One can easily understand Susan's sense of frustration in such a situation. If she truthfully answers the mother, she breaks the trust of the treatment team that expects a nurse to be a dependable team player. If, however, she puts the mother off with noncommittal comments or with lies, she jeopardizes the mother's trust and her own sense of personal integrity.

Patients, their families, and other health care providers all presume that nurses are personally honest, open, and loyal to them. But when a nurse cannot fulfill the conflicting expectations, when she is quite literally "caught in the middle," she cannot be entirely trustworthy to all parties. On the other hand, collaboration, in which nurses and other providers present their ethical arguments to one another, share information, and deliberate in a spirit of mutual respect, helps to solve the problem of being caught in the middle between a top-down hierarchical system and an inverse system based on patients' needs.

We are not saying that another health care provider must always agree with whatever a nurse thinks is ethically correct. Rather, we are suggesting that other providers and nurses must respect each other as autonomous moral agents. This requires, among other responses, addressing each other's ethical concerns, mutually deliberating and reflecting upon various courses of action, and in some cases agreeing with or adjusting to the ethical views of others. There is a sense in which we can respect someone as a moral agent even when we disagree with him or her and ultimately reject his or her decision—if we hear that person out, give reasons for our views, and make good-faith efforts to show why we believe our view is better.

Collaboration also can result in lower medical care costs by reducing burnout, a well-documented problem among hospital nurses in the United States. Problems of burnout among nurses underscore the dangers of continued conflict, stress, and loss of integrity. Indeed, this cause of burnout is so common as to have been given its own label—"moral distress." In a position statement on the topic, the American Association of Critical-Care Nurses defines moral distress as occurring when a nurse either (1) knows the ethically appropriate action to take in a given circumstance and is unable to act upon it or (2) acts in a manner contrary to her personal and professional values, which undermines her integrity and authenticity. The position statement identifies research indicating, among other things, "that nearly half the nurses studied left their units or nursing altogether because of moral distress." Replacing these nurses is costly, since nurses must be attracted to a hospital and oriented for a time. Consequently, hospital costs rise while continual personnel turnover causes the quality of care to decline. One identified cause of nursing burnout is the difficulty many nurses have maintaining personal integrity when their ideals conflict with the real world of health care.[56]

Suppose that, in Case 4.6, the nurses and physicians do not deliberate in a spirit of mutual respect; they do not discuss whether to continue aggressive treatment for the patient, Marsha Hocking. In addition, the nurse, Susan Cory, understands that if Marsha has a cardiac arrest, Susan will be expected to "call a code." Given her understanding of the case and her ethical views, Susan believes that calling a code would be morally wrong. Suppose, also, that Susan is caring for another patient with similar problems but who is under the care of a different physician who orders less aggressive treatment and leaves directions not to resuscitate. In caring for this second patient, Susan believes she can act morally in the event of a cardiac arrest. But, if Susan is the thoughtful, competent person described in Case 4.6, continued employment in such a unit, given the strikingly conflicting orders and expectations in medically similar cases, will certainly strain her sense of wholeness as a person. She cannot continue to think of herself as a nurse with integrity if situations continue to arise in which she must painfully face and agonize about inconsistencies in treatment policies.

Through collaboration among members of the health care team, the stress that nurses experience can be reduced. Positive results depend upon thoughtful, mutually satisfactory decisions, decisions that often require principled compromise among the various parties involved.

4. INTEGRITY-PRESERVING COMPROMISE

Compromise, construed as a settlement of differences in which each side makes concessions, must be clearly differentiated from being compromised, that is, being forced to give up one's interests, principles, or integrity. To compromise does not necessarily require that a person be compromised. Nurses and other health care providers who deliberate in a spirit of mutual respect may be able to reach a principled, integrity-preserving compromise. A well-grounded, integrity-preserving compromise is not to be confused with a lopsided "compromise" that merely repeats the doctor–nurse game in which a physician calls the shots and a nurse silently bites her lip.

Basic to a compromise that maintains integrity is an appreciation of the factual uncertainty and moral complexity of modern health care. In Case 4.6, it is not clear whether those advocating continued aggressive treatment or those advocating much less aggressive treatment have the more defensible position. Given moral pluralism (Chapter 2, Section 3), the complexity of many issues in biomedical ethics, and our limited knowledge and understanding of them, ethical disagreements often are not the result of simple conflicts between what is obviously right and obviously wrong. As Arthur Kuflik has pointed out:

> Individuals must often base their respective moral judgments on a picture of their situation that is relevantly, but irremediably, incomplete. Their differences of opinion may have less to do with deficiencies of moral sensibility than with uncertainties that are inherent in the situation itself. ... [Moreover] even individuals who are adequately informed and acknowledge the same fundamental principles can find themselves in disagreement when an issue engages several morally relevant considerations at the same time. In such cases the sheer complexity of the matter enables reasonable persons to form somewhat different assessments.[57]

Both of these factors, factual uncertainty and moral complexity, seem to be at the root of the disagreement in Susan Cory's case.

Susan Cory believes that no one would want to be kept alive in Marsha Hocking's condition. How can she be sure of this? Perhaps Susan and many of her acquaintances would not want to be kept alive in this condition, but what about Marsha? Susan would be on much stronger ground if she knew that before becoming ill Marsha had shared this view, but she does not have such knowledge. Similarly, those who are opting for continued aggressive treatment appeal to factors that are relevant to possible recovery—the patient's age, the sudden onset of the disease, her previously excellent health—but they have little else to go on when estimating her chances of survival. Perhaps more important, they cannot predict her future level of consciousness and activity even if she does survive. If they knew she would survive and that her ensuing condition would be good, or at least tolerable, they might be on stronger ground. They do not have such knowledge, however.

Moreover, apart from empirical uncertainty, each side can appeal to morally relevant considerations to support its view. Susan can appeal (although without full assurance) to the patient's right to autonomy, and perhaps to the inefficient use of medical resources. The latter appeal will be considerably strengthened if the ICU is full or if other patients in the ICU are likely to benefit from increased attention the staff can devote to them because they will not be doing so much for Marsha. Those taking the opposing view can invoke the value of each human life and the importance of their roles as protectors and preservers of life. Each side, then, may invoke legitimate ethical considerations on its behalf. If, in this case and in others similarly clouded by empirical uncertainty and moral complexity, health care workers can recognize the nature of their situation, they may be able to reach a well-grounded, mutually respectful accommodation that preserves the integrity of both sides.

First, each party may be persuaded to relinquish her or his original view and to replace it with a mutually agreeable new position. If both parties deliberate rationally and conclude that a third position is superior to their respective initial positions, they can adopt it with no loss of integrity. Strictly speaking, this would not be a compromise. Neither side would be making a concession to the other. Each would be embracing what is now believed to be the best position consistent with her or his own values and principles.

Collaborative discussion can also result in agreement when only one party changes positions. To change positions and to agree with another's views on the basis of ethical discussion does not lead to a loss of integrity if the new position is accepted autonomously and based on a reconsideration or reevaluation of the applicability of one's own moral principles. Such an accommodation might, however, lead to questions of "saving face," especially if both parties have publicly staked their reputations on their initial positions. In such situations, the person shifting positions could be supported if both disputants clearly explained to all involved that the agreed-upon position or action, although initially advocated by only one person is, on reconsideration, consistent with the moral views of both parties.

A compromise occurs when neither party gives up her or his original position but both agree to a decision based not only upon what they individually judge ought to be done but upon what they think ought to be done in light of their conflict and other values that they both esteem. Retaining one's original position and yet acting in accord with a compromise that makes some concessions to an opposing position may appear to present a difficulty. Does not this amount to being compromised; that is, having to give up one's principles or integrity?

To see how a compromise may be integrity-preserving it is important, following a suggestion of Kuflik, to distinguish (1) what Susan Cory or the physician believes ought to be done in this case, leaving aside for the moment that they disagree, from (2) what each judges ought to be done all things considered, when the things to be considered include their reasonable disagreement:

> When an issue is in dispute there is more to be considered than the issue itself—for example, the importance of peace, the presumption against settling matters by force, the intrinsic good of participating in a process in which each side must hear the other side out and try to see matters from the other's point of view, the extent to which the matter does admit reasonable differences of opinion and the significance of a settlement in which each party feels assured of the other's respect for its own seriousness and sincerity in the matter.[58]

These considerations reflect values and principles that many of us hold dear and that partially determine who we are and what we stand for. If we suppose that Susan Cory and the physician hold them too, then it is not so clear that agreeing to a compromise constitutes a threat to their integrity. On the contrary, taking into consideration *all* their values and principles, including a principle of mutual respect that recognizes the reality of reasonable moral pluralism, together with the fact that they reasonably disagree, a compromise solution may be more integrity-preserving than any available alternative. Such a compromise would be "principled" insofar as it is based on a principle of mutual respect and satisfies more of each person's entire set of principles than other possible courses of action.

The main point is that one's identity is constituted in part by a complex constellation of occasionally conflicting values and principles. In difficult cases it will not always be possible to act fully in accord with all of them. After as much consideration as the situation will allow, we will often pursue that course of action that seems, on balance, to follow from the preponderance of our central and most highly cherished values and principles. "Where ultimate values are irreconcilable," Isaiah Berlin has written, "clear-cut solutions cannot, in principle, be found. To decide rationally in such situations is to decide in the light of general ideals, the over-all pattern of life pursued by a man or a group or a society."[59]

Given the factual uncertainty and moral complexity characterizing the disagreement between Susan Cory and the physician, it seems unlikely that either can regard her or his position on the patient's treatment as more central or well grounded than the network of values and principles having to do with mutual respect, the acknowledgment of reasonable differences, not settling matters by force or rank, and so on. Thus, if integrity requires that they act in accord with the preponderance of their most basic values and principles, they may in this case agree to a proposed compromise.

Thus, if in Case 4.6 Susan and those wanting to continue aggressive treatment could find a position that more or less splits the difference between them and is in accord with the preponderance of their other values, they might be able to take this position without compromising their integrity. That is, such mutual accommodation would allow them to work together and respect each other while not requiring them to relinquish their original views. In so doing that would satisfy a principle of mutual respect that acknowledges the reality of reasonable disagreement.

In this case, an acceptable compromise might take the form of an agreement to continue treatment for a specified period and then to review the patient's condition and prognosis and the effective use of resources. If, after this period, certain changes made continued aggressive treatment appear to be a significantly more favorable option than it is at present, such treatment should continue. If there were no such changes, treatment should become less aggressive. If Susan Cory were to agree to this compromise, she would do so while fully preserving her ethical autonomy and personal integrity.

This is not, however, to say that the matter is fully settled. Although Susan Cory and the physician may agree that compromise at this point makes the best of a bad situation, they may try to ensure that the same situation does not arise in the future. Thus, each may make subsequent efforts to practice in settings where his or her colleagues are more likely to share his or her particular views on the treatment of patients like Marsha Hocking, or, each may continue to try to convince the other of the correctness of his or her view. If all coworkers agreed with their respective positions or if the decisions were ones they alone were qualified to make, they would act otherwise: Susan Cory would immediately call a halt to aggressive treatment while the physician would require that it continue indefinitely. As long as they must work together, however, and as long as neither can persuade the other of the correctness of his or her views, they may still arrive at an integrity-preserving compromise if they consider the full range of their important values and principles.

Such a compromise actually occurred in the real-life Susan Cory case. The nurses, respiratory therapists, and physicians agreed to continue treatment for a specified period and then to review the patient's condition and their resources. All agreed that, after this period, if no change had occurred, treatment would be less aggressive. Thus, all members, nurses as well as physicians and other health providers, were able to maintain their personal integrity.[60]

5. CONSCIENTIOUS REFUSAL

Placing a situation somewhere along the spectrum of urgency suggests one way for a nurse to begin to reflect upon when to question a physician's order. Further, as our previous discussion of the spectrum of urgency indicates, a nurse has the duty to override a medical order that is clearly outside acceptable medical practice and that may jeopardize a client in some way. In the following case, the nurse based her decision on her medical knowledge, discounted the risk that her actions might jeopardize her position as a nurse, and followed her own judgment without hesitation.

4.7 Emergency Room Action

When Valerie Workman graduated from a university school of nursing, she believed what she had been taught—when a doctor gives an order, follow it, but not unthinkingly. Over her 20-year nursing career, she has gained not only additional skills and knowledge, but confidence as well. She now questions doctors much more thoroughly, even though she recognizes that some often "aren't exactly thrilled that I question their judgment." In describing herself and other nurses, she says that, "the older we get, the wiser we get—sometimes."

A few years ago, when Valerie was working in a hospital emergency room, Mrs. Brown, a 24-year-old woman who was six months pregnant and in shock, was admitted following a serious automobile accident. The physician on duty was an older man who, Valerie felt, was not always competent in emergencies. Valerie, certain that the patient's life was in danger, suggested starting an IV, but the doctor rejected her suggestion. Alarmed, Valerie decided she must act, started the IV, initiated other emergency measures, and called for additional medical help. The physician was furious at Valerie's independent action, and she was extremely angry with him. Later, she remembers, she "got complete backing from the other doctors" and the matter was dropped.[61]

How did Valerie know not to accept the doctor's orders? Perhaps she reasoned that if a nurse believes that she has a moral obligation to meet a client's needs, then she must take risks, both by refusing to defer to a physician whose actions impede the delivery of adequate help and by taking independent emergency action. To Valerie, the young woman's chance to live must have seemed worth the risk to her own career. Had she chosen to obey orders, and had Mrs. Brown died, Valerie might not have been able to live with her conscience.

The doctor's decision against the IV differed so radically from usual emergency treatment that the other physicians in the hospital agreed that Valerie, not the doctor, had acted more appropriately. Moreover Valerie's action was justified by well-grounded medical and ethical considerations. A nurse may sometimes be in a situation, however, in which a physician's actions fall within acceptable medical practice but the nurse may believe that she cannot be party to the disputed procedure or treatment because to do so would violate her integrity. At times, even the most cooperative and thoughtful health care workers will be unable to agree upon a compromise position. In such situations a nurse can justify a refusal to carry out an order or to participate in a procedure only on the basis of conscience. The following case focuses on what may be called "conscientious refusal."[62]

4.8 Test for Sex Identification

Kalisha Hutton, a nurse practitioner with graduate-level education in genetics and counseling, is employed at the University Clinical Center. Among her

(Continued)

many duties, she explains to women seeking various medical tests what they can expect during the procedures. After results are known, she is the person who meets with the woman and her partner to discuss the meaning of the findings. At times she meets with them alone; at other times she invites health care team members who have knowledge about a particular genetic problem facing the family.

Generally, chromosome studies are done when parents, because of the mother's advanced age or a family history of a specific genetic condition, suspect that their fetus may be affected. Before joining the Clinical Center, Kalisha thought about the implications of such work, including the possibility that most women would choose abortion if tests indicated that a child might be severely mentally disabled. Until recently Kalisha opposed abortion, but she now believes abortion is permissible for parents who recognize that they do not have the strength, support, or money to rear a severely disabled child; she believes that abortion in such cases may also be in the best interests of society, which must bear the cost of a person who will require a lifetime of care.

Liming Lee has asked for karyotyping of fetal cells to determine the sex of her fetus. Prior to seeking assistance from the Clinical Center, Liming used a commercial blood test kit to determine the sex of her fetus, but she is unwilling to trust the results. Liming and her husband, both university post-doctoral students, plan to return home to China within the year. They want to follow their country's family planning policies and have only one child. They want that child to be a boy. And they plan an immediate abortion if the fetus is a female.

Dr. Milton Ely, who usually performs the test procedures, believes that the Lees are as entitled to choose abortion as any other family, and that they have the same right as other families to ask for technical information obtainable through medical tests. But Kalisha believes that the testing is not justified: the couple is highly educated and, she believes, should recognize that a baby's sex does not determine its worth as a human being. Kalisha believes that, in this case, to do the test—and a possible abortion—is sexist. Therefore, she has decided that she must refuse to participate in any way in determining the sex of the Lee fetus.

Kalisha's supervisor is aware of Kalisha's objections but has asked her to meet with the Lees, offer support, and perform her duties as usual. Dr. Ely has told Kalisha that her refusal to participate will not influence the Lee's decision in any way, so she may as well stop making a fuss. Kalisha fears that if she submits to pressure from her supervisor and Dr. Ely, she will have the death of a female fetus on her conscience, and she will have to admit that she is just one more spineless, manipulable nurse who has no meaningful convictions.[63]

In order to explore the question of when a nurse should (or may) use an appeal to conscience to refuse to participate in a particular procedure, we need first to analyze the notion of an appeal to conscience. For if appeals to conscience are to carry special weight, it is important to be able to distinguish them from appeals to self-interest or convenience. In a discussion of appeals to conscience, James Childress cites three cases which illustrate that "conscience is a mode of consciousness and thought about one's own acts and their value or disvalue."

1. On June 21, 1956, Arthur Miller, the playwright, appeared before the House Committee on Un-American Activities (HUAC) which was examining the unauthorized use of passports, and he was asked who had been present at meetings with Communist writers in New York City. "Mr. Chairman, I understand the philosophy behind this question and I want you to understand mine. When I say this, I want you to understand that I am not protecting the Communists or the Communist Party. I am trying to, and I will, *protect my sense of myself.* I could not use the name of another person and bring trouble on him....I ask you not to ask me that question....All I can say, sir, is that *my conscience* will not permit me to use the name of another person."

2. On December 29, 1970, Governor Winthrop Rockefeller of Arkansas commuted to life imprisonment the death sentences of the 15 prisoners then on death row. He said, "I cannot and will not turn my back on life-long Christian teachings and beliefs, merely to let history run out its course on a fallible and failing theory of punitive justice." Understanding his decision as "purely personal and philosophical," he insisted that the records of the prisoners were irrelevant to it. He continued, "I am aware that there will be reaction to my decision. However, failing to take this action while it is within my power, *I could not live with myself.*"

3. In late December, 1972, Captain Michael Heck refused to carry out orders to fly more bombing missions in Vietnam. He wrote his parents: "I've taken a very drastic step. I've refused to take part in this war any longer. *I cannot in good conscience be a part of it.*" He also said, "I can live with prison easier than I can with taking part in the war...I would refuse even a ground job supervising the loading of bombs or refueling aircraft. I cannot be a participant...*a man has to answer to himself first.*"[64]

In analyzing these cases, Childress suggests that an appeal to conscience is based on a desire to preserve one's integrity or wholeness as a person (see subsection in Chapter 1, Section 4, entitled "Developing a systematic framework"). These conscientious refusers are predicting that if they were to act in certain ways they would betray themselves as being certain kinds of people having certain personal ideals and standards of conduct. Insofar as their conceptions of themselves as particular people are determined by having and abiding by certain standards of conduct, what is at stake is, as Bernard Williams argues, nothing less than person identity.[65]

In addition, Childress suggests that appeals to conscience are personal and subjective, based on standards that one does not necessarily apply to others; are founded on a prior judgment of rightness or wrongness, since conscience itself is not a criterion of rightness or wrongness; and are motivated by personal sanction rather than external authority.[66] Kalisha's behavior in Case 4.8 seems to meet all of the conditions for making her act one of conscientious refusal. First Kalisha spoke only for herself in this case. She did not attempt to imagine what another nurse or physician might think or feel about using a medical test to determine sex. Nor would she oppose or try to prevent some other nurse from performing her duties. Second, she judged that her participation would be wrong because the test for what she regarded as a sexist reason could lead to the abortion of a healthy female fetus simply because she was a female. Kalisha used her conscience as a guide only to the extent that she debated with herself; that is, when she debated with her conscience about whether she should participate or not. Kalisha's belief that the abortion of a healthy fetus for "sexist" reasons is morally wrong was the basis for her appeal to conscience. A "conflict of conscience" arose because, although she believed in general that parents have the right to choose abortion, she rejected the grounds for the decision in this particular case. The conflict here is similar to one that might be experienced by someone who endorses a strong interpretation of the right to freedom of speech while also being opposed to its being exercised to further the cause of Nazism. (Consider, in this connection, a New Jersey baker who in 2008 conscientiously refused to write the name "Adolf Hitler" for a three-year-old child so named on a birthday cake ordered by the child's parents.[67]) Third, Kalisha, like Miller, Rockefeller, and Heck in the three passages Childress cites, felt first and foremost answerable to herself (Miller: "I am trying to, and I will, protect my sense of myself"; Rockefeller: "I could not live with myself"; and Heck: "A man has to answer to himself first"). Kalisha believed that if she participated in the test in any way she would have to acknowledge that she was a spineless person without the courage of her deepest convictions. Not only would she have felt guilt about the possible death of a healthy fetus, but she also would have felt ashamed of herself for not having had the strength to act in accord with her personal ideals of conduct—ideals that in part determine her identity.[68] That her participation in this procedure is perfectly legal and that the act is not punishable by any external authority have no bearing whatever on her deliberations.

We may now turn to the general question of under what circumstances and for what reasons a nurse may appeal to her conscience and refuse to participate in a particular procedure. As the discussion of Case 4.8 indicated, a nurse may make an appeal to conscience as a last resort when she has exhausted all other arguments for justifying her action. The appeal to conscience is personal or subjective although the moral standards on which it is based may or may not apply to other persons; it must *follow* a judgment of rightness or wrongness; and it must be based upon personal sanction rather than upon external authority. The individual nurse must determine the extent to which the act in question constitutes a rupture of her integrity or wholeness as a person or a particular self. Then she must determine whether the shame or "bad conscience" that would follow from her performance of the act constitutes a greater threat to her well-being than the possible punishment that may be forthcoming from whatever authority (agency or physician) may be displeased by her refusal. (A discussion of a nursing supervisor's response to a subordinate's appeal to conscience is included in Chapter 5.)

The question that the next case presents is whether a nurse's use of conscientious refusal is appropriate in a situation in which a physician's orders and a patient's wishes are in conflict.

4.9 Disagreement About a Do Not Resuscitate Order

Doris Winn, a staff nurse with two years' experience in a cardiac care unit, strongly wanted Dr. Farooqui to write a DNR (Do Not Resuscitate) order for Mr. Chester Saukin, an 87-year-old retired farmer with a history of three heart attacks and three years of cardiac failure. Mr. Saukin's written advance directive did not forbid resuscitation, so Doris wanted Dr. Farooqui to speak to Mr. Saukin about the issue. Doris believed Mr. Saukin was ready to die, for he had told her repeatedly that was all he wanted. When she told Dr. Farooqui this, he simply walked away from her. She knew he rarely wrote DNR orders. Doris understood, also, that legally she would have to participate in a resuscitation effort, but she thought it would be very hard for her to do.[69]

Could Doris make an appeal to conscience and not attempt a resuscitation? Before discussing this question, we need to return to two earlier discussions, one concerning the spectrum of urgency and the other concerning medical decisions. When Mr. Saukin was first admitted, Doris acted as if the implied disagreement between Mr. Saukin's spoken wishes and his written advance directive fell at the lower end of the urgency spectrum. She had time to tell Dr. Farooqui of Mr. Saukin's statements that he was ready to die, even though the physician did not initially allow her to discuss her unease concerning a Do Not Resuscitate order. Dr. Farooqui's behavior indicated his belief that as a physician his decision not to write a DNR order was indisputable given Mr. Saukin's advance directive.[70] The questions remains, is the decision for a DNR a technical medical decision? If the answer is yes, then the nurse has little recourse; the physician's superior

medical training gives him presumptive authority in technical medical decisions. If the answer is no, that the decision for a DNR order is a decision
in the medical context but not mainly a medical decision in the technical
sense, then the nurse may have something to contribute—especially when
she has some reason to believe that the decision does not reflect the values
and life plan of a conscious, competent adult.[71]

It is possible, however, that Dr. Farooqui's initial refusal to talk with
Doris has resulted not from a denial of her possible contribution but from
his adherence to Mr. Saukin's written advance directive and his awareness
of Mr. Saukin's transient confusion, especially in the evening. He believes
that Mr. Saukin is now not always fully competent. Without a written
request for a DNR order from Mr. Saukin's health care proxy or patient
advocate, he must follow Mr. Saukin's written directive.

A meeting between Doris or Dr. Farooqui or one of the health care provider staff and Mr. Saukin's patient advocate to consider Mr. Saukin's
remarks about being ready to die could be scheduled. Even if such a meeting is held promptly, however, the outcome may not support Doris's desired
DNR order for Mr. Saukin.

Doris strongly believes that the rights of patients should remain in force
to the end of their lives.

> I think patients should have the right to say if they want to live and if they
> want to die; I think that we, as nurses and doctors, should be able to respect
> that. We're all here to heal people, get them well, and send them home. And
> if we aren't able to do that, and the patient has suffered for a long time and
> wants to die, I think we have to deal with our own insecurities. Maybe I don't
> agree with that decision, maybe the doctor doesn't. But it's this patient's: it's
> his life. Who has more right?

Now the question is, what should Doris do in *this* case when, let us
suppose, (1) the patient, Mr. Saukin, repeats that he is ready to die, and
(2) Dr. Farooqui, after learning that Mr. Saukin's patient advocate senses
opposition from the rest of the Saukin family and therefore will not request
a DNR order, does not write a DNR order. On the one hand, Doris believes
she is morally required to respect Mr. Saukin's wishes and that her moral
views on the matter are well grounded. On the other hand, Dr. Farooqui's
well founded respect for the law requires her to override Mr. Saukin's
wishes by participating in resuscitation efforts.

Doris knows that some nurses pretend to follow the law by carrying
out "slow codes." That is, when a patient who is in a situation similar to
that of Mr. Saukin goes into cardiopulmonary arrest, some nurses take
the defibrillator into the room slowly and fumble getting the airway in
place, though in the end, as they know they must, they do the resuscitation

procedures. The patients survive sometimes, but "only to spend a few more days in agony before finally dying," according to Doris. Doris, however, does not want to compromise herself by carrying out a slow code in the guise of a full one.

In deciding whether to conscientiously refuse to comply with hospital policy requiring resuscitation, Doris needs to explore her reasoning with other people—other nurses, her nursing supervisors, Mr. Saukin and his patient advocate, and Dr. Farooqui if possible. Thoughtful discussion with others will help ensure that she has not overlooked certain important considerations; it may also change the views of others and possibly soften or eliminate Doris's dilemma. Above all, if she decides that she simply cannot participate in a resuscitation effort for Mr. Saukin, she must be sure that arrangements are made to ensure that her participation is not indispensable in carrying out a full resuscitation. Finally, she must realize that conscientious refusal carries risks, which range from simply antagonizing others to reprimands or possibly even to loss of employment. For, as the examples of Arthur Miller, Winthrop Rockefeller, and Michael Heck, cited above, indicate, the price of personal integrity in a complex world is often extremely high.

Late in 2008, a political controversy about conscientious refusal and the law developed in the last days of the presidency of George W. Bush. His administration announced new protections for health care providers opposed to abortion and related medical procedures, including contraception, on religious or moral grounds.[72] According to *The New York Times*, "The rule prohibits recipients of federal money from discriminating against doctors, nurses, and heath care aides who refuse to take part in procedures because of their convictions, and it bars hospitals, clinics, doctors' offices and pharmacies from forcing their employees to assist in programs and activities financed by the department [of Health and Human Services (HHS)]." In defending the new rule the Secretary of HHS, Michael O. Leavitt, said, "Doctors and other health care providers should not be forced to choose between good professional standing and violating their conscience."[73]

Seven states quickly challenged the rule and sued the federal government.[74] The states claimed the rule would override state laws protecting women's access to birth control, reproductive health services, and emergency contraception. National organizations and lawmakers also joined the controversy.[75] Those supporting this "11th –hour regulation" expected a battle with the new administration of President Barack Obama,[76] and, indeed, shortly after taking office Obama initiated the review process.[77]

As Mary Gallagher, president and chief executive of the National Family Planning and Reproductive Health Association pointed out, the rule would most likely affect poor and uninsured women who rely on family planning clinics for counseling, education, and contraception.[78] Such a rule might also affect Kathy Jorea, the young woman seeking information about abortion in Case 2.2 "Religious and legal considerations in conflict." In most cases, we believe, health care professionals are obligated to provide legal medical and nursing services to those who request them or, if they are conscientiously opposed, to refer those who request them to other professionals who are willing to provide them. If one assumes a particular professional role, one should be prepared to fulfill the obligations of the role or to refer patients to others who are willing to fulfill them. A Jehovah's Witness, for example, who is conscientiously opposed to administering blood transfusions should not assume a position as a physician or nurse in an emergency or operating room. So, too, pharmacists opposed to dispensing contraception, including emergency contraception, to those who seek it, or are opposed to referring them to pharmacists who will dispense it, should seek employment where such activities are not part of the job. And laws should, we believe, provide no protection to nurse Jean Lyons in Case 2.2 if, as the only professional nurse able to provide information about abortion sought by 17-year-old Kathy Jorea, she conscientiously refused to provide it or to refer Kathy to another source. Just as there are limits based on conscience to what health care professionals can be required to do, there are limits— based on patients' rights and the virtue of caring—to what heath care professionals can conscientiously refuse to do.

6. DETERMINING RESPONSIBILITY

Much nursing care occurs as part of team action that involves nurses and physicians as well as numerous other persons. The composition of various teams differs, depending upon their functions, as, for example, an operating room team, a resuscitation team, a primary care team, a rehabilitation team, or a dialysis team. As Edmund Pellegrino has pointed out, the common feature of the health care team is its collective action with final accountability belonging in one sense to each team member, and in another sense to the entire team.[79]

The following case raises questions relating to responsibility:

4.10 Child with a Fever

One hot summer Tuesday afternoon, Ami and Kevin Junkin brought their daughter, Emily, age five, to their pediatrician's office, as they had been instructed by Anwen Preuss, registered nurse. The Junkins had phoned the previous day to ask what they should do concerning Emily's fever of 103°F. After following Anwen's advice to keep her at home and how best to treat the fever, the Junkins had watched Emily's fever go down. But within 24 hours, it was up to 104°, and when they called again, Anwen told them to bring her in.

Carl Hoyt, physician's assistant, met with the Junkins to assess her condition. Emily had no complaints other than the high fever. Carl told the Junkins that Emily probably had a virus that was affecting other children in the area and that they should just keep treating Emily's fever as the nurse had directed the previous day.

Three days later Ami and Kevin brought Emily back to the office, and Carl again saw them. Emily was still having high fevers, but she still had no other complaints. She was eating and sleeping well, and was able to play happily when her temperature was down. Carl repeated that Emily probably had the virus that was going around.

When Anwen saw the Junkins as they were leaving the office, they told her they hoped Emily would soon recover from the virus that was going around. Anwen later spoke with Carl and was surprised to learn that he had not attempted to look for other possible causes of Emily's fever.

Five days later the Junkins were back in the office with Emily. Anwen privately, but pointedly in a loud and accusatory manner, told Carl to at least have Emily's urine checked this time. He was displeased with Anwen's rather intemperately telling him how to handle Emily's case, but he did follow her suggestion. Urinalysis showed that Emily had a severe urinary tract infection (UTI). Follow-up testing in the next few days resulted in a diagnosis of vesicoureteral reflux, which required long-term monitoring and treatment.[80]

This case raises questions relating to responsibility: What should a nurse do when she disagrees with a health care provider's actions? Or if she thinks that a provider is following an unsafe practice? Who is responsible for monitoring individual and team competence? To whom are lapses reported—the person making the error, the team, the institution?

A discussion of these questions must include both individual and team responsibilities. "Personal" physicians admit their patients to a hospital or clinic, and a patient quickly enters a relationship with that institution (through a team composed of the personal physician, hospitalist physician, resident physicians, consulting physicians, nurses, assistant physicians, therapists, dietitians, social workers, and other providers) which is very much like the relationship a patient has with his or her own physician. A patient's right to effective medical treatment obligates his or her physician to provide that treatment. When a patient is admitted to a hospital or clinic, he or she makes a similar claim upon that institution for safe, effective, morally responsible care, which the institution fulfills through the employment of health care workers, including nurses. One difficulty in a transitory team, which comes together to provide services for an individual patient and disbands when that particular person leaves the institution or agency, is in defining who is accountable for the care it provides. According to Pellegrino's view, one can interpret the responsibilities of a health care team in two ways. In one way, responsibility is allocated only to individuals. In the other, responsibility is allocated to the team and is not reducible to the individuals.

According to the interpretation of team ethics that allocates responsibility only to individuals, Pellegrino suggested that the problem of monitoring, correcting, and revealing a fellow team member's incompetence is an unavoidable complication. Unfortunately, when some member fails to perform competently, his or her failure blocks or compromises the actions of other team members.[81] In Case 4.10, the physician's assistant's failure to check the child for other causes of fever seriously compromised Anwen's attempt to provide high-quality health care. Therefore, Anwen's duty to provide care obligated her to act in a way that would make certain the competent functioning of another team member; thus, in order to meet her own professional obligations, Anwen had to convince Karl to assess Emily for a possible urinary infection.

Furthermore, according to the interpretation of the team ethic that allocates responsibility to the entire team, all team members are accountable for the patient's well-being. Therefore, in this situation, all were to blame when the team's total care (which included overlooking signs of a urinary tract infection) resulted in Emily's continued illness. In situations in which lapses in competence recur or bring discomfort or danger to a patient or in which optimal care is not given, the entire team may be morally (and legally) culpable.[82]

Anwen had two reasons for convincing the physician's assistant to assess Emily more thoroughly: First, as an individual professional, she was directly obligated to give the best possible nursing care, but the physician's assistant's lapse of competence compromised her efforts. Second, she was obligated as a team member for Emily's total care, which was frustrated by the physician's assistant's lapse of competence. Given these reasons, Anwen was obligated to obtain optimum medical care for Emily, which answers the first two questions the case raised. The actions a nurse should take, when she disagrees with another provider's actions or when she thinks that a provider is following an unsafe practice, must be based upon her responsibilities to the client both in her capacities as an individual practitioner and as a team member. The nurse may develop several strategies to meet her responsibilities. Anwen chose to confront Carl directly about his inaction.

If Anwen previously had brought Carl's attention to the need to assess children more thoroughly, her intense commitment to Emily's welfare and the seriousness of the situation mitigated any real or imagined errors in etiquette that she may have made. Although Anwen cannot *justify* the intemperate way in which she conveyed her objection, her conduct under the circumstances is in our view *excusable*.[83]

The answer to the third question, "Who is responsible for monitoring individual and team competence?" is based on the same dual interpretation of responsibility. Since each professional is responsible for his or her own actions, and since as a team member each professional is also responsible for the team's total effectiveness, each member of the team is obligated to monitor both the activities that affect his or her services and the outcome of the team's efforts. Of course, all team members cannot be aware of all aspects of one another's activities. Each professional, however, will be able to assess to varying degrees the effectiveness of other team members since the whole team focuses its attention on the same client.

Difficulty arises in answering the last question, "To whom are lapses reported?" The dual interpretation of responsibility suggests that insofar as responsibility can be allocated to an individual, that individual is also responsible for correcting his or her error. But to correct a problem an individual needs to learn of it.

Given the power structure of the health care professions, some persons—perhaps especially physicians—often view themselves as more important than other members of the health care team. Open communication in such situations is sometimes difficult. Ideally, a nurse should talk directly to the person who she believes made an error, but telling another person about a suspected lapse of competence is a delicate matter. When the nurse cannot trace the problem to an individual, she should share the information with the whole team. Within the health care team structure, the most effective course of action is usually for the nurse to report any lapse of competence to the person or persons who are directly responsible and to involve other people in the nursing and medical hierarchy only after attempting to solve the problem at its source.

5

Ethical Dilemmas Among Nurses

1. TENSIONS BETWEEN NURSES

In their practice, nurses work closely with other nurses. Since a nurse's activities normally overlap with those of other nurses, her practice affects and is affected by the practices of others. In addition, most nurses either supervise or are supervised by nurses. Given such interdependence, ethical dilemmas involving relationships among nurses are inevitable and understandable. The following case illustrates one such dilemma.

5.1 A History of Mistakes

Talk among night staff aides who worked with Lisa Jensen, R.N., on the 36-patient nursing home unit of a rural community hospital, centered on Lisa's recurring mistakes. A local woman with many relatives in the county, she had been out of nursing school four years and was the unit's lone registered nurse working nights. Joan Thurman, a recently hired aide who had just completed a nurse assistant short course, learned "it was common knowledge" that Lisa made many small mistakes, including medication errors. Joan, herself, had seen Lisa become distracted during busy times. She told the other aides that something ought to be done, but they told Joan that day nursing staff, Lisa's good friends, routinely took care of any small problems she caused.

Not satisfied, Joan worried whether she ought to tell the unit's charge nurse. She suspected that if coworkers thought she was a tattletale, she'd find herself in a very unpleasant work situation. But after a few days, Joan gathered her courage and spoke with the unit's charge nurse, Charlotte Bennett, who assured her of confidentiality. Charlotte said she appreciated Joan's concern and that obviously the nurse assistant course had done a good job in preparing her for work. She told Joan she was not troubled about Lisa, however, because she was kind to patients, well liked by everyone, and had not caused any real harm. She said the hospital tracked all medication errors. In

---

addition, she said, it was very difficult to find an R.N. willing to work the night position. She encouraged Joan to stick to her plans to become a registered nurse since there was such a local shortage of qualified people.

Several months later, Lisa misread an order for morphine and gave a huge overdose to an elderly patient between midnight and 2:00 a.m. At 7:00 a.m. the day nursing staff found him comatose, and in spite of efforts to revive him in the hospital emergency room, he died in the early afternoon. Investigation and legal settlement followed. Lisa quietly left the hospital's employ.

Reviewing her own responsibility for this tragedy, Charlotte Bennett questioned whether she should have excused Lisa's small mistakes. When Joan had brought the situation to her attention, had she failed to consider the problem adequately because Joan was a newly employed, inexperienced aide? Had she been influenced because Lisa was well liked and had many relatives in the community? Given Lisa's history of mistakes, did the difficulty in finding another R.N. to work nights justify keeping her in a position where she was the lone R.N.?

Although she knew about Lisa's reported medication errors, had she, Charlotte, been irresponsible when she missed knowing that other nurses, Lisa's friends, had covered for Lisa? What was the extent of underreporting Lisa's medication errors? And her other mistakes? What responsibility did Lisa's friends have in this tragedy?[1]

Among the questions this case raises are, To what extent, if any, should a nurse jeopardize her own professional position by admitting an error? And to what extent, if any, should a nurse cover up another nurse's error to maintain a smoothly functioning unit?

Some basic information about relationships among nurses is necessary for a discussion of this case. Various general factors, as discussed in the previous chapter with regard to conflicts between nurses and physicians, also affect relationships among nurses. These include remnants of the historical legacy of nursing; technological and social changes; the expanding scope of nursing practice; and the ideology of professionalism and increasing importance of education, especially with regard to baccalaureate and graduate degrees in nursing. We can see the effect of these factors on tensions in nursing relationships by examining personal variables among nurses and structural variables in nursing practice. Since both personal and structural variables tend to block and confuse efforts to engage in ethical inquiry, it is important to recognize them.

A. Personal Variable Among Nurses

Nurses differ from one another in many ways. Nursing is traditionally a woman's profession, but not all nurses are women. Some men have been and are nurses, even though as early as 1880 women nurses outnumbered men eleven to one and at present outnumber them seventeen to one. Like male nurses, ethnic minority nurses are fewer in number than their comparative percentages in the general population.[2] Desegregation of nursing schools did not begin until after World War II, and by 1951 only 3% of nursing students were Black/African American. To address imbalance of minority nurses in the profession, some schools have actively recruited minority students.[3] Sex and racial differences affect nursing relationships as they do relationships in other professions and in society generally. As the following discussion indicates, personal variables that add to tension in nursing relationships include a nurse's educational background, experience, view of nursing, and career goals.

All persons seeking to become registered nurses (RN) take the same licensure examination even though they may have graduated from one of three different educational programs varying in length from two to four years—associate degree, hospital-based diploma, or baccalaureate program. Discussion continues within the profession as to the comparative merits of various programs.[4] Persons seeking to become licensed practical or vocational nurses (LPN or LVN) study for approximately one year before taking a licensure examination for practical nurses.

Another personal variable is experience in nursing practice. We have seen that in certain circumstances an experienced and skillful nurse may have knowledge that an inexperienced physician lacks. So, too, certain situations will arise in which an experienced nurse who has kept up with new developments and has changed her nursing practice accordingly may know more about a particular nursing problem than a recent graduate from a prestigious nursing program. The quality and usefulness of nursing experience, like other personal variables, differ among individual nurses.

Given the variety of their educational backgrounds and their varying nursing experiences, nurses understandably vary in their views of nursing. As previously discussed (see Chapter 4, Section 1), nurses provide not only bedside nursing care; they also give physical examinations and teach health care. Common to nurses, however, is a shared legacy of belief as to what nursing is. Past nurse writers and nurse theorists today stress that (1) nursing assists both well and sick persons; (2) "health" is a general nursing goal; and (3) to accomplish the goal, nursing encompasses a wide range of activities based upon a problem-solving process that includes assessment, diagnosis, intervention, and evaluation.[5] Nurses, although they share a general historical view of nursing, emphasize various theoretical models of nursing and various activities involved in the nursing process differently.

A nurse's career goal is also an important variable that sometimes increases tension in nursing relationships. Some nurses pursue nursing as a lifetime career, while others prefer to work intermittently or part time.[6] Diversity of career options is reflected in the large number of active professional nursing organizations. As *Nurseweek* reported in 2001:

> No matter how you slice nursing—by specialty, workplace, geography, gender, heritage, ethnicity or eclectic interest—there likely is a professional organization for you, a place where RNs can find support and cohesiveness in a highly fractured profession. Organizations range from a few hundred members in highly specialized groups, such as the Pediatric Endocrinology Nursing Society, to 65,000 members in the all-encompassing American Association of Critical-Care Nurses. Sigma Theta Tau, the international nursing honor society that promotes standards and scholarship, dwarfs all with 300,000 members in 90 countries.[7]

To return to Case 5.1, notice that the educational backgrounds and experiences of the nursing staff involved are quite dissimilar; one is an RN with four years of experience, one is a recently hired nurse aide, one is an RN charge nurse (presumably experienced), and the others (unnamed) are RNs, LPNs, and UAP (unlicensed assistive personnel). They may or may not hold similar views of nursing or similar career goals. Note, however, that they all are responsible for providing safe care. In this one respect, they have been employed to carry out this same duty.[8] The dilemma of the case, "A history of mistakes," is made complex not only because of the personal variables involved but because of an equally important reason—the structure of nursing practice.

B. Structural Variables in Nursing Practice

The structure of nursing practice varies according to the setting and staff assignment model in which nurses practice. For most nurses, about 56%, the setting is a hospital.[9] Settings here include, for example, intensive care units, neonatal nurseries, medical inpatient care units, surgical inpatient care units, pediatric units, oncology units, in-service education programs, ambulatory care units, obstetrical units, emergency rooms, and outpatient units. For other nurses, the setting is an extended care facility. Still others are in clinics or the community, including, for example, nursing centers, offices, schools, and patients' homes. For some nurse practitioners, the setting is an independent practice.

In addition to practice setting, a nurse's employer determines his or her job responsibilities and assignments. Institutions use the following basic models for describing nursing staff assignments: (1) functional method nursing; (2) team nursing; (3) primary care nursing or some variation such as modular nursing; (4) patient focused care nursing; and (5) nursing with shared governance. According to the "functional method," a head nurse assigns staff members, RNs, LPNs, and UAP, specific tasks—as medication nurse, treatment nurse, bedside care nurse, and so on. In "team nursing," a registered nurse team leader assigns duties to each team member, plans and coordinates care, serves as a resource person, and sometimes provides direct patient care. In "primary care nursing," which generally requires an all-registered nurse staff, a primary nurse accepts responsibility for the total 24-hour care of a patient by interviewing the patient on admission, making a nursing diagnosis, issuing orders, and coordinating patient activities with the patient's physicians, family, and other health workers. In "modular nursing," a variation of primary nursing, several persons, such as two RNs, or an RN and an LPN, or two LPNs with the charge nurse as modular leader, are assigned to care for a small group of patients. In "patient focused care," a registered nurse serves as care manager, and UAP in various expanded roles undertake assessment activities such as drawing blood. In the "nursing with shared governance" model, emphasis is on nurse autonomy, medical-nursing collaboration, and shared decision making between nurses and managers.[10]

Whichever model or blend of models a particular institution uses to describe nursing staff assignments, safe and effective distribution of nursing tasks and activities is essential. The problem facing nurses is, as the ANA and the NCSBN (National Council of State Boards of Nursing) announced in their jointly published statement on delegation in 2005, "There is more nursing to do than there are nurses to do it." One outcome of this expanded workload is that nurses delegate tasks and activities to other workers. Most state nurse practice acts authorize RNs to delegate, but many states limit such authorization for LPNs. In an attempt to support nurses who must work with assistive personnel, the ANA and NCSBN determined that critical competencies for modern nurses must include ability to "delegate, assign, and supervise."[11] The document offers guidance for both RNs and LPNs and includes extensive discussion of the ANA's "Principles for Delegation," which states:

> The RN uses critical thinking and professional judgment when following the Five Rights of Delegation, to be sure that the delegation or assignment is: 1. The right task 2. Under the right circumstances 3. To the right person 4. With the right directions and communication; and 5. Under the right supervision and evaluation. Chief Nursing Officers are accountable for establishing systems to assess, monitor, verify and communicate ongoing competence requirements in areas related to delegation.[12]

Structural variables in nursing practice, combined with personal variables among nurses, including ability to delegate, assign, and supervise, tend to complicate and add significant tension to nurses' relationships. Therefore, in analyzing ethical dilemmas that are primarily disagreements between nurses, it is important to recognize the extent to which these variables underlie the issues.

To return to "A history of mistakes," we can see similarities in structural variables in that Charlotte, the charge nurse, Lisa, the RN, and Joan, the nurse aide, share the same rural hospital and nursing unit. It is reasonable to assume that Lisa delegates tasks and supervises Joan since they both work the night shift and Lisa is the only RN on duty, and that Charlotte is the top supervisory person in the unit's hierarchy. In addition, neither Lisa nor Joan work days with Charlotte and Lisa's nurse friends. Differentiation in terms of a personal variable, that is, the view of Lisa's "many small mistakes, including medication errors," appears between Joan and the rest of the staff—the other aides and Lisa's nurse friends. Tolerance for Lisa's small mistakes also seems to be Charlotte's view, although Charlotte may be inadequately informed about the extent of Lisa's errors. But while it is reasonable to assume that personal variables influence the nurses' and aides' perception of the situation and of one another, none of the variables changes the fact that their employer, patients, and other health care providers expect that Lisa, as well as the whole staff, will provide safe, effective, and responsible care. Further, nursing organizations have adopted codes of ethics to guide nurses in their conduct. For example, The Code for Nurses with Interpretive Statements adopted by the American Nurses Association states that "The nurse promotes, advocates, and strives to protect the health, safety, and rights of the patient." The Code underscores the nurse's primary commitment to the patient, directs her to express concern to any person engaging in a questionable practice, and to report to the responsible administrative person when a patient's welfare is threatened.[13] In terms of accountability, Lisa and the other nurses are responsible for their own acts.

In complicated cases, a number of different factors affect the situation. Therefore, in order to take a position on Case 5.1, we will make the following assumptions:

1. Prior to Lisa's final mistake, patients who received wrong medications or were affected by Lisa's small mistakes were in varying degrees wronged and possibly harmed.[14]
2. The overall cost of Lisa's small mistakes may have been negligible or, if those mistakes resulted in delays in assessment or treatment of other patients, may have added substantially to the medical care costs of other persons.
3. The overall productivity of the unit's nursing personnel was diminished by Lisa's small mistakes since time had to be spent correcting or covering her errors.

4. The nursing staff did not talk to Lisa or fully inform Charlotte about Lisa's small mistakes, perhaps including some or all of her medication errors.
5. By taking care of small problems that Lisa caused, the other nurses perpetuated an effective cover-up of her history of mistakes.
6. Charlotte lacked a thorough assessment of Lisa's skills, although she had a good opinion of Lisa in that she believed Lisa was kind to patients and well liked by other nurses. She also knew Lisa had many relatives in the community.
7. Joan, an aide, informed Charlotte that Lisa was distracted during busy times and made many small mistakes.
8. Charlotte, who knew Joan as an inexperienced but well-prepared aide, believed she was capable of becoming an RN and was, presumably, a responsible person.

Given the first three assumptions, use of the word "small" is misleading in the context of a history of making errors in the delivery of nursing care. Errors potentially harm patients and add costs. We are reminded of a college student who pleaded that his disciplinary, immediate removal from his university resident hall room was unfair because he had only started a "small" fire on another student's door. Like small fires that grow into blazing tragedies, a *history* of small errors is itself a large error and can potentially lead to serious errors and terrible outcomes. In Case 5.1, Lisa's last error resulted in great loss—the elderly patient's death, Lisa's loss of employment, and the rural hospital's costs of the investigation and legal settlement.

Assumption 4 raises questions about the general climate of trust among the nursing staff and administration and whether support exists for nurses who choose to report nursing errors since no one talked to Lisa about her mistakes, and Charlotte's long seasoned nursing staff, Lisa herself, and the other nurses on the unit, did not report fully that she made many small errors when she worked alone at night.

Assumption 5 points to questions about the day nursing staff. Like the choice of the word "small" to describe Lisa's errors, language is important. Characterizing the other nurses' behavior by saying they "routinely took care of any small problems she caused" directs attention to the immediate good that the other nurses provided. They kept the unit functioning and, we assume, they corrected as far as they could the effects of Lisa's mistakes. Their work of taking care of Lisa's mistakes can be supported by a utilitarian argument that a smoothly functioning unit resulted in the greatest happiness for all. Their activities can also be supported by duty-based arguments, such as the duty to provide optimum patient care. If, however, their actions are described in terms not of "routine fixing" but of a "cover-up," attention is broadened and questions arise as to what is being hidden. An occasional small, unfinished detail of a nursing activity another nurse catches and corrects is not termed a cover-up, but an error or a pattern of mistakes hidden from a supervisor is. In Lisa's case the other nurses covered not only her errors but her pattern of incompetence as well. Had the other nurses reported Lisa's repeated mistakes to Charlotte, their informing her could have been supported by utilitarian arguments that are more persuasive than the one supporting the good that results from a smoothly functioning unit. Had they reported to Charlotte, it is reasonable to assume that: nighttime nursing care might have improved; the unit as a whole might have operated as smoothly or even more smoothly than when the staff spent time fixing Lisa's errors; time and supplies would not have been wasted fixing problems stemming from her mistakes; and patients would have been safeguarded from her errors. Reporting Lisa's mistakes to Charlotte could also be supported by strong arguments based on the principle of respect for persons especially, as stated by the ANA Code, that a nurse's duty is to safeguard a patient when health care is affected by incompetent practice. Given these strong arguments in support of reporting, it is difficult to find additional arguments for not reporting. Perhaps some day shift nurses may have been motivated by friendship to fix Lisa's small problems, complete her tasks, and not report her, but personal feelings in this case do not override professional obligations. (The issue of friendship is discussed in Case 5.3.) Perhaps because day shift nurses routinely corrected night shift mistakes and kept the unit functioning smoothly, they did not think of their own personal actions in terms of a "cover-up."

Assumption 6 concerning Charlotte's superficial assessment of Lisa raises questions about the competent supervision of the hospital's entire nursing staff, including charge nurses such as Charlotte. It also raises questions about the chief nursing officer's competency.

Assumptions 7 and 8 raise another serious question: Why didn't Charlotte take some action, especially since she believed Joan to be a responsible person even if an inexperienced aide. Answers to the question involve both Charlotte and the nursing administration. First, either Charlotte was an unskilled supervisor or she apparently allowed Lisa's pleasant reputation to affect her judgment since she failed to assess Lisa's skills thoroughly. In addition, she may have allowed the real problem of the registered nurse shortage and the lack of potential replacements for Lisa to affect her judgment since she did not investigate, nor did she ask her supervisor to help her investigate whether Lisa was making unreported errors. Second, the hospital nursing administration may be inadequate or have problems of communication within its structure. Charlotte and her superiors did not know about Lisa's problem behaviors even though "it was common knowledge" among the nursing staff. Perhaps the nursing practice model employed in the hospital does not support and encourage the nursing staff to report errors. Perhaps the hospital needs to develop a different model of nursing practice. And, in addition, the nursing administrators, including Charlotte and the chief nursing officer, may need to examine their own management skills.

When Charlotte reviews her own responsibility in this tragedy, she should acknowledge that she ought not to have simply excused Lisa's pattern of small mistakes, and that she ought to have taken steps to investigate Joan's information. No excuse Charlotte may have for failing to investigate the situation and retaining Lisa in the lone RN night position—Joan's inexperience, Lisa's likeability and extended family, difficulty in finding an RN replacement—overrides her duty to safeguard patients by investigating and, if necessary, replacing Lisa. When Lisa's friends review their responsibility, they ought to acknowledge that arguments for reporting Lisa override arguments for continuing to take care of Lisa's mistakes. In addition, they should acknowledge that their not reporting Lisa resulted in harm to patients, to the hospital through increased costs, and to Lisa by isolating her from potential help. Although Charlotte did not question whether she herself had shortcomings in her own assessment and supervisory skills, or whether the nursing administration had any responsibility in the tragedy, questions remain. Ultimately, the chief nursing officer is responsible for the delivery of nursing care, and in this case, for its unsafe care and harm to patients.

One question this case raised initially was: To what extent, if any, should a nurse jeopardize her own professional position by admitting an error? Our analysis illustrates that, all things considered, the best course of action is to admit errors. While a small error is not usually in itself a cause for great concern, a pattern or history of errors needs attention.

Another question the case raised initially was to what extent, if any, should a nurse cover another nurse's error in order to maintain a smoothly functioning unit. Our analysis of Case 5.1 finds no justification, all things considered, for participating in a cover-up in order to support unit harmony. Participation in cover-ups may involve other motivations such as friendship. Questions concerning a nurse's obligations as a care provider and her desire to be helpful to a friend and colleague are discussed in Section 3. Professional Obligations.

2. RESPECT FOR PERSONS

Underlying the previous discussion, with its emphasis upon the nurse's decision about what she ought to do, is a presumption that the nurse is a self-determining person. A person cannot be held responsible for the consequences of her actions unless she is allowed to judge and choose for herself. Respect for persons, a principle discussed in Chapter 2, Section 1, and Chapter 3, Section 1, and which we will explore further in the following case, involves acknowledging people's rights as persons to do as they see fit within certain limits.

5.2 Judgmental Comments

Last week, public health nurse Mary Ann Rhoads went to a hospital to visit one of her clients, Debra Sharpe, who had just had her second baby. According to Mary Ann, "Debra is a 17-year-old, poorly educated, black person from the South so it's very difficult for me to understand her thick dialect. I went to the nursery to see the baby, and one of the nurses looked disgustedly at me and asked, 'How old is that mother, anyway?' I said, 'Seventeen,' and she sneered, 'I thought so.' I felt that she was placing a very negative judgment on Debra and her baby."

Mary Ann did not say anything to the nurse, but now she is bothered. "I realize I have some health values. I know that Debra's baby is going to be a high-risk child; in fact, the older sibling had lead poisoning. But the decision to have this second baby was Debra's decision; my own values about her child's future health are irrelevant. All people make decisions about their lives for one reason or another. If we don't know what those decisions and reasons are, and even if we do, we can't pass judgment on another person."

Mary Ann does not know what to do. She thinks she has two problems. First, she does not know if she should return to the nursery and attempt to talk to the nurse. Is it appropriate for her, a nurse from one agency, to advise a nurse who is employed in another agency? Second, she does not know whether she should try to force her own values on another person, specifically, the nurse who made the judgmental comment.

Before examining Mary Ann's concern about her relationship with the nursery nurse, we need to discuss the two nurses' views of the young mother, Debra. Mary Ann thinks her own values about Debra's decision to have a second baby are irrelevant at this point and that she cannot pass judgment on others. The nursery nurse implied that Debra was wrong to have the baby.

Mary Ann's statements indicate that she accepts a principle of respect for persons which holds that, generally and with certain qualifications, each person is in the best position to determine what will satisfy her or his interest, that is, each person is in the best position to determine her or his conception of the good and what means are most suitable to realizing it. According to this principle, a "person" is a being who is aware of herself or himself, not just as a process, happening, or thing but as an agent, making decisions that make a difference in the way the world goes, and able to determine and attempt to realize some conception of the good.[15] *Respect for persons* involves acknowledging a person's right to pursue her or his conception of the good so long as doing so does not interfere with the right of other persons to do likewise. In terms of the principle of respect for persons, Mary Ann acknowledged Debra's right to decide to have another baby, which, of course, would not interfere with the rights of others to have babies. Mary Ann treated Debra as a person since she did not interfere with Debra's choice to have a baby; that is, she responded in a fashion that respected Debra's decision by continuing to offer nursing care to her and her children and by refraining from passing judgment on her.

Although basically sound, Mary Ann's understanding of the principle of respect for persons is mistaken in one crucial respect. Mary Ann's recognition of Debra's personhood, which includes recognition of her self-determination, freedom, and dignity, does not mean that Mary Ann could not or should not engage Debra in discussions involving health risks to her children and other health-related topics. Rather, the opposite is true. Mary Ann's respect for Debra as a person is a reason to engage in health teaching and rational discussions about what Debra ought to do. Mary Ann, in holding to the principle of respect for persons, must, of course, take into account Debra's point of view; she must acknowledge Debra's prima facie claim to noninterference; and she must not use her special status as a nurse to impose her values on Debra.[16] Mary Ann is mistaken, however, in thinking that her health values are irrelevant. When Mary Ann engages Debra in health teaching, Debra may decide to adopt some of Mary Ann's health values and information in making her own decisions about the health of her children or herself. Further, since Debra's right to noninterference is a prima facie claim and not an absolute right, Mary Ann may override a particular decision of Debra's if she recognizes that it interferes with certain of the baby's rights. For example, a nurse might choose to override a mother's feeding plan if that plan would obviously lead to her infant's becoming dangerously overweight. In short, although Mary Ann's respect for Debra as a person requires that she not resort to manipulation or coercion, it does allow and perhaps requires that she engage her in dialogue and, where she thinks Debra is misinformed, attempt to educate her or alter her views with rational persuasion. Mary Ann's mistake here is in part attributable to a failure to realize that Debra's right as a person to decide for herself what she will do with her life does not imply that all decisions made in this fashion are the right or best ones. (See Chapter 3, Section 2, for an account of the distinctions between rational persuasion, manipulation, and coercion.)

The nursery nurse's behavior and remarks to Mary Ann, on the other hand, probably indicate that she does not regard patients in the same way as does Mary Ann. She may, like Mary Ann, believe in the importance of rights but believe that more important rights than Debra's are involved in the situation. For example, she may think that her right as a taxpayer to have lower taxes or to receive public services, which Debra's possible collection of public assistance would reduce to some extent, should override Debra's right to have a second baby. Or she may take a purely utilitarian view and believe that society's interest as a whole will be maximized if poor, uneducated, minority women like Debra are prevented from having a second child. Or she may simply be prejudiced and not have analyzed her feelings about Debra and her children.

Mary Ann's problems as she presented them in the case are, first, whether she should try to talk with the nursery nurse, an employee of another agency, and second, whether she should try to force her own values on another person. Both nurses should have as their primary concern the welfare of patients and, more specifically, Debra's and the baby's care. Mary Ann's worry about whether to discuss her concerns with the nursery nurse indicates that she views personal and/or structural variables as separating them as colleagues. Even though they may not be "peers," may not have equal standing in rank or class because of differences in educational background and other personal variables, and even though they differ in employment settings and nursing assignment responsibilities, both are equal as persons. As equal persons working to provide good nursing care to patients, each should be free to talk with the other about their practice of nursing; Mary Ann should feel free to tell the hospital nurse about her concerns that focus on a primary issue in nursing—patient care.

The second question, whether Mary Ann should try to force her values on another person, must be answered with a no. This does not imply that she cannot try to engage the other in dialogue and use rational persuasion to convince her of the soundness of her values. On the contrary, dialogue with the nursery nurse, as opposed to manipulating, coercing, or simply ignoring her, is the way for Mary Ann to show respect for her as a person. If Mary Ann is to be consistent in her dealings with others, she has to respect the other nurse's right to formulate and express views, opinions, and actions just as she respects her client's right to do so. Therefore, she must deal with the nurse as a rational being. But the nurse, like Debra and all persons, has only a prima facie right to noninterference. Mary Ann could question the nurse's actions (prejudicial comments about a patient) because she believes she can show that those actions could infringe upon a vulnerable patient's basic rights of self-determination, freedom, and dignity. In this case, however, the nursery nurse's disgusted look and her sneered "I thought so" are heavily nonverbal and would be difficult to discuss meaningfully a week or more later.

In summary, Mary Ann is free to talk as a person and colleague with the nursery nurse. In accordance with the principle of respect for persons, she could engage the nurse in a rational discussion about poor, young, minority mothers and their rights as persons. In discussing respect for persons, she could point out that judgmental negative comments may undermine a patient's dignity. The effect of such a discussion would depend upon the nursery nurse's ability and willingness to accept and use the information. Because so much time has elapsed since the incident, Mary Ann might well decide at this point not to revive the issue with the nurse. After thinking through this situation, however, she should now be prepared to deal with similar judgmental comments by nursing personnel if they occur.

3. PROFESSIONAL OBLIGATIONS

As we discussed in Chapter 4, section 6, each nurse is responsible in one sense for her own professional practice and in another sense for the practice of the health care team of which she is a member. The following two cases present questions relating to a nurse's responsibility as a member, not of a health care team, but of the nursing profession.

5.3 Working Extra Hours

Diane MacIntyre has two and one-half years' experience as staff nurse on a general medical unit that serves many diabetic and stroke patients. As a team leader, she both gives direct patient care and plans basic care for other nursing personnel to carry out. In the past, when she worked extra hours at home or in the hospital library writing procedures, the other nurses (especially another team leader, Arlene Estes, who is a single parent with three children) have said that Diane (who is single and without children) was foolish to work without pay. During the last few months, Diane's attendance at weekly meetings of a multidisciplinary team, composed of professionals from physical therapy, occupational therapy, and social service who are active in rehabilitation efforts on her unit, has strained her relationships with nursing coworkers. According to Diane, "The other nurses think I'm crazy to come in on my own time. I go to practically every weekly meeting, which are mainly on my days off. I get a lot of positive reinforcement from being with that group of people, and I think they have a little better impression of nursing due to my participation."

Diane's decision to participate with the multidisciplinary team stems from her desire to get more out of her job than just a paycheck and her conclusion that "nursing is one of those jobs that you really have to put a lot of effort into in order to get any satisfaction at all." She wants to show that "nursing is an important profession and nurses have something to contribute besides passing 'meds' and giving baths." Despite her justification for working extra hours, Diane nevertheless feels hurt by the other nurses' reactions, especially those of her friend Arlene, whose skills and integrity she has always admired.

This case raises the following questions: What are the obligations of being a member of the nursing profession? Do these obligations include attending meetings on one's own time and expense? Working overtime?

The American Nurses Association (ANA) Code for Nurses with Interpretive Statements addresses the question of responsibility to the profession. Provision 7 states that "The nurse participates in the advancement of the profession through contributions to practice, education, administration, and knowledge development." Discussion of Provision 7 states that "Nurses should advance their profession by contributing in some way to the leadership, activities, and the viability of their professional organizations.... by serving in leadership or mentorship roles or on committees within their places of employment.... through participation in civic activities related to heath care or through local, state, national, or international initiatives." Further discussion of Provision 7 states that nurses advance the profession "by developing, maintaining, and implementing professional standards in clinical, administrative, and educational practice."[17] In its discussion of collaboration in Provision 2, the Code states that "the complexity of health care delivery systems requires a multidisciplinary approach to the delivery of services that has the strong support and active participation of all the health professions. Within this context, nursing's unique contribution... needs to be clearly articulated, represented and preserved."[18] The Code clearly expresses the view that nurses have obligations not only to themselves, and to patients and the public, but to the nursing profession as well. While not stating that participation in activities to improve nursing as a discipline may require extra working hours, the Code implies as much.

Very few nurses have established independent nursing practices; rather, agencies (hospitals, nursing homes, community health departments, schools, industries, physicians, health maintenance organizations, etc.) employ the vast majority of nurses. A nurse contracts with an agency in order to carry out her primary obligation to the patient or client—provision of safe, effective, responsible nursing—in the words of ANA Code, "the promotion of health, the prevention of illness, the restoration of health, the alleviation of suffering, and the provision of supportive care to those who are dying."[19] An employment contract, either written or oral, specifies a nurse's obligations in terms of working hours and specific responsibilities, as well as an agency's obligations in terms of pay, benefits, vacations, and so forth. In addition, nurses often feel obligated to do more than contracts specify because they fall into the "compassion trap" by accepting the expectations of many agency employers, health care workers, and patients that nurses, being members of a "helping profession," will subordinate their own needs or desires to those of others.[20]

To return to the nurses in Case 5.3, both Diane and Arlene share high ideals about professionalism, and as dedicated nurses both are also affected by the "compassion trap," with its assumption that the nurse will sacrifice for others. Therefore, Diane is somewhat discouraged by Arlene's recent comments about working only for pay. Peggy Sayre, another nurse from a different unit in the hospital and a friend of both women suggested that Diane, Arlene, and she talk during a break about problems relating to Diane's working extra. After listening to the other two nurses describe the situation, Peggy asked each of them why she felt as she did about working extra.

Diane had no difficulty in pointing out that her involvement with the interdisciplinary team and working on hospital procedures would lead to better care for a larger number of patients. She also emphasized that her professional goals of high-quality nursing care and the hospital's current inclusion of her in the multidisciplinary team were in perfect agreement.

Arlene acknowledged that Diane's contributions to patient welfare were admirable but quickly shifted to her own feelings concerning Diane's extra work. Arlene believed that because Diane functioned as "super nurse," the head nurse looked upon Arlene and several other nurses, who could not devote extra time to hospital matters, as less than adequate professional nurses. Further, they themselves were beginning to feel inadequate. One way for them to restore their private as well as professional self-esteem would be for them to match Diane's work load by working extra hours. Arlene predicted that patient welfare would be negatively affected, however, since she and most of the other nurses would be worn out by the combination of home duties, regular job, and extra unpaid work.

Arlene also said that, perhaps more importantly, she believes the way a nurse feels about herself as a professional affects the way in which she approaches nursing care. Although Arlene did not think that her negative feelings about her current level of participation in nursing matters at the hospital had affected her practice, she thought that if her morale continued to deteriorate, her nursing might suffer. She also predicted that if the nurses continued to see themselves as inadequate, even though they did their best during every working hour, some of them would quit. The resulting nursing personnel turnover would cause confusion and a reduction of the high-quality nursing care now being provided. Further, Arlene believed that if a high turnover rate persisted, the good that Diane's work did would be undermined.

Peggy thought that both Diane and Arlene had missed the major issue. As for Arlene, Peggy did not believe that the decline in unit morale and the increase in nursing staff turnover would be as great as Arlene predicted, but she agreed that these were important concerns. More importantly, she believed that Arlene, who recognized that she must meet her basic duties as a nurse and honor her contract with the hospital, had not completely accepted the view that idealized commitments to professional nursing might be overridden by other more stringent and immediate commitments, such as those to her children. To Peggy, Arlene, like all nurses, had personal as well as professional obligations, and Arlene, as a single parent, need not apologize for not working more than a 40-hour week. Peggy illustrated her point by describing a public health nurse, whom they all knew, who had been extremely active in collective-bargaining activities in the county health department. When her mother had become seriously ill and needed her every evening, the nurse could no longer attend special nightly meetings. Her obligations to her sick parent, while not excusing her from her contractual obligations to the health department, did excuse her from the additional commitments she had previously taken on. Arlene's personal obligations, like those of the public health nurse, were more basic and thus took precedence over her less stringent professional obligations.

Neither was Peggy convinced by Diane's argument that her professional nursing goals were being met, and that the end result would be an overall improvement in patient welfare. Although she agreed with Diane that the initiation of a new program or change often required an initial period of voluntary effort, she argued that as soon as the program's value was recognized, it was necessary to press for its institutionalization. In Diane's case, Peggy believed Diane had amply demonstrated the value of what she was doing. Therefore, she should now take steps to make hers a paying, institutionalized position. Peggy pointed out that since Diane's work depended entirely upon one nurse's willingness to work extra, when she left her current position for one with more responsibility—which all three nurses agreed that a young, effective nurse like Diane would do within a short time—there would probably be no one to carry on her good work. Nor, since the hospital had gotten Diane's work free, would their employer believe that another nurse would not also step forward to give free time and effort to the hospital.

Peggy predicted that at Diane's departure, there would be no nursing contribution to the multidisciplinary team or to similar activities since no institutional changes to provide for participation by nurses would be made so long as Diane functioned as she did. Therefore, in the long run, patients would not be well served by nursing. Thus, Diane was not meeting her professional goals when the future was considered. Peggy summarized her position by saying that Diane's extra work was a problem because the nurses on the unit could not determine if Diane's special activities were merely an extension of her efforts to be professional by providing the highest-quality nursing care possible or if she had slipped into the hospital's institutionalized system of devaluing nursing, although the system was obviously more subtle than that which nineteenth-century hospitals had used to exploit nurses.[21] To Peggy, the major issue was that if Diane continued to attend special meetings without compensation, she would actually support the notion that her activities were not truly part of a nurse's employee role and that the hospital had no obligation to support nurses who work long hours to write procedures and attend multidisciplinary team meetings.

To return to the questions raised by this case, a nurse has certain obligations to the nursing profession as discussed in the ANA Code for Nurses. At times, those obligations may include working overtime and attending meetings on one's own time and expense. But as this case illustrates, when a nurse critically examines her obligations she may see that basic personal commitments sometimes override less stringent professional commitments that might be met by "working extra." She may also see that "working extra," while appearing to fulfil professional obligations and the ideal of compassionate service, may only superficially meet obligations to patients and may actually lead to a less desirable state of affairs not only for nursing colleagues and the nursing profession but ultimately for patients.

In the following case, a nurse faces an ethical dilemma somewhat different from that involved in the problem of working extra hours. The questions the case raises involve conflict between a nurse's obligations as a care provider and her desire to be helpful to her friend and colleague.

5.4 A Question of Friendship

Mitsuko Suzuki and Jerome White, RNs in an intensive care unit on the second shift, have been friends since they attended nursing school together five years ago. For the past few months Mitsuko has been concerned about Jerome, who has admitted to her that he has been having severe headaches and occasional fainting episodes. Jerome attributes the symptoms to stress because he has been working two jobs while trying to establish himself and his young family financially. Although Mitsuko understands Jerome's position, she has been encouraging him to see a physician because she fears that the symptoms may indicate something more serious than simple stress. She also worries that Jerome's physical symptoms may affect his ability to make rational decisions concerning patients in his care. Jerome is not convinced that his symptoms are serious and says, "Besides, I don't have time to be sitting around for a week while a dozen tests are being run. I can live on aspirin for a while until this thing blows over and I get used to the pace."

Over the past few weeks, Jerome has been making a few mistakes on duty. While the mistakes have not been costly, Mitsuko is afraid that Jerome will make an error that will harm a patient seriously. She wonders if she should discuss her knowledge of Jerome's problem with their supervisor before Jerome harms himself or his patients. At the same time, she feels guilty about betraying a friend who trusts her enough to share his problems with her.[22]

Engaging in ethical analysis can help a nurse like Mitsuko think more clearly about a troublesome problem because ethical analysis enables one to examine not only personal feelings but all aspects of a situation. By analyzing this situation in terms of ethical arguments, Mitsuko could step beyond personalities and feelings and thus develop a more critical and objective perspective.

Mitsuko does face an ethical dilemma: Should she tell the supervisor about her concerns and thus break the confidentiality implicit in her relationship with Jerome? Or should she maintain confidentiality and risk the harm that may result either to ICU patients or to Jerome himself? Either of these choices can be supported by ethical principles. On the one hand, telling the supervisor can be supported by role-based arguments, such as that a nurse's duty is to safeguard a patient when health care is affected by incompetent practice (as stated in the ANA Code for Nurses), as well as by utilitarian arguments, such as that provision of safe care in an ICU results ultimately in the greatest happiness for all. On the other hand, not telling the supervisor, and thus maintaining confidentiality, can be supported by appeal to friendship, privacy, and trust.

The importance of trust between friends provides a strong basis for an argument to support Mitsuko's not discussing her concerns about Jerome with the supervisor. In breaking confidentiality Mitsuko would not only be betraying Jerome in this one instance but she could damage Jerome's trust in their relationship. Mitsuko, too, would have to face her own feelings of inadequacy and guilt stemming from her view that good people, herself included, ought to keep their friends' confidences.

We value the keeping of confidences between friends. Our relationships with one another depend upon being able to trust that certain personal secrets will not be exposed; restricted information might lead to loss of self-esteem if made public. We all have shortcomings that we would rather not have widely known. We need the benefit of confidentiality when we seek advice and aid, and when we share intimate concerns. Sissela Bok points to four important considerations that support confidentiality: (1) respect for a person's autonomy and his right to his secrets; (2) respect for the relationship between two persons; (3) the implicit promise of keeping a confidence; and (4) the benefit that the security of confidentiality offers to us.[23]

Each of these considerations supports the argument that Mitsuko should guard Jerome's confidence. Keeping his problems to herself can be seen as confirming her respect both for him as a person and for their relationship. Mitsuko's worry that she will feel guilty about betraying Jerome suggests her belief that hearing a friend's troubles in confidence requires her not to reveal them. To reveal to others what Jerome has told her would cause her, therefore, to break an implied promise. Finally, Jerome and Mitsuko, like all of us, believe that they can explore ideas and questions with certain people in certain situations and not fear that such discussions will be used to hurt them. Mitsuko's silence would safeguard this important benefit of confidentiality.

A concern that may override the force of these reasons supporting confidentiality in this case is that Jerome's patients as well as Jerome himself face real dangers if he continues to make mistakes. Maintaining confidentiality because it preserves respect and trust, has been implicitly promised, or provides a general benefit are not convincing reasons if a consideration such as a potential danger to vulnerable patients is ignored. Given the danger of mistakes, Mitsuko could make three strong arguments for breaking confidence and discussing her concerns with the supervisor.

Briefly, the first argument centers on the welfare of patients who receive Jerome's care. Nurses, as nurses, have a duty to ensure that patients receive safe nursing care. An ICU is no place for even small mistakes. Given the serious condition of the patients and the fast pace of an ICU, mistakes can quickly lead to permanent damage. The clinical situation in an ICU is quite different from, say, a health care teaching situation in which a nurse can return the next day and correct erroneous information that she has given. Thus, Mitsuko ought to safeguard patients by reporting Jerome's problem to the supervisor.

A second argument that supports Mitsuko's breaking confidentiality is derived from concern for the greatest welfare for all. Mistakes that cause problems for a patient, even those that do not result in permanent damage, decrease an ICU's efficiency. Thus nurses and other providers are less able to give needed attention to other patients in the ICU, which limits the well-being of those persons. In addition loss in nursing time or supplies leads to increased health care costs, which, when passed on as increased costs to insurance companies or taxpayers, results in less well-being for those who must pay the bill.

The third argument that supports Mitsuko's discussing her concerns with the supervisor is that to do so would prevent Jerome from hurting himself. He risks losing his reputation as a dependable nurse if he continues making mistakes. Worse, if he makes a major error, he could face legal and professional problems. Since Jerome seems unable or unwilling to admit the seriousness of his situation, Mitsuko could protect him by discussing her concerns with the supervisor who, she assumes, will act to protect Jerome, even if it means removing him from the ICU. In other words, Mitsuko could treat Jerome parentalistically and act on his behalf, although not at his behest.

These three arguments in support of Mitsuko's discussing her concerns with the supervisor have some difficulties. First, Mitsuko does not know if Jerome's problem will increase or even continue. No one has been hurt yet. Jerome seems to be coping well enough so as not to make serious or costly errors. He seems to be able to concentrate on his work well enough to maintain a minimum level of competence.

Second, Mitsuko's acting parentalistically in this case may not be justifiable. As was discussed in Chapter 3, a parentalistic act can be justified if, and only if, it meets three conditions: the autonomy, harm, and ratification conditions. In terms of the first condition, Jerome seems to know he is making errors, and he is also apparently rational. Stress can cause errors, a fact he recognizes. According to his assessment, his situation should improve soon. In terms of the second condition, Jerome faces some danger. He has not, however, made a major error that could damage his career. Furthermore, all ICU nurses take risks every day because any one of them could make a mistake that could result in serious legal problems. In terms of the third condition, Jerome might ratify Mitsuko's discussing his problems with the supervisor if that discussion led to his recognition of a problem that could be treated or resolved soon. More likely, given the information in the case study, her discussion with the supervisor would lead to difficulties and even to a break in Mitsuko's and Jerome' friendship. In short, (weak) parentalism is not straightforwardly justified in this situation, at least according to these criteria.

This analysis of the case, while not clearly pointing out what Mitsuko should do, underscores both the high value we place on confidentiality and the probable dangers of Jerome's continuing to make mistakes. Thus, given the strengths and weaknesses of the various arguments, Mitsuko could propose to Jerome a plan that would address both the importance of maintaining confidentiality and of protecting ICU patients. Such a plan would require that Mitsuko first share her ethical analysis of the situation with Jerome. In other words, she could share with him her reasons for and against telling the supervisor about her concerns. She could also ask him to see the matter from her point of view and ask what he would do if he were in her shoes and why. If Jerome were not persuaded to make changes,

Mitsuko could tell him that, in view of the real danger of harm to patients, she will, after waiting a week for him to seek health care, be obligated to override his wishes to procrastinate and will discuss her concerns with their supervisor. By giving him a week to act, Mitsuko would confirm the high value she places on maintaining confidentiality, but by setting a definite time limit, she would minimize the period in which patients might be harmed by Jerome's mistakes (a period in which, incidentally, Jerome would probably be very careful).

Once Mitsuko had told Jerome of her intentions and given him ample time to act she could clearly justify discussing her concerns with their supervisor if Jerome failed to correct the situation. She probably could not persuasively argue that she should break Jerome's confidence for his own good, since the question remains whether he would ever ratify such a parentalistic act on her part. But she has two strong ethical arguments that support her telling the supervisor about Jerome's situation if he refuses to do anything about it: First, she has a role-based duty as a nurse to protect patients, and second, from the standpoint of utility a safe, efficient ICU increases the well-being of all.[24]

4. ADMINISTRATIVE DILEMMAS

Nursing administrators, whether directors, supervisors, unit managers, or head nurses, must decide how best to deal with nurses who are impaired, dishonest, or incompetent. The following is one such situation.

5.5 Employee with a Drug Problem

Maria Romero, Associate Director of Nursing, is responsible for daily nursing division operations of a 300-bed hospital. During the past year, she has met several times with Pam Altmann, a staff nurse with three years' experience in another city. According to Maria, "Last fall, Pam lived with a pusher and overdosed. She was very honest about her drug problem, and I wanted her to make it. I knew she needed a lot of support and trust." Impressed by Pam's honesty, Maria thought that she should have a second chance.

Maria had to face the questions: Ought a nursing administrator allow a nurse with a history of drug abuse to continue to work, and how ought a nurse resolve a conflict between her professional obligations and her personal desire to befriend a fellow nurse? As the Associate Director of Nursing, Maria has as her primary obligation the provision of safe, effective nursing care to all patients served by the hospital. Patients must be guaranteed that nurses will always be clearheaded and not under the influence of alcohol or mind-altering drugs. On the other hand, as a sensitive and compassionate person, Maria also recognized her desire to help Pam overcome her drug problem. Thus, there was a conflict between Maria's professional obligation to maintain standards and her desire to be a friend and helper to Pam.

Maria knew that Pam would have daily access to drugs and that consequently she would face extraordinary temptations to steal drugs for her own use. She also recognized that the length of Pam's previous nursing experience and the fact that she had not been found stealing drugs decreased the probability that drug-related problems would interfere with her effectiveness as an RN. Given these reasons, Maria thought it would be wrong simply to refuse to rehire Pam. Therefore, Maria encouraged her to attend weekly counseling sessions and waited until Pam's therapist submitted a written statement that she was able to work safely in a clinical setting before employing her again. Rather than sacrificing either her professional obligations or her personal desire, Maria apparently found a solution that satisfied both. The case developed as follows:

> To help as much as possible, Maria assigned Pam to work with a competent and supportive head nurse, where she did well for four months. Then the head nurse learned that fentanyl skin patches for pain control had been signed as given but had not been applied to a patient. The head nurse talked with the patient, who was coherent enough to verify that he had not had the patches changed on his back as scheduled, and with Pam, who admitted that she had taken them.
>
> When Maria met with her, Pam said something had happened that she could not handle. Maria was disappointed, for she had expected Pam to overcome her drug problem "not only for herself as a person but because she was a nurse." Maria has "higher expectations for people in certain roles." She believed that Pam was a good RN who was embarrassed by the difficulty she had caused.
>
> Maria knows she is obliged to report Pam to the State Board of Nurses, which will discipline her by rescinding her license to practice. Maria does not want Pam to go elsewhere to work, where she may steal drugs again but, because of her personal involvement, it is difficult for her to fire Pam and to make the report.[25]

Maria now faces the question, Ought a nursing administrator allow a nurse who has stolen drugs to continue to work? The law says that nurses as well as other people may not steal drugs. Although it is understandable that Maria feels a personal loss, since she sincerely wished for Pam's success and gave her practical support, the law and hospital policy require that Maria must discharge and report Pam because she has not fulfilled her legal obligations as a nurse. If Maria believes that Pam was unable to control her desire for drugs, she must acknowledge that Pam cannot fulfill the demanding responsibilities of a registered nurse. Thus, Maria must let her go and report her in order to protect patients from possible unsafe care. If, on the other hand, Maria believes that Pam was able to control her desire for drugs but nonetheless *chose* to steal the patches, Maria should still take the same action. Not to punish Pam would be to fail to respond to her as a person with the ability to make choices and to assume responsibility for the consequences of her own choices.[26] Finally, Maria could simply ignore the situation or forgive her for stealing the fentanyl skin patches. But either of these courses would have a number of undesirable effects: (1) Maria would be violating the law and thus involving herself in possible legal difficulties; (2) she would be disregarding professional nursing standards; (3) she would be ignoring a strong sign that Pam's future patients might be deprived of needed pain-relieving drugs; and (4) she would be contributing to Pam's continuing dependence on drugs. These possible consequences make it unacceptable for Maria—even given her desire to be a helpful friend—either to ignore the drug theft or to forgive it. Therefore, as argued previously, Maria should let Pam go and report her to the State Board of Nursing.

This case suggests two quite different approaches to the basic question of how a nurse ought to resolve a conflict between professional obligations and personal desire to befriend a fellow nurse. When Pam's situation appeared merely to be that of a person with a history of drug abuse and who posed no clear threat to provision of safe, effective care, Maria was able to identify a course of action that appeared to satisfy conflicting claims. At this point the case underscored a suggestion that it is sometimes possible to select a course of action that allows one to reconcile what may appear to be competing alternatives. At the point when the situation shifted from an episode of drug abuse to a matter of drug theft, professional obligations and legal demands clearly overrode person desires.

Does the fact that this case turned out badly imply that Maria's initial response was wrong? No, we think it does not. Sometimes it happens that the right decision in a particular case turns out badly. For example, a little more than 50 years ago, doctors and nurses appeared to have good grounds for believing that premature infants in respiratory distress needed oxygen-enriched air in order to thrive. What no one knew until later, however, was that excessive amounts of oxygen caused the tiny babies to be permanently blinded. Although, given the limits of medical knowledge at the time, doctors and nurses had conscientiously made the right decision, the results were unfortunate. With new knowledge and more refined methods of monitoring oxygen levels, this is no longer a problem.[27]

Another dilemma that nursing administrators face is deciding the best response to nurses who believe they cannot follow certain orders or rules because of conscience. The next case presents such a dilemma.

5.6 Working in a Bureaucracy: Special Favors

The only hospital in town, small Fairview Memorial, has a pediatric unit of eight beds, which is an extension of the general medical–surgical floor. Jason Campbell, 11-year-old son of Eric Campbell, a member of the hospital's Board of Directors, was admitted in the morning after a bicycle accident. He had minor surgery, was doing well, and was due to be released the next day. When Hilary Jones, evening charge nurse, learned that someone had ordered a special steak dinner for Jason, she protested. "Everyone should have the same care," she told Beth Otterson, the nursing supervisor. "Making sure that a certain child has everything—ordering a special meal, or giving special care, or providing the best nurse—goes against my grain. I think, being the nurse in charge, I should have control over what goes on here on the floor." The nursing supervisor told her the decision that Jason was to have a steak dinner had come from the "higher-ups" and so would not be changed. Anyway, she added, the cost of the dinner was small, no one else had to know, and Mr. Campbell would appreciate the nurses' special concern for Jason.

Hilary was not convinced that giving Jason the special dinner was right, and she said that she would lose her self-respect if she gave in and allowed some patients to receive "VIP treatment." Therefore, she explained, she would not serve the meal to the boy even if it were prepared and sent to the unit.

Hilary's position concerning the special steak dinner presents a problem to Beth, since she must decide how to respond to Hilary's insubordination. The basic question she faces is, How should a nursing administrator deal with a nurse's conscientious refusal?

In order to discuss this case, we must assume that in this hospital the authority to make decisions concerning the many small details involved in nursing care—including meal selection—rests primarily with the unit charge nurse but that ultimately she is under the authority of her supervisor and the nursing administrative hierarchy. Given this assumption, the nurse must follow her supervisor's directives or risk disciplinary action. We must also assume that the unit level nursing staff will support the charge nurse's nursing decision (i.e., in this case they will not serve the meal) unless a nursing supervisor intervenes. Beth can choose to respond to the immediate problem of Hilary's refusal by serving the dinner herself, by ordering another person to serve it, or by taking no action to get the meal served. But whether Jason gets the steak or not, Beth has to decide whether to report Hilary for insubordination.

Beth believes that all persons who are insubordinate should be reported and disciplined, so her first impulse is to report Hilary to the Director of Nursing. Beth also believes that she would cease to be a fair administrator if she did not deal with the nursing staff consistently, and she can cite reasons to support her position. If she did not insist that nurses at each level follow through on decisions and commitments made by persons at higher levels in the nursing and administrative hierarchy, discipline would break down. Further, if at a later date she reported another nurse for insubordination, that nurse could charge her with unfair labor practices.

However, a course of action very different from Beth's first impulse results if she recognizes her responsibility to a subordinate who disobeys because of conscience.[28] Therefore, Beth needs first to decide if Hilary's refusal to serve the meal is an act of conscientious refusal. To be recognized as an appeal to conscience (as discussed in Chapter 4, Section 5) the appeal must (1) be personal or subjective, although the moral standards on which it is based may or may not apply to others; (2) follow a judgment of rightness or wrongness; and (3) be motivated by personal sanction rather than external authority. Hilary's refusal passes all these tests: she spoke only for herself; she based her decision not to serve the meal upon her previous personal sanction—that she would lose self-respect if she served the meal. Once Beth recognizes that Hilary's refusal is based on such an appeal to conscience, she ought to rethink her initial impulse to report her. Having established that Hilary's apparent insubordination is motivated by conscience, Beth must consider a number of additional factors.

Mechanically responding to people who violate certain rules or directives without considering their reasons can lead to injustice, a fact which the legal system recognizes. For example, very often a judge or jury may select from a range of penalties when determining how severely to punish persons who, for different motives and under different circumstances, have committed similar crimes. In the present case, Hilary's conscientious refusal to serve the special dinner is quite different from a refusal based on her dislike of the child. Thus, for a supervisor to be fair in a case of insubordination involving conscientious refusal, the supervisor should take the nurse's reasons into account.

Another important consideration is that a nurse who conscientiously chooses to refuse an order is often representative of the more effective and thoughtful nurses in an institution. A nursing administrator needs to keep these valuable nurses employed in order to provide the best nursing care possible. Further, a hospital nursing organization will not collapse if it allows some room for the exercise of conscience. Hilary's refusal was not intended to undermine the authority of the nursing system. Nor was she refusing to provide needed nursing care. Rather she was attempting to strengthen nursing service by ensuring that it was fair to all patients. The nursing administration, given this view, has an obligation to support Hilary's independent nursing judgments based on conscientious refusal as long as the resulting actions fall within acceptable, safe practice. Beth should be relieved that Hilary is not going further by publicizing the hospital's preferential treatment.

Most important, since the nursing administration permits and even encourages nurses to make independent nursing decisions in questionable cases, it has the responsibility to try to reduce the risks that nurses must take in making such decisions. In the steak dinner case, a question remains as to what is the right course of action concerning the provision of a special dinner to a child of an influential person. Both Hilary's and Beth's positions have something to recommend them. Hilary's position is that Jason's preferential treatment is unfair to other children on the unit who would enjoy, or who might even be helped by, a dinner they especially liked instead of having only "regular" hospital food. As the charge nurse, Hilary believes that she is in the best position to assess nursing care needs and that the nursing administration is attempting to override her skills and judgment in such a way that her other patients will not be treated fairly. Hilary's Kantian appeal to equality and fairness does not, however, diminish the force of Beth's utilitarian appeal to the possible consequences of preferential treatment in this case. Since Mr. Campbell is in a position to influence the hospital's resources, it is likely that the hospital and especially nursing service will stand to benefit. Thus, there are good reasons on both sides, and the best course in the steak dinner situation is uncertain. Since the nursing administration encourages its nurses to think for themselves, it ought to be reluctant to discipline nurses who make well-grounded conscientious decisions. A possible negative consequence of disciplinary action in this case is that it will have a chilling effect on independent thought and judgment among the nursing staff.

In conclusion, if Jason is given the steak, his father will probably learn of the meal. If he is not given the steak, his father will probably not ever know that it was ordered, but some people in the nursing and/or hospital administration will be displeased, including Beth. Since Beth believes that giving Jason the special dinner is in the hospital's best interest, she may decide to serve the steak herself or ask another person to serve it.

Yet, she still must answer the basic question the case raised: How should a nursing administrator deal with a nurse's conscientious refusal? As the discussion has shown, the administrator must first recognize whether the nurse's position qualifies as conscientious refusal. Once she has determined that it does qualify, as it does in Hilary's case, she must not decide too hastily for disciplinary action. In determining how she ought to respond, she must consider the reasons in favor of the refusal, the value of thoughtful, conscientious nurses, the capacity of the institution and the profession to allow some latitude for conscience, and the extent to which an indiscriminately harsh response will repress independent judgment. On balance, we believe that the reasons for not reporting Hilary in the case outweigh those in favor of reporting her.

Administrators may face a similar dilemma concerning how best to respond when nurses refuse to provide nursing care during a highly infectious disease epidemic. In Case 3.11 "Refusal to care for SARS patients," Mary Duncan-Keilman told Crystal Mahorn, a nurse manager, that she would leave her position if she had to care for patients in the special SARS unit.

Crystal believes that nurses who refuse to accept assignments should be dismissed. Yet she also believes in respecting a nurse's appeal to conscience or personal integrity. Thus, like the nursing supervisor in Case 5.6, she believes she must first decide whether Mary's refusal to care for SARS patients is an act of conscientious refusal; if it is, she will try to make accommodations to support Mary.

Mary's refusal, however, fails to meet the three tests of an appeal to conscience: Mary's claim that the assignment violated her rights may have been based on a personal or subjective moral standard; she did not, however, mention what that standard might be, although she did say that her life and the lives of her husband and children were worth more than her job. The appeal did not follow a judgment of rightness or wrongness; that is, Mary did not say that providing nursing care to SARS patients was morally wrong. She did not claim that she was motivated by personal sanction; that is, she did not say, for example, that she would lose her self-respect if she gave nursing care to patients on the SARS unit.

Before dismissing Mary for refusing to accept an assignment, Crystal needs to make certain that she, as the nurse manager, has met her obligations as a nursing leader; that is, that she has provided Mary as well as the rest of the nursing staff assigned to the SARS unit with support—adequate education, supplies, and protective equipment. She also needs to make certain that adequate numbers of nurses competent in the use of protective equipment and required special procedures are assigned to the unit. Assuming that Mary is a skilled and reliable nurse with emergency room experience, Crystal needs to determine whether Mary's refusal is related to inadequate information about SARS and/or the use of the special equipment and procedures. A nurse manager can combat staff nurses' fears of contracting potentially fatal diseases by providing staff (or having others provide) up-to-date instruction on epidemiology and procedures for self-protection. A nurse manager can also insist that all nurses in the hospital have adequate employee health services as further tangible support.

Assuming that an ongoing and adequate education and support program for nurses is in place as part of the hospital's program of preparation for man-made or natural catastrophes or epidemics, Crystal needs to determine whether she is being unfair to Mary in assigning her to the SARS unit rather than to another unit in the hospital. Patients on the SARS unit present a challenge, but Mary has the skills, education, use of protective equipment, and hospital special procedures to lower her personal risk level to that more routinely found in other units. Being assigned to care for SARS patients, while potentially difficult given the need to use special protective equipment and procedures, is no more risky in terms of contracting SARS than caring for other patients on other units during the epidemic.

In summary, Crystal has no choice but to let Mary go for her refusal to care for the patients on the SARS unit. First, Mary's refusal fails to meet the three tests of an appeal to conscience. Second, adequate educational, support, and employee health programs are and have been available to Mary. And, finally, the assignment to the SARS unit is fair, that is, it is no more risky than an assignment on other units during the epidemic. Of course, Mary, if she carries through her threat to walk off the job, will herself sever her employment immediately.

Asking nurses to volunteer to care for SARS or other highly contagious patients may, of course, be an adequate option for a short period of time. It may even be necessary until a nursing staff can be supported and well educated to care for such patients. A problem, however, could develop if assignments continued to rest upon volunteerism because a nurse manager could reinforce the perception that caring for a patient with a highly contagious and potentially fatal disease is somehow different than caring for other patients. Thus, the manager could unwittingly be emphasizing fear of such patients among the nursing staff. The number of nurses prepared to provide care to highly contagious patients in such a situation could remain dependent upon volunteers rather than upon a well-developed education, support, and health services program coupled with institutional and community preparedness that would prepare all nurses in an institution to care for patients during a pandemic or catastrophe. Given the threat of new, potentially fatal diseases such as avian influenza in humans, sufficient numbers of nurses, not just a few volunteers, must be prepared to provide nursing care to patients with highly infectious and potentially fatal diseases.

6

Personal Responsibility for Institutional and Public Policy

1. THE SCOPE OF INDIVIDUAL RESPONSIBILITY

Up to this point, we have been discussing ethical issues that involve identifiable individuals; ethical inquiry, however, may lead us beyond specific individuals to social structures. For what reasons, if any, do ethical considerations require us to identify faults in social structures and then attempt to remedy them?

6.1 Turnover among Unlicensed Assistive Personnel

David Page, RN, has made a career change to nursing after managing a fast food restaurant for six years. The transition has been long and difficult, requiring many hours of study and effort, commuting to evening prerequisite courses, and juggling his working schedule to fit class hours of nursing theory and clinical courses. His wife and two children are proud of him, and now, after working as an RN for three years, he believes that he made the right decision.

But his latest position at a privately owned nursing home is troubling. He is frustrated not with his workload or patients but with the UAP (unlicensed assistive personnel) who are ever-changing. He has told his wife that the unlicensed staff seem to appear and disappear through a revolving door. He has to depend upon nursing assistants to answer lights, relay patients' requests and needs to him, help patients transfer from chairs to beds, and in general do many nursing care tasks. In addition, he has to depend upon several part-time dietary helpers, usually high school students, to get evening meals to patients promptly since only lunch is served communally. Sometimes, trays are left on bedside tables when patients are stuck in chairs across their rooms, and with food getting less palatable by the minute. This is because dietary helpers are not allowed to move patients, and UAP don't deliver food.

When he tried to analyze why he was so frustrated, David thought of his past. As a fast food manager he had successfully trained and supervised many unskilled workers to become a smooth functioning team. But in this situation, personnel come to him already trained—at least they have met minimum nursing assistant training standards that allow the nursing home to qualify for Medicare/Medicaid payments. And in fact, some of them do give good care. But as a group they are not dependable because so many leave their jobs before they really learn how to work together. He finds that having continually to orient and assess so many new UAP detracts from the overall level of nursing care he and the staff can deliver.

David likes being in charge, has no complaints about his salary and work schedule, and thinks he has executive skills. He believes that the nursing home administrator is pleased with his work. And he especially enjoys geriatric nursing. But his staff, in general, does not enjoy working in the nursing home.

Where are the people who might like working with geriatric patients? Why do so many UAP leave so quickly?[1]

David's exasperation and distress arise not only from the way he is limited by the nursing home's high turnover of nursing assistant staff but also probably from an apprehension that the situation may be beyond his—or perhaps anyone's—control. What may underlie his feelings of frustration is the sense that his difficulties result not so much from the deliberate intentions and choices of identifiable individuals but from the impersonal and complex interplay of social forces and structures—"the system."

This situation, of course, is not unique to nursing. Yet it does raise the question, To what extent and for what reasons should David try, first, to determine why the UAP turnover is chronically high and, second, to do something about it?

According to the rules and principles defining the institution of nursing, nurses have social as well as individual obligations. The ICN Code of Ethics for Nurses states that "the nurse shares with society the responsibility for initiating and supporting action to meet the health and social needs of the public, in particular those of vulnerable populations." (Appendix A). Provision 9 of the American Nurses Association Code of Ethics for Nurses states that the "profession of nursing, as represented by associations and their members, is responsible for articulating nursing values, for maintaining the integrity of the profession and its practice, and for shaping social policy."[2] We believe that concern expressed in the codes with questions of social as well as individual ethics is well grounded.

Generally, an obligation to provide a certain level of care to individuals entails as a corollary an obligation to take steps to ensure that conditions exist for providing that level of care. As John Ladd has pointed out,

> A parent's responsibility for the health or welfare of his child implies, for example, that if he does not have the power (e.g., the money) or the competence (e.g., the knowledge) to take care of his child, he should forthwith try to get them. There is no reason to think that the same logic does not apply to participants in a social process: if they do not have the power or competence to fulfill their responsibilities they should take all the necessary steps to obtain them.[3]

In the nursing context, this line of reasoning implies that in Case 6.1 David's obligation to provide standard nursing care to patients under his care entails a further obligation to try to identify the sources of the staffing problem and to correct them. Since the grounds of this obligation are not limited to nursing, however, it is important to note that the responsibility in question does not fall solely on David's shoulders. Nursing home administrators, teachers of nurse assistants, persons who determine educational standards, nursing home owners, persons who determine health care service payments (private or public), and possibly others are also obligated in various, and in some cases greater, degrees to attend to the problem. But if they do not appear to be fulfilling their responsibilities, David's responsibility, though perhaps not increased, is not thereby diminished. He still owes it to his patients to make reasonable efforts to determine why the nursing home faces high nurse assistant turnover and then to try to do something about it.

If we agree that David has a prima facie obligation to contribute to improving the situation and that the situation may involve a complex network of social structures, how does he discharge his obligation? Before addressing this question directly, we must explain what we mean by "social structures."

Social structures include organizations (like nursing homes), institutions (like medicine and nursing), and practices (like fee-for-service or third-party-payment modes of financing health care). A particular combination of social structures dealing with a more or less restricted set of goods may be called a "system," as, for example, the health care system.

Following Etzioni, we take *organizations* to be "social units (or human groupings) deliberately constructed and reconstructed to seek specific goals."[4] Standard examples are corporations, armies, schools, churches, prisons, and hospitals. Organizations differ from other kinds of social structures in having more explicit goal-directedness and greater control over their nature and destiny. The prominent characteristics of organizations are (1) explicit divisions of labor and power; (2) one or more power centers that control members' efforts and direct them toward the organization's goals; and (3) substitution of personnel.

Institutions, as we understand them, are social structures that differ from organizations principally in having less control over their nature and destiny. Examples of institutions are property, marriage, the family, nursing, and medicine. Social institutions fulfill certain functions in society, and they are characterized by certain rules that fix roles and determine relationships in particular contexts. Nursing and medicine, for example, circumscribe different roles for patients and providers and presume different though complementary roles for nursing and doctors. Finally, although institutions as such do not exert direct control over their own nature and destiny, organizations may be created and maintained that are aimed at shaping and strengthening particular institutions. Thus, the American Nurses Association (ANA) and the American Medical Association (AMA), both organizations, have as their goal the shaping and strengthening of the institutions of nursing and medicine, respectively.

Practices are made up of rules that coordinate and regulate behavior in determinable ways. Common examples are the "-isms," like racism, sexism, capitalism, and socialism. Controversies over the merits of capitalism and socialism are mirrored in health care controversies over the merits of fee-for-service versus a nationalized health service. Practices often involve and relate different institutions and can be supported or opposed by various organizations. For our purposes, what is important about practices is that, like organization and institutions, they explain various patterns of human behavior.

If we are to understand, for example, why the nursing home in Case 6.1 faced high nursing assistant turnover, we must try to identify, first, the organizational causes of this state of affairs and, if necessary, the extent to which the conduct of the organization in question—the nursing home—is itself restricted by social institutions and practices. If it turns out that the actions of the organization are restricted by certain institutions and the institutions are, in turn, limited by certain practices, then the organization can be fully understood only in terms of its role within the practices. In this event, by placing the action of the institution (e.g., nursing home) within the context of a practice (e.g., for profit, fee-for-service, or third-party payment for health care) we obtain a deeper understanding of its conduct and are, as a result, in a position to intervene more effectively (perhaps by joining or forming an organization to do so).

Returning to Case 6.1 and David's obligation to make some effort to identify the source of the problem and to correct it, we suggest the following. Since our concern is not simply that nurses be able to explain situations such as David's but that they be able to help change them, a helpful rule of thumb is to examine the *most alterable* possibilities first. In David's case this means restricting his initial inquiry to the nursing home and to its sub-organizations, such as the nursing service. In discussions with the nursing administration, David could explore alternatives based upon nursing management programs for ways to increase his skills in supervision as well as methods to increase employee satisfaction. If that fails, he could then enlist the support and expertise of another organization, such as his state nursing association. The next step, if the problem is rooted in practices governing UAP education or the distribution and financing of nursing home care, might be to become politically active at the local, state, or federal level.[5]

Apart from these schematic rules of thumb, David should also be sensitive to the detailed history of the situation and personalities of those involved. He should recognize that although his efforts may be necessary for a satisfactory resolution of the problem, they are unlikely to be sufficient. Change in the situation may require the action and resources of the hospital administrator, hospital owners, and local nurse assistant training programs. Thus David must be careful not to alienate other parties by being overly self-righteous or condemnatory. Problems attributable to the unintended or unanticipated workings of complex social structures often require social solutions, and individuals who may be credited with initiating changes are unlikely to achieve their ends without the support and cooperation of others.

2. INSTITUTIONAL POLICIES AND STRIKES

Suppose that David is able to identify the source of the staffing problem but that efforts by the nurses to persuade those empowered to correct it are unsuccessful. Would they then be justified in shifting from rational persuasion to a more coercive mode of achieving their ends, such as a work stoppage or a strike? Before examining the ethical implications and possible justifications of such measures, we should briefly review the history and legal status of strikes and other forms of work stoppage by nurses.

Collective bargaining by nurses to change organizational policies has a short history, and the use of strikes and other work stoppages, an even shorter one. A movement for collective bargaining began in California during World War II, and in 1946 the ANA created an economic security program that endorsed state nurses associations as bargaining agents.[6] But the 1947 Taft-Hartley Labor Management Relations Act (LMRA), which specifically exempted nonprofit organizations from recognizing bargaining rights of employees, and the no-strike pledge made by the ANA in 1950, made collective bargaining difficult. Basically, nurses had to depend upon public relations campaigns and moral suasion when negotiating with health care organizations.

The 1960s brought changes. When collective bargaining became a right for federal employees in 1962, civilian nurses employed by the government gained the right to choose a bargaining agent. In 1966, when nurses in the San Francisco Bay area threatened to submit mass resignations after long, unproductive negotiations with area hospitals, the California Nurses Association revoked the ANA no-strike policy and the nurses negotiated successfully. Nurses also struck successfully in Youngstown, Ohio, during that year, and the threat of resignations or strikes led to successes elsewhere. The ANA repealed the no-strike pledge in 1968, as did the National Association of Practical Nurses in 1969.

In 1974, the LMRA was extended to employees of nonprofit health care institutions so that at long last these hospitals were obligated to bargain with nurses. In 1990, the Supreme Court ruled that nurses could organize their own separate RN bargaining units. Four years later, a Supreme Court decision ruled that persons who directed the work of less skilled workers are supervisors and are not protected by federal labor law. Therefore, such nurses are not to be included in collective bargaining units. Given this ruling, the issue of whether "charge nurses" are supervisors led to years of legal battles between nurse employers and nurse unions and resulted in multiple decisions by the National Labor Relations Board (NLRB) and the courts. In 2006, the NLRB ruled that, in general, charge nurses are supervisors. For a nurse to be deemed a supervisor, however, requires that the nurse meet certain criteria since the title alone does not automatically make a charge nurse into a supervisor.[7]

In addition to defining who may be included in a bargaining unit, federal labor law specifies dispute-settling and strike procedures by requiring time limits for notification of intent to modify contracts and, if no settlement is reached, notification of the Federal Mediation and Conciliation Service. Further, the law provides time limits for no-strike, no-lockout periods and requires a ten-day strike or picketing notice. Even though legal dispute-settling and strike procedures exist, not all nurses, as the following case illustrates, agree that strikes, mass resignations, or other work stoppages are appropriate.

6.2 Proposal for a Strike

For the past nine months Alice Byrum, RN, has worked evenings on a 20-bed medical-surgical unit in Batavia Community Hospital. She believes that the quality of nursing care she can provide is being compromised by the

(Continued)

hospital's choice to systematically understaff her unit. Alice wants the nursing administrator to find a solution to continual understaffing. The hospital's frequent use of "casual nurses" who work per diem for a private agency has not lessened the problem.

Alice is frustrated because, as she says, "You are behind before you start. You can't give adequate care and you can't expect your aides to give good care. It's frustrating knowing patients aren't getting the care they are supposed to get. I must spend so much time giving 'meds,' making time-consuming rounds with one particular surgeon who insists that I accompany him (the other doctors are more flexible), checking IVs and doing the paper work that I can't do anything else."

Most aides rarely get two days off each week because the administration routinely calls them to cover a shortage when they are off duty. Needing to keep a steady job, they comply. Alice, too, has been called to work extra days, but she has repeatedly reminded the caller of her problems in making last minute babysitting arrangements. She has asked administrators not to call her because refusing makes her feel guilty (which she assumes they want her to feel).

When Alice complained about the overworked nursing staff, her supervisor told her that the hospital's staffing practices met all required standards. Alice was offended at being told that the hospital met required standards; she knew that when she was overworked, the quality of her nursing care suffered. Alice suspects that her supervisor, a sympathetic listener, never reports her complaints to higher authorities.

Monthly "group gripe" sessions with hospital nursing staff and nursing administration have brought no results—the same complaints have elicited the same answers. Alice has come to believe that the only solution is for nurses to organize and, acting together, stage a walkout strike the next time staffing is hopelessly bad. She has suggested a strike to hospital evening personnel, who all have the same problems, but no one has supported her. Alice believes that the nurses may "not be the type to do anything, but in any other situation you can bet people would not put up with that kind of staffing. So a strike is not going to happen here. But I am hoping that somehow and in some way..."

Alice believes that both nurses and patients would benefit from a strike. Her two main arguments for a nurses' strike appear to be that it would benefit clients by producing changes that would improve the quality of nursing and benefit nurses by reducing job stress and requests that they work overtime. In an ideal situation, nursing care that a hospital demands of its staff does not conflict with nursing care that nurses believe they should provide. But Alice and other nurses repeatedly find themselves in situations where they can only provide what they regard as substandard care because of being overworked. In Alice's view, the hospital's substandard health care is related to its exploitation of the nursing staff. The question now is whether a strike aimed at correcting the situation is ethically justified.

Deciding to initiate or participate in any form of work stoppage—sit-downs, mass resignations, strikes, and so on—is difficult for nurses. Strikes are especially problematic because they amount not only to withdrawing services but also to using the resulting distress as a lever to coerce a hospital or agency into meeting the strikers' demands. Even if efforts are made to provide warning and to staff certain units, such as intensive care, emergency rooms, and a minimal number of general nursing units, the strike will still force some people to wait for care, at the very least inconveniencing and possibly even harming them. Since nursing strikes by their very nature require nurses to threaten patient services, such strikes bear a heavy burden of justification.

The presumption against nursing strikes, like presumptions against parentalism, deception, and coercion discussed in Chapter 3, is very strong. Not only may strikes inconvenience and possibly harm clients, they are also likely to backfire. As with strikes by other groups providing vital social services, like police and fire departments, the public is likely to respond negatively when striking nurses seem to be using the sick and infirm as hostages to better their position. Such public perceptions may be detrimental not only to the strikers but also to the entire nursing profession. Moreover, even if a nursing strike is successful, lingering acrimony between strikers, on the one hand, and hospital administrators, other providers, and the public, on the other, may seriously compromise whatever gains the strike achieved.

Although the presumption against nursing strikes is very strong, we do not think that it is impossible to justify a nursing strike. Like presumptions against parentalism and deception, it can at least in principle be overridden by appeal to certain ethical considerations. We turn now to a brief survey of arguments that attempt to justify such strikes.

A. Utilitarian Arguments

A utilitarian argument in favor of a strike aimed at improving chronically substandard care is that while the strike will to some extent inconvenience and possibly harm *presently* hospitalized patients, it will in the long run contribute to significant improvement in the care of a much larger number of *future* patients. This assumes that the good of an improved response to the needs of future patients outweighs the bad of continued failed response to the needs of presently hospitalized patients. On the other hand, a nurse choosing to respond to the needs of presently hospitalized patients in such a situation would be making a decision based on short-term interests rather than on the long-term effects of perpetuating poor nursing care.

To increase the net balance of good over bad consequences of a nursing strike, those making a utilitarian argument could suggest that strikers not withdraw all services to presently hospitalized patients. Care for all who would be directly and severely harmed by the strike could be provided. Advance warning of an impending strike would allow prospective patients to choose between seeking other sources of care or tolerating delay.

A less direct utilitarian defense of a nursing strike might focus on the long-term benefits to patients of a highly qualified nursing staff with a fairly low rate of turnover. Continued employment of a well-trained staff depends largely on the level of its salaries and working conditions, including respect as professionals. If these fall well below those offered by other health care organizations or even other occupations, the hospital or agency will be unable to attract and retain good nurses. Thus, nurses may argue that collective bargaining, strikes, and the threat of strikes aimed at improving their working conditions will indirectly, but significantly, benefit patients.

Whether such arguments can justify nursing strikes depends on two factors: the extent to which one accepts the principle of utility and the conclusions of arguments based on it as decisive on such matters, and the extent to which the utilitarian calculations of overall benefits and harms favor a strike. The first requires a review of the strengths and weaknesses of *purely* utilitarian arguments in this context. Is maximizing overall utility the only or most important consideration in this context? The second requires taking into account *all* of the probable consequences of a proposed strike and not simply those that support one's predispositions. Thus, the long-term gains of a strike must be balanced not only against short-term losses but also against possible long-term losses, such as negative public perceptions and lingering acrimony between (and possibly among) nurses and other health professionals.

One final utilitarian argument against a strike merits special consideration. It is often maintained that nursing strikes weaken the profession itself when staff nurses become adversaries of nurses in administrative positions. This objection, however, may ignore the possibility of the profession's being equally weakened by the submission of the rank and file to prevailing practices. Further, it assumes that an adversarial relationship, with its conflict and stress, results only in harmful consequences. Such a relationship may, however, also offer certain benefits, such as mutual goal setting and the incorporation of diverse ideas and points of view resulting in improved nursing services.

Therefore we conclude that utilitarian considerations may, in certain circumstances, support a nursing strike. Whether in any given situation a strike is justified must be determined by careful efforts to predict, weigh, and balance all of its likely consequences. In most cases, however, utilitarian considerations alone are unlikely to override the presumption against a nursing strike because the short-term negative consequences will always be more certain than the possible long-term benefits. Moreover, as moral pluralists, we have some misgivings about relying solely on utilitarian considerations in this as well as in other settings. Some obligations or rights whose justification is independent of appeals to the overall social good may also have a bearing on nursing strikes.

B. Care-based Arguments

At first glance, it appears that we can construct a clear and unconditional care-based argument against nursing strikes. A nurse's primary duty is to provide for the care and safety of her patients. Assuming the patients in question are present rather than future patients, nurses would have to assure all patients of safe and adequate nursing care during a strike. But this, of course, would undermine the very point of a strike, which is to coerce management into altering its policies by withdrawing (or threatening to withdraw) nursing services. Therefore, if a nurse is professionally obligated to provide for the care and safety of her patients, and the patients in question are present patients, participation in a nursing strike will always be wrong because it requires abrogation of the primary virtue of nursing—caring about and for one's patients.

This argument presents a plausible alternative to utilitarian approaches to the question of nursing strikes. Its strength, however, depends in part on two important assumptions, which may not always be true. First, the argument assumes that the nursing care that would be withdrawn during a strike is safe and adequate. There may, however, be situations when nursing care in a particular hospital or nursing home is so substandard that patients would be better off if, during a strike aimed at changing these conditions, they returned home or were transferred to another institution. If, for example, a patient in Case 6.2 were hospitalized for elective surgery and the understaffing problem significantly compromised the safety and adequacy of his or her nursing care, one could argue that the nurses would not be "uncaring" in withdrawing their services. On the contrary, the patient would probably benefit from either postponing the operation or having it performed at another hospital. Moreover, it could be argued that, *under these circumstances*, providing seriously substandard nursing services is less caring than not providing them.

The second assumption underlying care-based arguments against nursing strikes is that the patients who may presently be harmed by the strike and the patients who would, in the future, benefit from it are entirely different groups of people. In a number of cases, however, especially when the patients in question are suffering from chronic illnesses requiring periodic hospitalization or continued nursing home care, those harmed or inconvenienced by the strike and those benefited may be one and the same. In such circumstances, when the benefits appear to significantly outweigh the harm or inconvenience, it could be argued that a nurse's duty to adequately care for these patients justifies her taking limited risks with their present interests by engaging in some form of withdrawal of services. There would be no group whose care would be sacrificed for the benefit of others.

Thus, although care-based considerations provide a strong presumption against nursing strikes and other forms of withdrawal of services, we have tried to show that there are circumstances under which such actions might be justified within a care-based framework. And again, as moral pluralists we are reluctant to restrict our deliberations to care-based arguments. Considerations of utility, respect for persons, and perhaps other values, principles, and virtues may also come into play.

C. Respect for Persons-based Arguments

As persons, it may be argued, nurses have a right to the same respect as other people, and when employers violate this right, nurses are entitled to defend themselves. When, for example, nurses are continually required to work overtime because of personnel shortages, are paid considerably less than people performing comparable tasks for other hospitals or agencies, or are denied a voice as professionals in determining the conditions under which they work, they have a right to do what is necessary to improve their situation. If less drastic means fail, and nothing short of a strike appears likely to induce the organization to acknowledge their rights, then they have a right to strike.

A difficulty with this argument, however, is that the nurse's right to strike appears to conflict with the patient's right to nursing care, and the latter, on the face of it, seems more important than the former. Most patients receiving nonelective treatment would be likely to prefer substandard nursing care to no nursing care at all. So it is unlikely that even patients who sympathize with the nurse's concerns would be inclined to waive their rights to care.

In response, we must distinguish *special* from *general* rights.[8] Special rights are conditional, limited in scope, and grounded in special *relationships*. The rights to the repayment of a debt or the keeping of a promise are special rights. Such rights are conditional in two ways. They are held not against everyone but only against the person who borrowed the money or made the promise, and they depend on the nature of the special relationship between lender and debtor, promisee and promiser. General rights, on the other hand, are unconditional, unrestricted in scope, and grounded simply in one's being a person. The right to life and the right to liberty are general rights. The sense in which they are unconditional is the obverse of the sense in which special rights are conditional. Thus, they are held against everyone and depend on no special relationship between right-holder and those who have the corresponding obligation to respect the right. Although only people who have borrowed money or made promises are obligated to repay debts or keep promises to an individual, everyone is obligated not to kill others or to restrict their liberty.

The question now is whether a "right to nursing care" is a special right, a general right, or both. To say, for example, that the right to nursing care is a special right is to say that it is grounded in the special relationship between particular nurses and particular patients. Once a nurse assumes care for a patient, she acquires an obligation to the patient and the patient acquires a right against her, just as the making of a promise creates special rights and obligations between promisee and promiser. But in both cases, once the respective obligations are fulfilled, the special relationship is ended and further rights and obligations are contingent upon reentering into the special relationship. If the right to nursing care is of this kind, then a nursing strike that results in the abandonment of patients who have already come into the health care system and established a relationship with a nurse or nurses is likely to violate their rights to continued care. If, however, the strike is announced well in advance and makes provision for honoring commitments to those already in the system and to those requiring emergency care that can be provided by no other hospital or agency, the extent to which it violates the special rights of patients may be considerably reduced.

If, in addition to such special rights, there is a general right to health care, including nursing care, which has the same status as the rights to life and liberty, health professionals probably could never justify withdrawing their services. Whether there is such a general right, however, and exactly what it requires is a matter of great controversy. A right to health care, unlike the rights to life and liberty, is a positive rather than a negative right. Whereas the latter requires only that one not be interfered with, a right to health care requires that the right-holder be provided with certain services. And it may be difficult to satisfy this as well as other positive general rights without requiring others to provide time or money which may conflict with their negative rights to liberty and property. For this reason, it is a matter of much debate whether there is a general as well as a special right to health care and, if so, exactly to how much health care. Therefore, an appeal to a general right to health care does not, at least at this time, provide a strong basis for opposing nursing strikes, especially when the strikers scrupulously honor the terms of existing relationships with patients and continue to staff facilities providing emergency care that cannot be provided elsewhere.

To return to Case 6.2, we believe that Alice's suggestion for a walkout strike is at least premature and perhaps could never be justified on the basis of rights grounded in the principle of respect for persons. First, since the monthly meetings between the nursing staff and administrators are unproductive, a reasonable next step would be for the nursing staff to ask for help from a bargaining agent, such as the state nurses' association, and to negotiate a contract that would address staffing problems.[9] Labor law obligates the nursing and hospital administration to negotiate with such an agent in good faith. If these collective bargaining negotiations failed, the nurses could then decide whether to strike in support of their demands. Until then, however, a strike is untenable. Without further attempts at rational persuasion, a strike cannot be supported by considerations of utility, caring, or respect for persons.

If further efforts are unsuccessful, it is possible, though not likely, that utilitarian reasoning could justify a walkout strike. So too might care-based reasoning if the strikers could show that current considerations prevent them from providing minimally adequate care for their present patients and that the situation can only be remedied by a walkout strike. On a respect for persons rights-based view, however, the special rights of presently hospitalized patients to even substandard nursing care are stronger than the nurses' rights or the questionable general rights of the population at large to more adequate care. Indeed, insofar as such strikes require nurses to violate the special rights of those for whom they have already assumed care, it may be impossible to justify any *walkout* strike on the basis of the rights of nurses or patients.[10]

3. INSTITUTIONAL ETHICS COMMITTEES

An awareness of the interplay between institutional policies and standards of nursing care focuses attention not only upon institutional faults that impede nursing practice but also upon the need to create and use new institutional structures to address new problems.[11] Many ethical dilemmas confronting nurses cannot be resolved by nurses alone. They involve questions that may require the joint deliberation of patients, physicians, lawyers, social workers, administrators, other health professionals, clergy, and others, as well as nurses. The next case points to a need for a nursing home to employ an institutional ethics committee composed of such individuals to address matters of ethics.

6.3 Withdrawing Necessities of Life

Abby Wilson, staff nurse, can barely contain her frustration. The issue is whether a feeding tube should be removed from a permanently comatose patient. Melvin Thompson, 20 years old, was in an automobile accident a year ago and has never regained consciousness. His doctors, including a board certified neurologist, say he is in permanent vegetative state—he is totally and permanently unconscious. Because the damage to his brain is restricted to the cortex and his brain stem is largely intact, he is able to breathe without the assistance of a respirator and is being fed through a gastric feeding tube.

Abby is frustrated because she sees the family continue to agonize over an issue that is not being adequately addressed. Melvin's physicians, including the neurologist, have met with the family repeatedly and recommended that Melvin's feeding tube be withdrawn and he thus be allowed to die. Melvin's parents understand that their son will die without tube feedings, and they were beginning to agree with the physicians' recommendation until they consulted with their minister. When he learned of the situation, the minister said that to agree to have Melvin's feeding tube removed was "unthinkable," since food and water were not medical treatment, but rather necessities of life, and removing them did not fall under the right to refuse treatment. Food and water are what all "decent human beings" owe to each other. To remove them is to deliberately kill—"murder"—the patient just as if one were to chain someone to a basement wall and deliberately starve him or her to death. Besides, there was no documented evidence that Melvin would have wanted the tubes removed. Perhaps if he knew about the situation or had considered the possibility of it before the accident, he would have wanted treatment to continue regardless of whether he was totally and permanently unconscious or not. Furthermore, the minister said, many people in their generally more deeply religious part of the state thought as he did and they would be appalled if the parents were to allow the tube to be removed, an act possibly leading to their being ostracized.

After this, Melvin's parents were plagued by doubt. They now said they were not certain that removing the tube was right, and they began to fear that their ordeal would become a nationally televised nightmare like the politicized case of Terri Schiavo in Florida some years ago.[12] They were modest, private people and did not want to subject their son or themselves to being seen in everyone's living room on the evening news.

Abby remembers, though not in detail, of some court decisions in which tube-administered hydration and nutrition were classified as medical treatment falling under the right to refuse such treatment. But she has had little opportunity to discuss this with the family, and there is still the question of whether Melvin would want the tube removed in present circumstances or, given the circumstances, whether his parents should have the right to make

(Continued)

the decision. Abby is not certain that she understands or has thought through all relevant aspects of the situation; neither is she certain of how much weight ought to be given to the minister's or the community's views of the matter. So far the family has resisted meeting with the nursing home ethics committee. Abby is frustrated because she does not see a way for all parties to work through this difficult situation.[13]

Abby needs access to a structure within the nursing home that could help her, the Thompsons, and the Thompsons' physicians address the ethical questions raised by this case. Like nearly all hospitals and some nursing homes, hers has an ethics committee, but, like many hospital ethics committees, it is generally underutilized, especially with respect to specific cases. As a recent report puts it, "The use of ethics consultation services varies widely from hospital to hospital, but physician experts and ethicists agree that they frequently are underused. That leads, they say, to increased medical costs and ugly disputes among physicians, patients, and families." Moreover, many physicians regard ethics committees as somehow interfering with their ethical obligations to the patient. The report mentioned above quotes Richard E. Thompson, a retired neonatologist who has written a book on ethics committees saying, "The physician thinks, 'I've got this license, and it says that I'm supposed to be making the decisions, and now I've got these nurses and preachers and social workers who want to make these decisions.' It's a feeling of displacement."[14]

But as Abby seems to realize, the problem is an ethical one, and ethical problems in health care are, as a rule, not generally physicians' problems alone. They are multifactorial and multidisciplinary. Hence a multidisciplinary ethics committee composed of nurses, physicians, other providers, clergy, social workers, patients or patient representatives, and so forth, ensure that all relevant perspectives are brought into discussion. And if a committee includes someone with special training in bioethics and a command of the relevant literature, it will be even better informed.

In Case 6.3, for example, an ethics committee could be especially helpful to Abby, to Melvin's family, and to the family's minister. The committee might help the family and minister explore the ethics of terminating treatment in such cases, including a brief summary or review of relevant court cases and decisions. The minister is not, of course, alone in thinking removal of medically administered hydration and nutrition does not fall under the refusal of treatment. But in 1990 the Supreme Court in the case of *Cruzan v. Director, Missouri Department of Health* decided that medically administered hydration and nutrition constituted medical treatment (which makes sense insofar as it seems clear a nonphysician trying to administer such treatment could be charged with practicing medicine without a license). The more relevant and serious question is whether there was reason to believe that the patient, Melvin Thompson, would have wanted it ceased. Unfortunately, like most Americans, especially those in their twenties, Mr. Thompson has not filled out an advance directive expressing his wishes or authorizing someone to make a decision for him in a situation like this. So the issue is not clear-cut. (See, in this connection, Section 5.) Perhaps, after talking with the physicians, Abby may be able to persuade them to convene the ethics committee, and the committee could in a fair, respectful, and dispassionate manner consider the various issues and provide some helpful information and guidance to those involved. Committee members, as part of their responsibilities, should be up-to-date on the most recent literature and court cases having to do with the issues raised by the case. Not every individual can keep up with all the ethics literature and related court cases, but, in fulfilling their responsibilities, the ethics committee, or at least a member of the committee specializing in bioethics, could. In other instances, the committee might be able to show physicians, family members, and others that their uncertain ethical intuitions were or were not supported by good arguments in the relevant literature. The committee could also either point out additional viewpoints or arguments, or assure the parties that they had not overlooked something of importance.

Perhaps, after continued discussion, the family and their minister could agree at least that medically administered hydration and nutrition were medical treatment and could be refused or removed without constituting murder. The question might then turn to whether there was any reason to believe that Melvin Thompson would not want to be kept "alive" in this condition, or whether those who knew him best, his parents, were entitled to make the decision whether to remove the tube. An ethics committee could identify the different perspectives from which his parents, their minister, and the physicians were viewing the patient and, thus, enable each party to see and understand the other's position.

In such cases, informed, mutually respectful dialogue is most important. The committee could also be helpful by discussing whether the family would be harmed by public opinion in their community and whether the minister could play an important role preventing such harm. Insuring absolute privacy and emotional support to the family throughout the deliberations could be critical to the outcome.

To conclude, nurses and others troubled by ethical questions may find it useful to enlist the support of institutional ethics committees when thinking them through. It is important, too, that the nursing perspective be represented on these committees and, indeed, an aim of this book is to enable nurses to more effectively serve on them. Institutional ethics committees can provide educational forums, develop policy, and provide informed, thoughtful advice and support to patients and health professionals puzzled by or at odds over ethical questions in health care. Finally, institutional ethics committees can be more sensitive to nuance and the details of specific cases than can courts of law, and they can provide support and information not otherwise available in many hospitals and nursing homes.

4. BLOWING THE WHISTLE

What should a nurse do if correcting a dangerous or unethical practice seems to require that she go outside routine institutional channels? The term "whistle-blower" has been coined to refer to members of organizations who sound an alarm externally to call attention to internal negligence, abuses, or dangers that threaten the public. A civil servant, for example, whose attempts to correct corrupt or unsafe practices in his agency by proceeding through established channels are repeatedly frustrated, may feel there is no alternative but to "go public." This may take the form of writing a letter to an elected official or making a public revelation and accusation through the press. Nurses, too, may be tempted to blow the whistle on what they regard as slovenly, dangerous, unethical, or illegal care in hospitals. Although a nurse is expected to have a certain amount of loyalty to colleagues and coworkers, codes of nursing ethics stress her responsibilities to clients and the general public. And in cases of conflict, it is the latter that are supposed to prevail. The following case, taken nearly word for word from a newspaper article, implies that a student nurse blew the whistle on a rather egregious instance of unethical and illegal conduct by a physician.

6.4 "MD Suspended from Operating Room"

A…urologist who had his 14-year-old son assist him in an operation on a 50-year-old woman has been prohibited from working in an operating room for two weeks.

The Michigan Board of Medicine reluctantly imposed the sanction Wednesday after [the physician] admitted that the incident occurred and that he had violated state law.

"He didn't err very much," argued…a board member from Detroit, who opposed any limitation of the doctor's license. "In the operating room, it's not a solemn wake. It's more like M*A*S*H. People walk in and out. Jokes are made. I can understand how this doctor could get carried away, not only as a teacher but as a father."

But [the] vice chairman of the board argued for the sanction. "We are here to protect the public. If this had been my mother, and he had allowed his

14-year-old son to assist with a major operation, I would be extremely upset. If we let this go by the board, I think we are telling the public that we are not here to protect them, we are here to protect the physician."

The incident occurred in March 1983…while [the physician] was performing a bladder operation. He had his son scrub and come into the operating room because [he] said his son was interested in medicine and had asked repeatedly if he could watch an operation.

During the operation [the physician] instructed his son to insert his gloved hand inside the woman's abdomen and feel a catheter balloon in her bladder. As [the physician] was sewing together a layer of tissue over the muscles, he had his son put in two stitches, despite the objections of the anesthesiologist.

The woman, who recovered uneventfully, was not told that [the physician's] son participated in the operation. [The physician], former chief of staff at [the hospital], said he realized his mistake immediately after the operation and apologized to the anesthesiologist and the chief nurse.

A nursing student reported the incident to the Board of Medicine. State law requires that the board take disciplinary action in such cases.[15]

This case raises a number of interesting and important issues. Most important for present purposes is that it appears that the incident never would have come to light, and the physician never would have been suspended, had it not been for the student nurse. Neither the anesthesiologist nor the nonstudent nurses who must have assisted in the operation took any action. Of course, at least one person objected at the time and that person and others may have tried to pursue the matter through the hospital's internal channels. But, in addition to compromising his coworkers and being unethical with his patient, the physician also violated state law. Although there was no legal obligation to report this transgression, there was an ethical obligation to do so.[16] No one except the student nurse appears to have had the courage to bring the incident to light.

We would, of course, like to know more about this central figure who receives only one brief line in the newspaper article. Did the nursing student observe or participate in the operation? Or did she simply hear of the incident through the hospital's grapevine? In either case, she appears to have shown more concern for protecting the public than did the other nurses, the chief nurse, and the anesthesiologist who participated in the surgery. Although state law requires the Board of Medicine to take disciplinary action when such incidents are reported, no one is legally obligated to make such reports (though there is an ethical obligation to do so).

Blowing the whistle is often a risky business. As an insider, one is presumed to have a certain loyalty to one's colleagues and organization. The whistle-blower, as Sissela Bok has pointed out, though he is neither referee nor coach, blows the whistle on his own team. His insider's position carries with it certain obligations to colleagues and clients.... When he steps out of routine channels to level accusations, he is going against these obligations. Loyalty to colleagues and clients comes to be pitted against concern for the public interest and for those who may be injured unless someone speaks out. Because the whistleblower criticizes from within, his act differs from muckraking and other forms of exposure by outsiders. Their acts may arouse anger, but not the sense of betrayal that whistleblowers so often encounter.[17]

In the present case, the student nurse was accusing the urologist and, by her act of disclosure, was also implicitly criticizing the other doctors and nurses who knew of his action but refrained from reporting it to the Board of Medicine. We cannot help but wonder how they responded to her action. Did they regard her as a heroine or a snitch? Did the other nurses celebrate or condemn what she had done? Honor her or shun her? And how was she later regarded by doctors in the hospital? If no reprisals were taken directly against her, were new restrictions placed on subsequent groups of nursing students? As the newspaper account reveals, at least one member of the board was reluctant to sanction the urologist, even though he admitted that the urologist had violated state law and he was charged with enforcing it. Surely this sympathetic attitude was shared by other physicians who could subsequently exert both direct and indirect pressure on the student nurse.

Although there is a sense in which the whistle-blower's being a student made it more difficult for her to do what she did (because of her inexperience and academic vulnerability), there is also the possibility that this made it easier. As a student she was probably not close to the practicing nurses and physicians. She was probably not dependent on their continued friendship and goodwill. She may not have had time to develop close relationships with the others and, assuming her assignment was only temporary, she would not have to endure for very long the prospect of subtle—or perhaps not so subtle—harassment and reprisals from the urologist's friends and colleagues. It is the whistle-blower's inside position, his or her personal loyalty to the members of the group, together with a deeply rooted, widely shared antipathy to tattletales, that render blowing the whistle so psychologically difficult.

Despite its hazards, the practice of whistle-blowing has received guarded general endorsement. Bok has pointed out that

evidence of the hardships imposed on those who chose to act in the public interest has combined with a heightened awareness of professional malfeasance and corruption to produce a shift toward greater public support of whistleblowers. Public-service law firms and consumer groups have taken up their cause; institutional reforms and legislation have been enacted to combat illegitimate reprisals. Some would encourage even greater numbers of employees to ferret out and publicize improprieties in the agencies and organizations where they work.[18]

However, the oppositions involved are not simply between personal risk and public good. Not all acts of whistle-blowing are justified. Like parentalism, whistle-blowing is a descriptive notion. Having identified an action as whistle-blowing, we must then determine whether we can justify it.

All organizations require a certain amount of trust. "There comes a level of internal prying and mutual suspicion," Bok points out, "at which no institution can function."[19] Groups and societies riddled with members eager to curry favor with an external authority by informing on other members are in grave danger of disintegration. It is especially destructive of intimacy and trust when totalitarian regimes encourage family members, particularly children, to report various forms of private behavior to the authorities. Moreover, the motivation of a whistle-blower may often be impure. Accusations made by those holding grudges or who are paranoid, malicious, resentful, jealous, and so on may be aimed more at settling scores or hurting certain people than at protecting the public. Some who blow the whistle may also be more concerned with getting pubic recognition and acclaim than with correcting a serious wrong. The use of internal channels is often more effective than going public. Thus the motivations of one who blows the whistle too soon—who regards whistle-blowing as a first rather than a last resort—are suspect.

There are important lessons to be drawn from the above discussion of whistle-blowing on the part of nurses. First, nurses should do all that they can to establish routine, internal channels for reporting and reducing the incidence of impaired, dishonest, and incompetent practice, and for resolving various ethical disagreements. Whistle-blowing should be used sparingly and reluctantly, and then only to deal with a serious problem. Sound, everyday procedures will often minimize the need for it. Second, guidelines or criteria, as precise as the subject matter allows, should be developed for determining the conditions under which whistle-blowing is justifiable. Third, changes should be initiated to protect from reprisal those who justifiably blow the whistle. The remainder of this section expands on each of these.

In 1983, the Department of Health and Human Services (DHHS) issued a revised set of "Baby Doe" regulations that required hospitals receiving federal funding to place a notice in "each nurse's station" prohibiting the failure to feed and care for handicapped infants. The notice (which was required to be at least eight and one-half by eleven inches in size) was to include a toll-free, 24-hour-a-day "hot line" number. Individuals with knowledge that any handicapped infant was being denied food or customary medical care were encouraged to use this number to prompt an outside investigation.

Apart from one's personal position on the question of when, if ever, aggressive treatment may be withheld from seriously ill newborns, this particular proposal for institutionalized whistle-blowing was premature and bound to breed alienation and mistrust. As George Annas suggested at the time, it was likely to drive a wedge between doctors and parents on the one hand and nurses on the other:

> The nursing station requirement…makes sense only in the light of [D]HHS Secretary Margaret Heckler's comments at her confirmation hearing. Without citing any evidence, she testified that the Baby Doe regulation was needed because nurses were afraid to report cases of child neglect to the appropriate authorities. Her department seems to believe that nurses have been unwilling but passive participants in child abuse. Nothing short of supplying them with a hotline number that they can use anonymously and with immunity will induce them to take their role of child abuse reporters seriously. This view of modern nurses is extremely demeaning, and at odds with their role as team members in most specialized pediatric units.[20]

The hot line, like the policies of totalitarian governments that encourage family members to turn each other in to the authorities, would have, if allowed to continue, promoted unnecessary, excessive fear and distrust, especially in view of the complexities of the issues and the failure at the time to explore less draconian, internal means of addressing them.[21] The policy was, under the circumstances, unwarranted. It put nurses at odds with the care, concerns, and deliberations of the parents of seriously ill newborns and their physicians.[22]

Certainly, there are circumstances in which nurses are justified in blowing the whistle. What general considerations should a nurse take into account in deciding whether a particular instance of whistle-blowing is justifiable? It is important, first, to determine if there is sufficient evidence of negligence, abuse, or danger to the public to warrant action. Hearsay or intuition is usually not enough. If one is about to make a serious accusation, fairness to the accused and maintaining one's own credibility require that it be well grounded. After getting the facts straight, a prospective whistle-blower should be very certain that relevant internal channels and procedures have been adequately explored. As Bok has pointed out:

> It *is* disloyal to colleagues and employers, as well as a waste of time for the public, to sound the loudest alarm first. Whistleblowing has to remain a last alternative because of its destructive side effects. It must be chosen only when other alternatives have been considered and rejected. They may be rejected if

they simply do not apply to the problem at hand, or when there is not time to go through routine channels, or when the institution is so corrupt or coercive that steps will be taken to silence the whistleblower should he try the regular channels first.[23]

A prospective whistle-blower should also analyze his or her own motives and make sure that personal bias, settling a score, jealousy, and so on are not the driving force behind the action and that protecting the public is the paramount concern. Finally, even after all of the foregoing conditions have been met, a prospective whistle-blower must carefully consider the likelihood of success, the negative effects on what we will suppose is an otherwise worthy organization, and various personal repercussions.[24] With regard to the last, there are, we believe, times when retaliation by the accused is so certain and so powerful that a person cannot be blamed for refraining from blowing the whistle, even if his or her action is otherwise justified.[25]

This brings us to our final topic, structural protections for those who blow the whistle. Whistle-blowing is a risky undertaking. A number of individuals whose acts of blowing the whistle have been met with public acclaim also have lost their jobs, have lost large amounts of money and have had their families disintegrate, or have been reassigned to meaningless, dead-end positions in their organizations. Others, however, although undergoing some hardship, have fared better.[26]

Apart from structural changes to reduce the need for whistle-blowing, we should also consider structural changes that protect those who find it necessary to blow the whistle. A number of laws have been enacted to protect certain federal, state, and corporate employees who blow the whistle. For example, Michigan's "Whistleblowers Protection Act," which went into effect in 1981, allows courts to award back pay, reinstatement to their jobs, and the costs of litigation to whistle-blowing corporate employees who can demonstrate improper treatment.[27] Two difficulties, identified by Bok, with laws of this type are the availability of more subtle modes of retaliation against whistle-blowing employees that fall beneath the threshold of such laws and the difficulties encountered by courts in distinguishing legitimate from spurious complaints.[28] According to the ANA, state nurses associations along with the ANA continue to promote whistle-blower legislation on the state level. Whistle-blower laws, with varying degrees of protection and provisions for health care employees, exist in 20 states in 2008.[29] "However, current whistleblower laws remain a patchwork of incomplete coverage."[30] We believe that nurses ought also to continue devising effective institutional protections for justifiable acts of whistle-blowing. In so doing, however, they must be aware of various limitations and pitfalls. A set of protections may, for example, turn out to be too strong, encouraging a degree of whistle-blowing that reduces openness, trust, and cooperation to a point where a basically good institution can no longer effectively function.

There is no simple solution to the problems of whistle-blowing; there is no simple list of do's and don'ts that will tell us what we should do in every case.[31] There are, of course, easy cases at either end of the spectrum—cases in which we can say with confidence that the whistle should or should not be blown. In between is a vast range of cases that require detailed knowledge of the particular circumstances and a sensitive, probing application of the various considerations outlined above.

5. PUBLIC POLICY: ADVANCE DIRECTIVES

In addition to a concern for what goes on in the particular organizations within which they work, nurses' obligations to their patients may also require them to participate in shaping public policy. When, for example, an analysis of barriers to adequate nursing care reveals a recurring problem, nurses as well as other health professionals have a responsibility to help address it.

Although conscious, mentally competent adults have a right to accept or refuse medical treatment, including treatment to preserve or prolong life, what do we do if illness or injury renders a formerly competent patient unable to exercise this right? This is, in part, the problem raised in Case 6.3. Who makes the decision in such cases? And on what basis?

Beginning in the mid-1970s, individual doctors, nurses, legislators, and bioethicists, as well as organizations such as the ANA, the AMA, and the American Bar Association, began to address these questions. The eventual result was legal recognition of the "advance directive," a document in which an adult provides direction for decisions about his or her medical treatment if due to illness or injury he or she is unable at the time to make them. If Melvin Thompson in Case 6.3 had filled out such a directive, some of the problems may have been avoided.

There are two types of advance directive: (1) a "living will" in which written instructions are given for one's care (one might, for example, write that if one is ever in permanent vegetative state like Melvin Thompson in Case 6.3, medically administered hydration and nutrition should be removed) and (2) the appointment of someone whom one knows and trusts as one's health care agent, an individual authorized to make treatment decisions on one's behalf if one is unable to do so oneself. All 50 states and the District of Columbia now have laws recognizing and governing the use of advance directives, although specific provisions of these laws vary from state to state.

Individual nurses as well as representatives of nursing organizations contributed to the development of public policy on this matter. As a member of a Legislative Task Force on Death and Dying of the Michigan House of Representatives, one of us (M.B.) observed the valuable contributions of nurses and the Michigan Nurses Association to the Task Force's deliberations and the eventual passage of legislation on advance directives. Yet, the work of public policy on this matter is not done. Despite the fact that signing and putting into effect an advance directive does not require a lawyer and is cost-free, only 18%–30% of adults in the United States have done so.[32] Policies must now be developed and implemented to better inform citizens of the nature and availability of advance directives and to encourage them to make use of them.[33]

Moreover, the following case identifies a need for an additional kind of directive.

6.5 CPR and POLST

Joan O'Brien is the evening charge nurse on a small, busy cardiac care unit. Mr. Joseph Mesick, aged 81, has been hospitalized for three days following a severe episode of angina and his call for an ambulance. For almost a decade Mr. Mesick has suffered from serious cardiac disease. As requested by the hospital near the time of his admission, Mr. Mesick's daughter submitted a ten-year-old copy of his advance directive to be attached to his medical record. It included the general statement, "I authorize all measures to prolong my life." Mr. Mesick is a retired lawyer who is much respected in the community. He plans to return to his daughter's home in the morning.

Although Mr. Mesick passively accepted treatment (including nasal oxygen and IV therapy during the first 24 hours), he later told Joan that he did not want to be treated again with "tubes and machines" and that "he had made his peace and was ready to die." However, Joan was quite busy at the time and was not able to discuss his wishes with him at any length.

A few hours later Joan responded to an urgent cry for help from his roommate and found Mr. Mesick slumped in his bed. She could not detect a pulse, and he did not respond when she called his name. She believed that if she did not start cardiopulmonary resuscitation (CPR) immediately, death was imminent. Joan also knew that hospital policy in such cases was to initiate resuscitation and call immediately for help. But she believed, too, that she should honor Mr. Mesick's wish not to be treated with "tubes and machines." Mr. Mesick's physician had made no comment or notation whether to withhold aggressive treatment in an emergency. And since Mr. Mesick was pain-free after the first day and planned to return home very soon, Joan had not discussed the question of withholding resuscitation with other persons involved in his care or in detail with Mr. Mesick himself.[34]

Joan's dilemma is quite clear. If she is to respect what Mr. Mesick says are his overriding wishes, she should not start CPR. If she is to act in accord with hospital policy and his ten-year-old advance directive, she must start it. Given the facts of the case, there is no clear resolution. The situation is a bad one, and Joan must quickly determine which alternative is, all things considered, best.

Although we agree that patients in Mr. Mesick's position have a right to refuse treatment with "tubes and machines," we believe it is important that health care providers and others be reasonably sure that such refusals are genuinely autonomous.[35] Perhaps Mr. Mesick's decision was genuinely autonomous, but at this point Joan cannot yet be sure that it was. Even if she were sure, it is questionable whether her word alone would be sufficient to override the hospital's policy to initiate immediate resuscitative measures in such situations. That this specific situation has apparently not been adequately discussed not only with Mr. Mesick but also with his daughter, his physician, and others involved in his care further complicates an already complicated problem.

The National POLST Paradigm Initiative Task Force is working to provide a solution to the problem facing Joan O'Brien in Case 6.5.[36] POLST is an acronym for "physician orders for life-sustaining treatment." The Task Force has developed a uniform POLST form that represents a way of summarizing, authenticating, and ratifying the wishes of an individual like Mr. Mesick regarding life-sustaining treatment. Its aim is to bridge the gap between patient goals and preferences—expressed directly or by means of an advance directive—and the actual care plan as reflected by physician orders. The form is intended for any individual with an advanced life-limiting illness. The form has two major purposes: (1) to document and "translate" the wishes of an individual into actual physician orders and (2) to be portable from one care setting to another. Prior to filling out the form, the patient and his or her family or health care agent discuss relevant end-of-life treatment options with one or more health care providers involved in the case. Then the patient's wishes are incorporated into the doctor's orders by being documented in a standardized POLST form. Once filled out, the form serves as the cover sheet on the patient's chart or medical record and is recognized as a set of physician orders as would be any physician's orders. It is an advance planning tool that reflects the patient's here-and-now goals for medical decisions in a specific context in the more or less immediate future.

The form has four main sections: A. CPR; B. Medical Interventions; C. Artificially Administered Nutrition; and D. Signatures and Summary of Medical Condition. Section A, CPR, which is directly relevant to Case 6.5, has two check boxes: one for "Attempt Resuscitation CPR;" and one for "Do Not Attempt Resuscitation/DNR (Allow Natural Death)." Once fully executed, the POLST form is to be recognized across medical settings, including those involving emergency rooms and emergency medical technicians. The POLST form is not a substitute for an advance directive like a living will or the appointment of a health care agent. It is, rather, a useful supplement for implementing such a directive. Moreover, a POLST form may be used in the absence of either a living will or the appointment of a health care agent; neither is necessary for the use of a POLST form.

Implementation of POLST Paradigm Programs varies among the states. As we write, there are endorsed statewide programs in six states, developing programs in 17 states, and no programs in the remaining states. On July 8, 2008, Governor David Paterson signed Medical Orders for Life-Sustaining Treatment (MOLST) into New York state law. On August 4 of the same year Governor Arnold Schwarzenegger signed Assembly Bill 3000, ensuring that Physician Orders for Life-Sustaining Treatment (POLST) would be honored by all health care professionals in California.[37] A recent article strongly shows the need for such programs in all states.[38]

If Case 6.3 had occurred in a California hospital that had signed on to the program after the law had gone into effect, Joan O'Brien's dilemma could have been avoided. Soon after Mr. Mesick was hospitalized, if not before, he and his physician, daughter, and perhaps Joan O'Brien as well, would have discussed his wishes regarding life-sustaining treatment, including CPR. If Mr. Mesick had indicated, as in the case he later indicated to Joan, that he did not want to be treated with "tubes and machines" and that "he had made his peace and was ready to die" and there were no grounds for questioning his understanding and autonomy, the POLST form could have been filled out with a check in the "Do Not Attempt Resuscitation/DNR" box and signed by the physician. Then when Joan O'Brien found Mr. Mesick slumped in his bed and without a pulse, she could—indeed, *should*—have ethically and legally refrained from starting CPR. In so doing she would have been following the physician's well-grounded orders.

If, to go back to the original situation, Joan lives in a state that has no program or task force for implementing the POLST Paradigm, she ought, after her unfortunate experience with Mr. Mesick, do what she can to help start one. She cannot resolve dilemmas like the one she encountered by herself. It requires a policy, not a personal, solution. As nurses contributed to the development and legal implementation of advance directives from the mid-1970s to the 1990s, they must now participate in the development of policy regarding POLST. To some extent this has already occurred, as 2 of the 14 members of the National POLST Paradigm Task Force are RNs.[39]

Concern to meet obligations to patients and families facing end-of-life decisions has led nurses as described above to participate in shaping public policy. More recently recognized barriers to adequate nursing care, such as workplace violence, also present requirements for nurses to participate in activities to remove them.

6. PUBLIC POLICY: WORKPLACE VIOLENCE

Violence against nurses not only harms them but negatively impacts staff retention and patient care. Unfortunately, however, violence in the health care workplace is covert; it is generally underreported.[40] Hidden or not, nurses and others have a responsibility to address the problem.

6.6 Workplace Violence

Harriet Clark, worried about her safety, questioned whether she ought to continue as an emergency room nurse at the city hospital. She enjoyed her job and believed she gave skillful nursing care to many sick and injured patients. Recently on her shift another patient attack occurred. The emergency room was crowded and an angry woman, one of many persons who had waited for service, suddenly lashed out, slapping and scratching coworker Sally King as she was taking the woman's blood pressure. When the staff discussed the incident later, Harriet was disheartened, first, because Sally's opinion was that slaps and scratches simply came with the many challenges of being an emergency room nurse caring for angry, distressed people. Sally pointed out that the city police person assigned to the emergency room protected her from real danger. Harriet was disheartened, second, because Sharon Thurman, another emergency room nurse with 14 years of experience, reminded every-one that the emergency room served more persons than in the past, although the nursing staff level had not increased. During some shifts the unit actually had fewer nurses on duty than in the past. Sharon also reminded the other nurses that the city hospital administration had not responded to staff per-sons who had been victims of violence in the emergency room and who, with their nursing supervisor's support, had voiced their concerns. Harriet was left with her original dilemma. What course of action might she take short of quitting her job?[41]

Harriet has several possible courses of action. The basic choice she must make, of course, is whether to leave her position as an emergency room nurse. As previously discussed in Chapter 3, Section 4, she is not required to risk her own personal health and safety while providing patient care. By staying, she could continue to be a valuable asset to the hospital emergency room. By leaving, she could protect her own health and well-being and perhaps find another nursing position in a more protective environment. Whatever she decides is right for her, she still has several additional courses of action she ought to take. First, given the covert aspect of violence against nurses, Harriet ought to fully report the violent episode to her nursing supervisor. Second, if she and other nurses in the hospital are represented by a professional nurses association in contract negotiations, she ought to fully report the incident to the local representative of that organization. Third, if she remains employed at the hospital, she ought to make a reasonable effort to assist nursing or hospital committees that address workplace violence.[42] Fourth, she ought to make a reasonable effort to work with her state nurses association or other professional nurses associations on initiatives designed to reduce workplace violence. And fifth, she ought to make an effort to support the work of persons interested in addressing public policies and laws that contribute to workplace violence; for example, financial policies that affect emergency room crowding and overuse.

As long as barriers to adequate nursing care such as workplace violence can be tied to various public policies and laws relating to access and payment of health care, nurses have an obligation to make reasonable efforts to alter those policies and laws. As was pointed out earlier in this chapter, obligations that we have to others generally entail as a corollary a requirement that we take steps to ensure that conditions exist for fulfilling these obligations. In the present case, this means that Harriet's recognition that workplace violence against nurses is a barrier to adequate nursing care entails a further obligation to do what she can to alter institutional and public policies that may contribute to the situation.

7. PUTTING IT ALL TOGETHER

We mentioned at the beginning of Chapter 3 that, although we would be examining various sorts of questions, issues, and concepts separately, individual cases often raise more than one of them. In everyday life, considerations of parentalism, deception, confidentiality, and so on frequently overlap.

The same holds true of many of the topics covered in different chapters of this book. Although separate chapters are devoted to the relationships between nurses and clients, nurses and other professionals, and nurses and other nurses, and to questions of personal responsibility for institutional and public policy, these topics too are often interrelated. The following nationally publicized case provides a rich and interesting illustration of this important point.

6.7 What Would You Do?

Shortly after coming on duty on a mid-September evening in 1983, Thomas P. Engel, RN, walked into the room of Joseph Dohr, a patient at St. Michael Hospital in Milwaukee. Eighteen days earlier, the 78-year-old man had collapsed at his home, the victim of a stroke. Mr. Engel had cared for him since then.

The patient's brainstem was severely damaged, and despite extensive high-technology care, his condition was worsening each day. Earlier that morning Dr. Allan Kagen had told Mr. Dohr's wife and daughters that Mr. Dohr had suffered irreversible brain damage and would soon die. The family then asked the doctor to disconnect Mr. Dohr's life-support system, but he refused. Although hospital policy would have permitted this and Dr. Kagen later acknowledged that he could have acceded to the family's wishes, he decided not to because he believed that, even with life support, death was imminent.

Entering the patient's room, Mr. Engel found himself alone with Mr. Dohr. Mr. Engel proceeded to turn off the alarm systems on the patient's heart monitor and on the respirator. He disconnected the oxygen supply and waited for 6–8 minutes until there was no heartbeat. Then he reconnected the oxygen supply and summoned a doctor, who pronounced Mr. Dohr dead at 6:10 p.m. Shortly after, Mr. Engel notified the Dohr family that their husband and father had died peacefully and without pain.

The nurse's surreptitious role in this case would probably have gone undetected had Mr. Engel not spoken about it. Eight months later, however, he talked of what he had done with some of his colleagues, one of whom was married to a police officer. As a result, he was formally charged in a criminal complaint with practicing medicine without a license, a misdemeanor.

He pleaded guilty to this charge and received a 20-month suspended sentence in 1984. Then on March 19, 1985, his license was revoked for a period of one year by the Wisconsin Board of Nursing. The board said that although Mr. Engel had acted with "altruism" and that his patient should have been allowed to die, his action fell outside the scope of the nursing profession. In addition, however, the board recommended that a separate disciplinary panel investigate the professional conduct of the doctors involved in the case for their refusal to withdraw treatment from the patient despite his family's request to do so. The board's recommendation implies that other doctors besides Dr. Kagen were involved.

In an interview in December 1984, Mr. Engel explained his action by describing a bedside scene with one of Mr. Dohr's daughters:

> She was standing there by her father's bed stroking his arm and his cheek and crying and talking to him. He was in a coma, in a steady decline. The only thing keeping him alive was the ventilator breathing for him. "This isn't right," she said. Then she looked across the bed at me, right in my eyes, and she said "If I could do this thing, I would."

"Now what would you do?" Mr. Engel asked the interviewer.[43]

This case raises many of the questions discussed in this chapter. If patients or their families make a legitimate request for an action that is permitted by hospital policy, and yet an attending physician refuses to comply with it, what recourse should they have? Is it their responsibility to seek a different physician who is inclined to honor their request? Should it be the attending physician's duty to find such a physician? Should a patient representative or an Institutional Ethics Committee play a role in the situation? If a similar medical situation were to occur now and the patient had signed an advance directive authorizing his wife or one of his daughters to accept or refuse medical care on his behalf, would the doctor have been legally obligated to disconnect the life support system? What should be a nurse's role in such a case? Since the Dohr family was aware of no policy for dealing with situations of this kind, they appealed to Mr. Engel, or so the quotation at the end of the case presentation would lead us to believe.

When one of the patient's daughters looked across her father's bed and said, "This isn't right....If I could do this thing, I would," it could be interpreted as implying that if Mr. Engel wanted to do the right thing, and if he knew how to disconnect the ventilator, then he should do it. Mr. Engel's description of the event and his question to the interviewer, "Now what would you do?" suggests that this was, indeed, his interpretation. The question remains, however, whether Mr. Engel subsequently did the right thing.

Let us consider, first, the relationship between law and ethics. Mr. Engel probably knew that what he was doing was, strictly speaking, illegal. Hospital policy permitted the ventilator to be disconnected, but neither hospital policy nor the law permitted a nurse to do it. There would have been no problem of law had Dr. Kagen or some other physician done so.[44] From an ethical point of view, Mr. Engel's disconnecting the ventilator was not a terribly serious offense. It was not as if what he did was absolutely forbidden. Given these circumstances, we, like the Wisconsin Board of Nursing, can understand how Mr. Engel would have been tempted, from noble motives, to perform such an action.

That Mr. Engel deceived the family and his colleagues and that his action was covert are, however, at least as troubling as the fact that his action was illegal. Would it have been better if, shortly after disconnecting the ventilator, Mr. Engel had admitted that he had done so, and then blown the whistle on Dr. Kagen as a dramatic way of trying to prevent such occurrences in the future? Questions of personal prudence aside, which is more justifiable from an ethical point of view—going public in this way or maintaining a deception? We must also ask whether more justifiable ways of trying to effect a change in policy were available to Mr. Engel. Did he exhaust regular internal channels for bringing a complaint against Dr. Kagen? Would such channels have been effective? Was there time to pursue them? Could he have threatened to call a local newspaper as a means of coercing Dr. Kagen or others to comply with the family's wishes? Would it have been likely that Dr. Kagen would have responded punitively to any overt attempts to alter his behavior? These are only some of the questions that can be raised about Mr. Engel's conduct.

Let us turn now to the other nurse involved, the one who blew the whistle on Mr. Engel. What would you do, we might ask, if you were sitting around the coffee pot and one of your colleagues revealed that eight months earlier she had done what Mr. Engel had done? In the actual case, one of the nurses apparently told her spouse and Mr. Engel was charged as a result. We do not know whether the nurse encouraged her spouse to report the case. We may still ask, however, whether a nurse should, in such circumstances, report an act of this kind, and why.

Finally, note that many of the problems raised by this case—and much more can be said about it than has been said here—cannot be resolved by individual nurses or the nursing profession alone. The issues involve maters of law and policy and of relationships among nurses, other providers, and patients and their families. Mutually satisfactory, well-grounded resolutions to these broad issues require disciplined ethical analysis and reasoning by all the parties involved. Ethical problems in health care are often public problems; they cannot be resolved by one individual or by one profession. Nurses have much to contribute to this ongoing process, and a principal aim of this book is to enable them to do so more effectively.

7

Cost Containment, Justice, and Rationing

As health care costs continue to soar, nurses find themselves pulled in contrary directions. The traditional patient-centered ethic stresses the health care professional's commitment to particular patients, irrespective of their ability to pay or the cost of their care to society. At the same time, pressures to contain costs occasionally require health care professionals to limit treatment or even turn away some patients who could benefit from their care. Consider, in this connection, the following case.

7.1 Ideals and Reality

During her 27-year career in nursing, Gail Crain, RN, MSN (Master of Science in Nursing), has earned a reputation as one of the most committed nurses in her city. She now owns and operates a home health care agency. As her own boss, she is able to provide the high-quality nursing care that she thinks her patients should receive. In the face of spiraling health care costs, however, she finds herself confronted with a difficult dilemma: she can no longer continue to accept nonpaying patients if her agency is to remain financially solvent, yet she knows that if she were to declare a moratorium on accepting clients who could not themselves pay for her agency's services, they would probably not find another source of home nursing care. She knows from experience that some patients would soon be forced to leave their homes for institutionalized care. Institutionalized care, though ultimately more expensive for society and less satisfying for these patients, is publicly funded. The thought of restricting her services to those who can personally pay for them is repugnant to Gail Crain; allocating health care services based on ability to pay violates her sense of justice. But how can she provide home care to anyone if providing it to some without payment will force her to close her doors?[1]

The dilemma facing Gail Crain reflects a larger problem facing the health care system and society. Deciding how to allocate access to care in the face of limited resources raises difficult questions of social justice. Should ability to pay be the principal criterion for access to care? Or should health care be rationed so as to guarantee a basic minimum of care to all? If we elect to ration, how do we determine the basic level of health care to which everyone is entitled? How do we pay for making this care available to all? And what will be the costs to the system as a whole in terms of overall quality and professional integrity and autonomy?

These questions are related to the problems of resource allocation that troubled Alice Byrum in Case 6.2. Whereas Alice was concerned about what economists call *micro*-allocation (the allocation of particular resources at the level of the clinic or hospital), Gail Crain is concerned about matters of *macro*-allocation (determinations at the societal level about how much money should be allocated to health care—as opposed to other social needs—and exactly how this money is to be apportioned among needs for acute care, chronic care, prevention, education, and so on). Nurses, if they are to meet their social obligation to provide high quality nursing care, must understand and address questions of macro-allocation as well as questions of micro-allocation. An obligation to provide a certain level of care to individuals entails as a corollary an obligation to do what one can to ensure that conditions exist for providing that level of care (Chapter 6, Section 1).

The problems facing Alice Byrum and Gail Crain are not new. "Nurses who responded to an ethics survey conducted in 1985 by the Minnesota Nurses Association," wrote nurse educator Mila Ann Aroskar, "identified the allocation and rationing of scarce resources as 'the most important ethical issue facing nursing today'."[2] But, Aroskar added, this is an issue that cannot be adequately addressed by individual nurses or by the profession of nursing itself. It requires cooperative efforts and interdisciplinary understanding among many affected parties, as well as a new perspective on nursing ethics:

> Our society is confronted directly with issues such as the allocation and rationing of resources in health care. It becomes clearer that much of the work in bioethics, and even in nursing ethics, that has focused on the intricacies of individual decision making and rights of individuals is not adequate to the challenges confronting us today—that is, making sense of how we as a society are going to use and pay for societal benefits, including nursing and health care.[3]

It is an indication of the difficulty of the issues that Aroskar's words are no less important today than they were when she wrote them.[4] The aim of this chapter is, therefore, to expand the focus of nursing ethics by incorporating questions of cost containment, social justice, and the possibility of health care rationing.

We begin by identifying problems created by limited resources. The problems are deep and unavoidable. Proposals for reducing waste and inefficiency in the health care system, while softening the problems, will not, as many seem to think, eliminate them. Considerations of justice then lead to the concept of rationing—a widely used but frequently misunderstood term. We examine a plan for rationing health care developed by the state of Oregon and suggest an ethical framework for assessing the ethical justification of various rationing proposals. Finally, we show that nursing care has a special role to play in any justifiable rationing scheme.

The set of issues discussed in this chapter will frame ethical inquiry in health care for the foreseeable future. Traditional interpersonal ethical concerns such as informed consent, patients' rights, allowing to die, and so on will continue to be important, but they will be inseparable from issues of macro-allocation having to do with limited resources and the justice of the health care delivery system as a whole. Debates about continued care for those in *permanent* vegetative state (patients determined to be *totally* and *permanently* unconscious) must, for example, consider that there may be many thousands of patients in this condition.[5] And the cost per patient ranges between $220,000 and $283,000 per year. If, then, we conservatively suppose that there are about five to ten thousand such patients in the United States at a cost of about $250,000 per patient per year, the total cost would range between approximately $1.25 billion and $2.5 billion per year for patients who are not, and will never again be, conscious. Are there, one may reasonably ask, more just and effective uses for these funds in the health care system? It is therefore important that nurses understand current debates about limited resources, justice, and rationing in the health care system so that they can contribute their insights and understanding, both individually and as a profession to the resolution of these debates.

1. COST CONTAINMENT AND THE CLAIMS OF JUSTICE

Thoughtful nurses are already aware of questions of macro-allocation as they are raised by efforts to contain health care costs:

7.2 Limiting Health Care

Akilah Griggs, Chairperson of the Professional Nursing Practice Committee in her 200-bed community hospital, is increasingly concerned about possible

---

(*Continued*)

limits on health care spending. She believes that nurses like herself should become involved in community grassroots organizations to make their views known to legislators. At such a community meeting, Akilah met Toni Gonzales.

Akilah believes that every person of any age should have access to the best health care money can buy. Toni, however, advocates limiting expensive, marginally beneficial efforts to prolong life—efforts undertaken mainly for persons in their eighties and nineties—and she reminds Akilah that money spent on such care is money that cannot be spent on other important care such as preventive and prenatal care and that money spent on health care in general cannot be spent on other important needs such as education. She encouraged Akilah to read Daniel Callahan's *Setting Limits: Medical Goals in an Aging Society* and Leonard Fleck's *Just Caring: Health Care Rationing and Democratic Deliberation*, and she emphasized the need to balance the costs of high technology, marginally beneficial, end-of-life care with long-term care expenses when considering health care for the very old.

For several weeks, Akilah pondered Toni's position. Should she modify her own views and agree that some very expensive treatments for end-stage cancers and other fatal diseases in the aged be limited? And if she modifies her position about the elderly, should she also modify her views that all newborns, no matter their size and the expense incurred, should be treated? Or can new ways be found to increase funding for health care?[6]

Akilah Griggs is asking the right questions. There are, however, no easy answers.

The increasing cost of health care in the United States is a matter of great concern. Expenditures on health care in 2007 totaled $2.2 trillion and accounted for 16.2% of the Gross Domestic Product (GDP).[7] An earlier edition of this book cited figures for 1989, in which total expenditures on health care totaled $600 billion (up from $121 billion in 1980) and accounted for only 11.5% of the GDP. Even controlling for inflation, this is a large increase, particularly in percentage of GDP devoted to health care, which increased by nearly 50%. Projections by the Centers for Medicare and Medicaid Services (CMS) indicate that growth in national health care expenditures will average 6.7% until 2017, at which point the health share of GDP is projected to be 19.5%.[8] The United States, according to many commentators, cannot continue to spend this much on health care without neglecting other pressing societal issues such as education, housing, poverty, environmental protection, alternative and sustainable sources of energy, disposal of toxic wastes, and maintenance and repair of the nation's infrastructure (roads, bridges, sewers, etc.).

A number of factors have contributed to the increasing cost of health care. Advances in, and more frequent use of, medical technology accounts for a significant percentage of the rapid rise in health care costs. Many of these new technologies, such as CAT and MRI scanning and ultrasound, provide greater benefits with even lower risks than their predecessors. But they come at a cost not only for research, development, and manufacture but also for the larger number of highly trained and consequently better-paid health care professionals required to employ them. The same is true of new fertility technologies and care and treatment of very low birth weight infants as well as complex life-extending surgical procedures such as organ transplantation. To this we can add improved and more frequent use of expensive prescription drugs. A second important factor is our aging population. The number and percentage of Americans 65 years of age or over is projected to rise dramatically over the next 20 years. Health care costs for this part of the population are considerably higher than among other age groups. In 2004, for example, per person personal health care spending for the 65 and older population was $14,797, 5.6 times higher than spending per child ($2,650) and 3.3 times spending per working-age person ($4,511). Compared to children and those of working age, the elderly were the smallest population group—12% of the population—but accounted for 34% of health care spending in 2004. As the percentage of elderly population increases, so too will its percentage of health care spending. The aging of the "baby boom" generation is projected to double the size of the population age 65 and older by the year 2030.[9]

It appears, therefore, that something must give. Either the society explicitly limits or forgoes certain types of beneficial health care to all or some members of the population, *or* it ignores or gives short shrift to other important needs, such as education, housing, energy, climate change, and general economic well-being (as determined, for example, by the nation's ability to compete in the world marketplace). Before coming to grips with the dilemma between either limiting health care or limiting other important social goods, let us examine two proposals for dissolving it. The first argues that there is no need for a societal decision on the matter; health care, like other goods and services, is a matter of individual decision, not public policy, and should be bought and sold according to free-market principles of supply and demand. The second proposal suggests that we can eliminate the problem by reducing waste and inefficiency in the health care system. Once the "fat" in the health care budget is cut, we will no longer be faced with having to choose between cost containment and the claims of justice. Neither of these proposals, however, nor some combination of them, can extricate us from the dilemma.

A. Health Care as a Consumer Good

Some argue that the conflict disappears when health care is conceived as an ordinary consumer good. Like cars, television sets, music lessons, and membership in health clubs, health care should, on this view, be distributed according to general market principles to those able and willing to pay for it.[10] The government, the argument goes, has no special role in paying for or distributing health care. If those who desire and can afford to pay for expensive health care are willing to pay for it, the market will respond to their demands. Those lacking either the desire for certain forms of health care or the ability to pay for it will go without. This is the principle of distribution most compatible with individual choice and liberty and which governs the distribution of most other goods and services in the society.

The difficulty with this view is its assumption that health care is simply another consumer good or service such as an iPod or a personal trainer. Health is importantly different from ordinary consumer goods or services because, like education, it is necessary for maintaining fair equality of opportunity among members of society. Individuals can no more exercise their capacity to lead decent and meaningful lives or compete for other social goods if they are restricted, through no fault of their own, by preventable or treatable ill health than they can exercise these capacities if, due to parental poverty or neglect, they are deprived of a good basic education.[11] It is for this reason, and perhaps others, that we are rightly reluctant to allocate health care resources solely in accord with market principles. A commitment to preserving equal liberty, understood as equal opportunity for leading a decent and meaningful life, provides the justification for a system of publicly funded, equally accessible health care, as well as for a system of publicly funded, equally accessible education; thus, for example, our deeply rooted, well-grounded reluctance to allow parental poverty or neglect to foreclose a child's access to both basic health care and basic education.

Problems remain, however, in determining the *level* or *amount* of health care to which citizens should be equally entitled. Establishing a basic minimum for health care is, for reasons examined in Section 3, more complex than establishing a similar minimum for education.

B. Reducing Waste and Inefficiency

A second proposal for eliminating the conflict between cost containment and the claims of justice centers on reducing waste and inefficiency in health care. According to James Roosevelt, president and CEO of Tufts Health Plan, "a staggering $760 billion—more than the $700 billion bailout of the US banking system [in 2008] and a full third of the $2.3 trillion in annual health care spending—is wasted on things like medical mistakes, hospital-acquired infections, medication errors, overuse of emergency departments, and unnecessary lab tests and medical imaging."[12] Reducing this and, among other things, inefficient processing of health claims (due largely to multiple insurers with multiple criteria and forms for reimbursement) and ineffective use of technology can significantly reduce the conflict between increasing access to care and reducing—or at least holding the line on–health care costs.

Research on Medicare records conducted by the Dartmouth Institute for Health Policy and Clinical Practice reveals significant differences in health care spending between one geographic area of the United States and another with no corresponding differences in patient outcomes, even after adjusting for differences in local prices, and the age, race, and underlying health of the population. "Patients who live in areas where Medicare spends more per capita are neither sicker than those who live in regions where Medicare spends less, nor do they prefer more care. Perhaps most surprising, they show no evidence of better outcomes."[13] Thus, for example, Medicare spending per capita is significantly lower in Minnesota, New Mexico, or Virginia than it is in southern New Jersey or Texas, but Medicare patients in southern New Jersey or Texas are not necessarily sicker than those in Minnesota, New Mexico, nor Virginia, nor do they necessarily receive better care. Overall costs, with no loss in quality or effectiveness of care, the research shows, are likely to come down if the organization and delivery of care in the more expensive states becomes more like that in the less expensive states.[14]

The Mayo Clinic, for example, is identified as among the organized systems of care that has been able to improve the quality of care while containing costs without denying patients needed, effective care. "Using the Mayo Clinic as a benchmark," a Dartmouth Institute White Paper writes, "the nation could reduce health care spending by as much as 30 percent for acute and chronic illnesses; a benchmark based on Intermountain Healthcare [in Utah] predicts a reduction of more than 40 percent. Substantial savings in Medicare spending on surgery—perhaps as much as 30 percent—are also possible if demand for elective surgery were based on informed patient choice."[15] It is clear from what James Roosevelt and the Dartmouth Institute for Health Policy and Clinical Practice say that reducing waste and inefficiency in the delivery of health care will enable us to provide better care to a larger number of patients at the same cost we are now paying to deliver a lower quality of care to fewer patients.

Although efforts to reduce cost and inefficiency in the health care system should certainly be undertaken, they will at best soften our dilemma. They cannot eliminate it. The demand for increasingly sophisticated, expensive high-technology medicine is largely inexhaustible. No matter how carefully and efficiently we use what we now have, a new set of budget-busting medical miracles will invariably appear on the horizon.

The concept of "medical need" is notoriously elastic. What counts as a medical need varies in part with the possibility of medical treatment. As new treatments become available, the class of "medical need" expands accordingly. "How many coronary angioplasties," Leonard M. Fleck asks,

> did we "need" in the United States in 1970? The correct answer is that we needed none because the technique had not been invented. How many of these procedures did we "need" in 2006 in the United States? We apparently needed about 1.2 million of them at a cost of about $35,000 each. There have been thousands of these examples in our health care system over the past 40 years.[16]

And there is no natural limit to the development of medically beneficial knowledge or technology. The edge of medical progress is, as Daniel Callahan illuminatingly observes, invariably "ragged" rather than fixed or definite:

> Imagine that you are trying to tear a piece of rough cloth and want to do so in a way that leaves a smooth edge. Yet no matter how carefully you tear the cloth, or where you tear it, there is always a ragged edge. It is the roughness of the material itself that guarantees the same result; a smooth edge is impossible. No matter how far we push the frontiers of medical progress we are always left with a ragged edge—poor outcomes, with cases as bad as those we have succeeded in curing, with the inexorable decline of the body however much we seem to have arrested the process. Whether it be intensive care for the premature newborn, low-birthweight baby, or bypass surgery for the very old, or AZT therapy for AIDS patients, the eventual outcome will not likely be very good; and when, eventually, those problems are solved there will then be others to take their place. That is the ragged edge of medical progress, as much a part of that progress as its success.[17]

In health care, especially if one focuses on preventing death and eliminating or mitigating pain and suffering, there will always be a ragged edge to the available treatments and therapies. Mortality is an "illness" for which, in the end, there is no cure.

Still, if we are willing to spend the money, further research and development will always promise new knowledge and technology that can forestall death—even if it is very expensive and only for a day or two. Even if, in other words, it is only *marginally* beneficial. Yet, to change metaphors, no matter how many battles we may win, we can never, so long as we remain mortal, win the war. "We cannot," as Callahan puts it, win the struggle with the ragged edge. We can only move the edge somewhere else, where it will once again tear roughly, and again and again. If this is so, and if the effort to defeat the ragged edge assures ever-rising costs (for many of the easier, clearer tears were made earlier in history), when will we know when and how to stop? Not when and how to stop because further progress cannot be made—further progress can *always* be made; we have no reason to disbelieve that. But knowing how and when to stop because further progress entails either too great an economic or social price or too little likely improvement in the human condition, or both, is a far harder decision.[18]

Eliminating waste and inefficiency in the health care system will not, therefore, eliminate the conflict between cost containment and distributive justice. Though such efforts can do much to mitigate the problem and should, where feasible, be undertaken, we will still be confronted with hard choices about limiting cost while justly distributing access to care.

2. ACCESS TO CARE

Despite the United States' spending a much higher percentage of its GDP on health care than other Western industrialized nations, its overall health status is not significantly higher. On the contrary, according to epidemiologist Ichiro Kawachi, health status in the United States "ranks near the bottom among the 13 most economically advanced countries of the world."[19] This includes ranking thirteenth for percentage of low birth weight infants, thirteenth for neonatal mortality and total infant mortality, and thirteenth for years of potential life lost. Why, if we spend so much more on health care than other nations, is this not reflected in health care statistics? Waste and inefficiency provide part of the explanation. But there are other factors as well, including differences in access to care and, Kawachi persuasively argues, economic inequality.[20] Despite the billions spent—much in the form of public funds—on state-of-the-art, high technology medical care, a disturbingly large number of Americans have little or no access to it.

About 47 million Americans are without medical insurance. Many of these are what are called the "working poor" and their families. If they were unemployed or poorer, they would be eligible for Medicaid. Too "rich" to qualify for Medicaid, but too poor to pay for or receive employer provided health insurance, they "fall through the cracks" of the system. In 2007, 46 million workers were uninsured because not all businesses offer health benefits, not all workers qualify for coverage, and many employees cannot afford their share of the health insurance premium even when coverage is available.[21] While the official poverty level for a family of four in 2009 was $22,050, the average annual premium that a health insurer charged an employer for a health plan covering a family of four averaged $12,700 in 2008.[22] The cost of this insurance would, presumably, be higher if a self-employed head of household or one whose employer did not provide health insurance had to pay the entire cost him- or herself. How can a self-employed head of household of a family of four earning just over the poverty level be expected to spend more than half of the family's income on health insurance?

The consequences for the health of the poor are, in many respects, scandalous. "The uninsured are 33% more likely to report their health as fair or poor and spend one-third more days in bed than the insured do," reported the President's Commission for the Study of Ethical Problems in Medicine and Biomedical and Behavioral Research.[23] Lack of care, for this and other reasons, "can have serious health, economic, and social consequences for both society as a whole and for individuals. The most obvious of these is that people affected by lack of access may go without needed services and suffer the consequences."[24] An editorial in the *New York Times* commented on two studies presenting "the most comprehensive evidence yet that the lack of health insurance is seriously harmful to a patient's health." Uninsured people, the studies confirmed, "suffer significantly worse outcomes from cardiovascular disease, diabetes and cancer than those who have coverage." Uninsured near-elderly (under 65) individuals suffered more from heart disease, stroke, high-blood pressure, or diabetes than when they turned 65 and became eligible for Medicare. Lack of adequate insurance was also associated with poorer outcomes for cancer patients. "The uninsured were less likely to receive recommended cancer screening tests and more likely to have their cancers diagnosed at a later stage, when they are less curable. They had lower survival rates than those with private insurance for several cancers for which there are screening tests and effective treatments, including breast and colorectal cancer."[25]

To remedy this situation, many see the need for providing access to health care for all with certain medical needs, regardless of their ability to pay. Yet intense, widespread resistance to increasing taxes together with pressure to contain health care costs make it unlikely that the problem can be solved simply by additional infusions of public funds. Moreover, the inexhaustible demand for increased medical technology—what Callahan characterizes as the "ragged edge" of medical progress—limits what may be gained by reducing waste and inefficiency. This is where the disagreement between Akilah Griggs and Toni Gonzales in Case 7.2 is joined. For if, as Toni believes, the claims of justice require that society provide everyone with equal access to a certain level of health care, regardless of ability to pay, she must, with Akilah, face up to the prospect of rationing.

3. THE CONCEPT OF RATIONING

Rationing implies a just and efficient allocation of limited goods or services. The paradigm is, perhaps, allocating food among soldiers at a battlefront. When food supplies are limited, every soldier is entitled to a certain fixed amount. The allotments of food are in this context dubbed "rations," as in C rations, K rations, and so on. Other items may in wartime be rationed as well. During World War II, gasoline, sugar, coffee, and so on were rationed among the civilian population both to conserve supplies and to assure that what was available was distributed equally.

An illuminating, frequently overlooked feature of the term *rationing* is its Latin root. *Rationing* is (or should be) an essentially rational undertaking, the Latin word *ratio* having to do with reason and rationality.[26] Rationing, therefore, is something undertaken deliberately and in the name of reason or rationality. This is not to say that all existing or proposed rationing schemes are in fact justified or the most rational, but rather that rationing policies are explicitly adopted and defended for the sake of reasons having to do with justice or fairness. Strictly speaking, then, it is a misnomer to talk of "tacit," "invisible," or "unintentional" rationing or of "rationing by default" (in contrast with "rationing by design"). Not all processes that allocate a limited supply of goods or services can be said, strictly speaking, to ration them. Medical economist Victor Fuchs therefore obscures an important distinction when he writes:

> The United States has always rationed medical care, just as every country has and always will ration care. No nation is wealthy enough to supply all the care that is technically feasible and desirable; no nation can provide "presidential medicine" for all its citizens. Moreover, medical care is hardly unique in this respect. The United States "rations" automobiles, houses, restaurant meals— all the goods and services that make up our standard of living.[27]

What Fuchs calls "rationing" is more accurately described as allocation by supply and demand. To allocate automobiles, houses, and restaurant meals in accord with market principles is not thereby to ration them. To ration health care is, as in rationing among soldiers, to apportion or allot a fixed amount of a limited resource *for reasons* of fairness or overall efficiency or both. To allocate health care in the same way we allocate restaurant meals is not to ration health care; it is, on the contrary, to *ir*ration it.

Access to a certain level of health care is necessary for maintaining fair equality of opportunity, which is in turn necessary for everyone's having more or less equal liberty to lead a decent and meaningful life in a society that repeatedly affirms this liberty as an important defining value. Yet health care is a set of goods and services for which supply falls, and will always fall, short of demand. Money alone, even if, contrary to fact, the society were willing to raise taxes so as to increase access for the poor, cannot itself solve the problem. There is, therefore, a strong prima facie case for rationing health care. (Indeed, most nurses are already familiar with rationing within their own caseloads or assignments, given the extensive demands on their time and energy.) The question is whether we can determine what ought to count as an appropriate portion or allotment of health care to which everyone ought to have access. Where, in other words, are we going to draw the line in determining a basic minimum level of health care?

This is a vexing question. Health care differs from the customary objects of rationing, such as food or gasoline, in a number of important ways. First, health care needs, unlike nutritional needs, vary widely among individuals. Some, through good fortune, live entire lives requiring very little in the way of health care. Others, through decidedly ill fortune, consume health care resources totaling hundreds of thousands of dollars. It is, therefore, difficult to specify an equal allotment, perhaps, in terms of number of dollars worth of care to which each person should be entitled over a lifetime. Second, it is more difficult to distinguish needs from wants in rationing health care than it is, say, in rationing food or clothing. One's craving for caviar carries no weight in determining a basic level of nutritional need; nor does a longing for an individually tailored expensive suit determine what counts as sufficient clothing. But whether the basic level of health care provided by a system of rationing should include, for example, experimental, possibly life-saving surgery, attractive wigs or hairpieces for chemotherapy patients, or *in vitro* fertilization and embryo transplantation for childless couples is harder to say. Third, the very complexity of health care—including tensions between extending the quantity of life and improving its quality, or competing claims for the benefits of basic research, health promotion, prevention, palliation, rehabilitation, supportive care, or acute care—places added burdens on determining a coherent rationing scheme. Finally, health care's open-endedness—the shifting sands of medical progress and resulting changes in what medicine can provide—makes it difficult to determine, once and for all, what counts as a basic level of health care to which everyone ought to have access.

4. THE OREGON PROPOSAL

The state of Oregon was the first unit of government to publicly address the problem of justly distributing limited health care resources. In 1986, 400,000 Oregonians were without any health insurance—one person out of six under 65.[28] Of these, 120,000 were employed but earning below the federal poverty level; 260,000 were adults and families earning above the federal poverty level; and 20,000 were high-risk individuals who were denied insurance and others. Acknowledging that optimal health care for all—that is providing everyone with everything that may benefit him or her—was not a genuine possibility, Oregon began developing a plan for distributing some of its health care resources as fairly as possible. The aim was to set a floor in terms of access to health care below which no Oregonian would fall.

In 1983, a prescient organization called Oregon Health Decisions initiated a statewide series of "town meetings" to inform Oregonians of ethical and economic issues in health care and to elicit informed citizen opinion on these issues.[29] Similar groups subsequently developed similar programs in other states.[30] Then in 1987, faced with a very tight budget, those administering Oregon's Medicaid program decided the program should, for reasons of justice and efficiency, no longer fund heart, liver, bone marrow, and pancreas transplantation, which at the time were not nearly as cost-effective as they are today. Funds that had previously been spent on these very expensive transplant operations for no more than 30 Medicaid recipients would be shifted to prenatal care. The *rationale* was that the same sum of money would purchase more in the way of effective health care for the Medicaid population as a whole if devoted to 1500 pregnant women—thereby reducing the number of low birth weight and disabled infants—than if spent on a very small number of expensive transplant operations of (then) limited effectiveness.

This first instance of governmental rationing attracted national attention when seven-year-old Coby Howard died of leukemia. Coby's last weeks were spent helping family and friends desperately trying to raise 100,000 dollars to pay for a bone marrow transplant that would have had some chance of saving his life. His family and friends had managed to collect 70,000 dollars when Coby died. A year earlier, before implementation of the limited rationing program, the state of Oregon would have paid for this operation without question. Coby Howard and his family were the first identifiable individuals to feel negative effects of Oregon's decision to ration Medicaid benefits.

In 1988, despite heated criticism, the Oregon legislature reaffirmed the Medicaid program's controversial decision to limit funding for transplants. The next year the legislature, led by senate president (and emergency room physician) John Kitzhaber, extended and systematized this decision by passing a three-part Basic Health Care Act seeking to do the following:

1. Expand Medicaid to cover everyone at or below the federal poverty level. (Like many states, Oregon had been containing its Medicaid

budget by the politically expedient but ethically questionable practice of raising eligibility standards by lowering the income level needed to qualify for Medicaid. This meant the state provided the full range of benefits but made them available to a declining portion of the poor. Thus, in 1988, Medicaid benefits were available to only slightly more than half of those falling below the official federal poverty level.)

2. Require nearly all employers who did not already provide health insurance to their employees to do so.

3. Establish a state-sponsored insurance pool to provide coverage for all who, because of preexisting severe illness, were uninsurable.

The Basic Health Care Act would thus require the state to assume broad responsibility for providing a basic minimum of health care to all falling below the federal poverty level, and the private sector would be required to cover nearly all who were employed. Extending Medicaid coverage to all falling below the poverty level would, however, involve an explicit trade-off. The state could not provide access to all if it meant access to nearly everything. So instead of extending a fairly generous level of benefits to slightly more than half of this population, the Medicaid program would subsequently provide a more limited basic minimum of health care benefits to *all* falling below the federal poverty level. The next step in the process was to determine this basic minimum. Once specified, it would provide the standard for coverage in all three categories.

Implementation of Oregon's Basic Health Care Act called for the creation of an 11-member Health Services Commission (HSC) to develop a priority list ranking health care services in terms of cost-effectiveness and the extent to which they are valued or deemed important by the community. The HSC was to do this by collecting data on the effectiveness of various medical procedures and their costs. It would also collect data on values and what citizens regarded as important as revealed through town meetings and surveys. Combining these kinds of data, the HSC would rank order medical services in terms of their costs, benefits, and perceived value. The most cost-effective, highly valued services would be at the top of the list, the least cost-effective, least-valued services at the bottom. This list would then be given to the legislature, which would use it to define the basic level of health care. The legislature would not be obligated to follow the list mechanically (e.g., take a fixed amount previously budgeted for health care and go as far down the list as this amount would cover and then simply draw a line) but could use the list to inform its judgment as to how much money to allot to health care. It was conceivable, though perhaps unlikely, that legislators could, in the light of where the line would be drawn (given a fixed dollar amount previously budgeted for health care), elect to increase the Medicaid budget by diverting funds initially allocated for other purposes or even by raising taxes. Wherever and however the legislature drew the line in determining the basic minimum, it would then have the opportunity to redraw it two years later (Oregon's legislature meets biennially), taking into account changes in the health of the state's economy, the size of the state budget, the development of new technology, new knowledge about the cost-effectiveness of various procedures, competing claims on the state treasury, and so on.

An initial ranking of priorities issued by the HSC in the spring of 1990 encountered heavy criticism and was returned for revision. Then, when the priority list finally received approval from the state legislature, the federal government refused in 1992 to grant a needed waiver to Medicaid laws on the ground that items on the list discriminated against the disabled and, hence, violated the Americans with Disabilities Act of 1990. In particular, the administration of George H. W. Bush argued, the list discriminated against alcoholics with cirrhosis of the liver and infants weighing less than 500 grams, or about 18 ounces) by placing both so far down on the list that the alcoholics would not receive needed liver transplants nor would the infants receive aggressive life support.[31] There were, moreover, political difficulties in achieving the comprehensive coverage that the plan hoped to achieve.

Oregon's employer mandate, which was beset by business opposition and hampered by the election of a conservative Republican legislative majority in 1994, never received the federal waiver necessary for its implementation. Consequently, Oregon's aim of achieving universal coverage, which is something that no US state has yet attained, was not met. Yet the state's Medicaid reforms, after considerable national debate, were approved by the Clinton administration and the OHP [Oregon Health Plan] began operating in 1994.[32] A 10-cent increase in the cigarette tax helped fund the additional $400 million needed to implement the program.

By 1998, however, the OHP had encountered major problems. In addition to the failure of the requirement that employers provide insurance for all their workers, physicians were finding ways to bypass the rationing restrictions, and friction with federal Medicaid regulators was blocking efforts to deny less cost-effective treatments. The cost of the plan was increasing greatly and the higher taxes did not meet the added expenses. The plan's partial success in terms of reducing the percentage of uninsured Oregonians to 11% in 1996 from 18% in 1992 was offset by the fact that there were still approximately 350,000 people with no insurance. Matters then went from bad to worse. An economic downturn led to rising unemployment and decreasing state revenues. In early 2004, voters rejected an increase in taxes that would have provided additional funds for the OHP.

This led the state to reduce the OHP budget, and Medicaid coverage fell from about 120,000 people to fewer than 25,000. The decline, as reported by Jennifer Fisher Wilson, continued:

> The OHP closed to new enrollment until 2008, when Oregon conducted a lottery to award 3000 new slots. More than 90,000 uninsured Oregonians vied for a slot. Because of a high unemployment rate during the early part of this decade [the first of the twenty-first century] and health care coverage cutbacks, the number of people in the state lacking insurance has almost returned to pre-OHP levels.[33]

As we write, Oregon is attempting to renew its efforts at reforming its health care system for the poor. Its goals, as reported by Wilson include,

> lowered costs, improved quality, and health care coverage for all Oregonians. The job of achieving these goals goes to the newly created Oregon Health Fund Board, a public board of 7 citizen leaders. The Board is currently formulating the key concepts for health reform and is expected to present a comprehensive plan in the 2009 legislative session.[34]

The ultimate fate of this renewed effort is uncertain. What is important for our purposes, however, is the example that Oregon has set. It is the first significant unit of American government to actually come to grips with the dilemmas of rationing health care, and there is much to be learned from its efforts even if they have yet to be fully successful. As Wilson rightly observes of the initial plan, it "at least as idealized, held a promising formula for both containing costs and providing health care to more people who need coverage."

This is not the place to undertake a detailed assessment of the Oregon plan's past shortcomings and future prospects. Identifying difficulties with aspects of the Oregon plan before its latest alteration is fairly easy; supporting the existing health care system in the United States or resolving the growing conflict between cost containment and the claims of justice is, however, much more difficult. Those responsible for the Oregon proposal should be commended for directly confronting a deep and important problem that most Americans still deny exists. They should be commended, too, for at the outset conducting their deliberations in full view and striving to involve the citizenry through the Oregon Health Decisions project. In making its work public, those developing the proposal received a great deal of criticism. But much of the criticism was helpful and resulted in a number of refinements as the proposal developed. This sort of improvement is a significant benefit of a public process and should serve as a model for future efforts.

It is important, in concluding our brief account of the Oregon proposal, to emphasize that nurses were intimately and importantly involved in the policy-making process from the beginning. Two Oregon nurses, Cecilia Capuzzi and Jeanne Bowden, have written an account of the "Oregon story" that details their own and other nurses' involvement in the OHP. Bowden became involved when asked to serve on the nine-member Oregon Health Council in 1986. In 1989, Capuzzi had a legislative internship and represented a nonprofit advocacy group at the session of the Oregon legislature where the beginnings of the Oregon plan were introduced. She subsequently did research on aspects of the plan, including managed care, cost-containment strategies, and quality of care. Their account tells of nurse involvement in various aspects and phases of the development and implementation of the OHP, including, for example: testifying at legislative hearings and presenting their concerns; providing expert knowledge about the difficulties their patients had in gaining access to health care; providing data about the effectiveness of having nurses provide certain types of health care services; and "meeting with key policymakers and providing information about the nursing profession, nurses' roles in the health care system, and the cost-effectiveness of health and nursing care delivered by nurses."[35] Overall, Capuzzi and Bowden conclude, many nurses have contributed to efforts to shape health policy in Oregon and they "need to continue to be actively involved" in shaping health policy at both the state and national levels.[36]

5. TOWARD ETHICAL RATIONING

Debates over health care rationing are likely to continue for a number of years. Continued, informed participation of nurses in these debates will prove important both for the public and for the profession of nursing. In what follows, we provide an ethical framework for developing and assessing specific policies for rationing health care.

A realistic, ethically justifiable rationing system must, in the first place, acknowledge that we will occasionally have to deny patients types of care that could in some sense possibly benefit them, despite our best efforts to eliminate waste and inefficiency in health care. The combination of a growing aging population; advances in medical knowledge and technology (with emphasis on what Callahan calls its "ragged edge"); competing claims on the health care dollar for research, prevention, and public health; other pressing social needs such as education, housing, maintaining the infrastructure, global warming, alternative sources of energy, and so on makes this inescapable. The question is not whether we can avoid having to limit possibly beneficial health care—a realistic understanding of limited resources and the unlimited possibilities of medical benefits makes this inevitable—but whether, when we are forced to do so, we can do so fairly and without violating the integrity of health professionals.

A rationing scheme threatens the integrity of health care professionals when it forces them to sacrifice or betray their traditional commitment to the health or welfare of particular patients for the sake of some overall social good. This is part of what troubles nurse Gail Crain in Case 7.1, "Ideals and reality," as she considers the ethics of restricting her services to those who can pay for them. How, then, can the traditional patient-centered ethic of nursing and medicine be reconciled with the aims of justly and efficiently allocating limited health care resources?

A. Fairness in Allocation

It is useful in responding to this important question to distinguish a result's being unfortunate from its being unfair. Suppose, to take a comparatively straightforward example, we have what everyone agrees is a fair system of allocating a limited supply of transplantable hearts among a large number of potential recipients:

7.3 Unfortunate but Not Unfair?

Three patients—Mr. Jackson, Ms. Chang, and Mr. Herrera—of roughly the same size, age, and blood and tissue type are each in desperate need of a new heart. As the rules of the allocation system (perhaps some combination of "first-come, first-served" and medical efficiency) are scrupulously followed, the first heart to become available goes to Mr. Jackson. A week later a second donor heart becomes available and is successfully transplanted into Ms. Chang. Then, while awaiting a donor heart for himself, Mr. Herrera dies of heart failure. Has the system treated Mr. Herrera unfairly?[37]

Assuming that the scarcity of donor hearts in this case was unavoidable and that the system of allocation was more just than any alternative, we conclude that Mr. Herrera's dying before receiving a life-extending heart transplant was not unfair, though certainly unfortunate.[38] The question now is whether this distinction can be extended from micro- to macro-allocation; a rationing scheme for the entire health care system. That a patient who could benefit from one or another type of medical treatment does not receive it is always unfortunate. But it is not necessarily unfair. Although there may be little we can do to eliminate scarcity and the need to ration health care, we can try to ensure that the principles guiding our rationing policies are just or fair.

The best criterion of the justness or fairness of such a rationing scheme may be that all to whom it applies have at some earlier point agreed to abide by its results or would have so agreed if given the opportunity. This agreement is similar in some respects to the consent one gives in buying a raffle ticket. If a person fully understands all the rules of the raffle and voluntarily engages in it, and the rules are scrupulously followed, the person can hardly claim to be a victim of injustice if he or she loses. That the person loses is perhaps unfortunate—he or she has been unlucky—but it is not, under these conditions, unjust or unfair. A guiding thought, therefore, as we evaluate proposals for rationing health care should be whether we can reasonably expect a particular rationing scheme to be agreed upon by those to whom it applies, especially those who would, on its terms, be denied access to possibly beneficial care.

B. Contractual Justification

We already have a model for contractually justified rationing in cases in which members of a voluntary, cooperative, prepaid health plan must jointly determine whether coverage should be extended to an expensive, modestly successful treatment for a disease affecting a small number of participants. Paul T. Menzel presents an example, based on an actual situation, involving adult liver transplantation. (The specifics of Menzel's example are somewhat dated because liver transplantation is now much more cost-effective than it was in the 1980s. Still, the general point remains relevant and instructive. A realistic, future-oriented example could replace liver transplants with the totally implantable artificial heart, now in clinical testing, which is projected to cost about $300,000 per implantation and to be of possible benefit to *millions* of cardiac patients. Total cost of funding this technology will be many magnitudes greater than funding liver transplants because unlike the supply of transplantable livers, which will always be limited by nature, we will be able to manufacture as many implantable hearts as money can buy.) To continue with Menzel's example,

> After surveying the membership and a variety of discussions at different levels, the plan decided not to cover them [liver transplants]. At a cost of nearly $300,000 per transplanted patient in first-year care and $6,000 to $7,000 per year per patient for follow-up costs, and with a five-year survival rate of 65 percent, in effect this is a decision that $600,000 could be better spent on other things than five- to twenty-year additional life spans. The decision is publicized to the plan's current and prospective members and some other plans that cover this procedure are available to the community. Under these

circumstances, who would really want to argue that the plan's doctors and nurses are violating their moral oath to patients if they subsequently cooperate with this decision?[39]

Justifications of this sort place a premium on prior informed agreement and are, accordingly, called *contractualist*.

As formulated by philosopher T. M. Scanlon, the contractualist criterion of moral justification states that an act can be justified if it follows from a system of rules that, on reflection, cannot reasonably be rejected by anyone seeking informed, unforced, general agreement about the matter in question.[40] That agreement be *informed* presupposes that the contracting parties are aware of their circumstances. In the present context, this would include full knowledge of the increasing costs of health care, Callahan's "ragged edge" of technology, competing social needs, and so on. *Unforced* agreement rules out coercion as well as being forced to accept an agreement by being in a weak bargaining position; for example, in this context by being forced by one's desperate medical condition to settle for a particularly low minimal level of care on threat of otherwise receiving none at all. To say that the system of rules to which one agrees *cannot, on reflection, be reasonably rejected* presupposes the need or desirability of finding principles or a policy that could be the basis of informed, unforced general agreement. It is not reasonable, on reflection, to reject a principle or policy simply because its application has some untoward or unfortunate results if the consequences of any alternative principle or policy or of having no applicable principle or policy at all would be worse. We must in the present context compare the unfortunate consequences of a sound rationing policy with the unjust consequences of the status quo, as identified above in Section 2. Finally, in placing a premium on prior *agreement*, contractualists hope that even when principles or policies so chosen turn out to work against the interests or desires of some individuals, these same individuals will nonetheless acknowledge the justification of what is being done.

Applied to health care rationing, contractualism directs us to develop a set of criteria that, given unavoidably limited resources and the need for general prior agreement, cannot reasonably be rejected by anyone *seeking a fair, efficient, and workable system* for allocating access to care. Foremost in our mind should be patients who are likely to be denied possibly beneficial care under the proposed rationing scheme. Assuming they acknowledge the facts (e.g., limited resources, the "ragged edge" of medical technology, other pressing social needs, and so on) and the need for general agreement on a fair and efficient rationing policy, we must ask whether we can reasonably expect them, at a point optimal for this kind of decision making, to have endorsed the specific criteria by which they lose out.

C. Respect for Persons

The previous example involving payment for liver transplantation shows that a contractualist justification of health care rationing can resolve the integrity-threatening conflict between a health care professional's commitment to individual patients and his or her role as an agent of a more impersonal rationing scheme. Nurses who, as directed by a contractually justifiable rationing policy, withhold possibly beneficial health care from patients would, in effect, be doing it *at the direction of these very patients*. The point has been well expressed by Menzel:

> If individual patients beforehand would have granted consent to the rationing policies and procedures in question (or more clearly yet, if they actually have consented to them), then the appeal of those policies and procedures will rest not merely on attachment to the morally controversial goal of aggregate welfare, "efficiency"; such policies will gain their moral force from respecting individual patients' own will.[41]

A health professional who, in the name of a rationing policy to which all members of society have directly or indirectly given their informed agreement, withholds a possibly beneficial type of treatment would not, therefore, be betraying the patient's trust. On the contrary, such a health care professional would be doing exactly what this patient and all other potential patients have, at some earlier time, optimal from the standpoint of policy making, directed him or her to do. The health care professional would, in this respect, be an agent of the patient's autonomy. That the policy directs that the patient not receive the treatment would be, to recall the distinction illustrated by Case 7.3, "Unfortunate but not unfair?"

One may, at this point, raise an objection. Granted, the patient may have agreed, well before he or she became sick, that treatment for this comparatively rare, very expensive illness should be limited to competent, compassionate palliative care, but include no system-supported efforts to cure. But that was then; this is now. Having contracted the illness, the patient at this point desperately wants the treatment, and for health care professionals to withhold it is to betray and deny the autonomy of the actual, flesh-and-blood person before them.

The response to this objection provides further illumination of contractualist justification. If we are concerned with cost containment, we will have to place some restrictions on access to care; if we are concerned with fairness, we will have to do so without discriminating against identifiable individuals. These considerations, together with the fact that health care needs vary among individuals and within an individual's life, require that the standpoint from which we seek the sort of unforced, informed, general agreement characteristic of contractualism be either prior to or abstracted from that of a concrete individual suffering from a particular illness.[42]

The reason health care professionals would not be violating their commitments to particular patients in the foregoing case involving liver transplantation is that they would, in withholding access, be respecting the patients' prior informed, unforced agreement to the policy requiring them to do so. In so doing they are, Menzel suggests, actually respecting the autonomy of these patients if we construe this as respecting the informed, unforced decisions of the whole person and if "whole person" is understood to include informed, unforced decisions made at an earlier time in a person's life and intended to apply to later times as well.[43] This, by the way, is the sense of respecting a person's autonomy to which we appeal in overriding, on parentalistic grounds, the actual, here-and-now, suicidal request of one who is temporarily aggrieved, depressed, or insane (Chapter 3, Section 1). Before experiencing the grief, depression, or loss of sanity, we presume, the person wanted to continue to live—even during the period in which he or she is expressing suicidal desires—and it is this prior decision, not the present one, that we must honor if we are to respect the whole person's capacity for rational choice.

D. Expanding the Model

The question now is whether the contractualist model represented by Menzel's example of informed choice by members of a voluntary, cooperative, prepaid health plan can be extended to the nation and its health care system as a whole. This is an enormous undertaking, beset with numerous obstacles.

The implementation of a contractually justified system of rationing will, for example, require major changes and restructuring in the health care system. Funding for the level of care to which everyone has access would have to be centralized and prospectively budgeted in a "closed" system—one in which funds withheld or withdrawn from one type of care could, with assurance, be redirected to another type of care that is, from the standpoint of justice and efficiency, more important.[44] The transition to such a system will assuredly encounter significant opposition and resistance from powerful, deeply entrenched elements of the medical establishment and industries and institutions profiting from present arrangements.

There will be problems of design as well as implementation. Defining the basic level of health care remains a great difficulty. Given vast differences in individual circumstances, it will be difficult to draw the line simply in terms of categories of treatment. Cost–benefit ratios for various therapies differ widely from patient to patient, and developing guidelines taking account of all relevant variables is a formidable task.[45]

Moreover, although Menzel has made a useful beginning, the notion of prior consent as applied to health care rationing needs to be developed in much more detail, and on a larger scale, taking account of additional complexities. (Leonard Fleck's emphasis on the nature and role of democratic deliberation is, in this connection, a promising development.[46])

Yet, despite these and other difficulties, there is no more promising model for devising a realistically just and effective health care system than that based on contractualism and prior consent. It must, as we proceed, serve both as an ideal and as a benchmark for assessing the adequacy of various steps toward its realization.

6. RATIONING AND THE IMPORTANCE OF NURSING CARE

We cannot forecast the details of the long period of contentious national debates and experiments that will, we hope, eventually lead to a contractually justified system of health care rationing, one providing access to a decent minimum of health care for all, regardless of ability to pay.[47]

If, however, the process is to be democratic, it will have to involve the sorts of community consciousness-raising educational forums that were instrumental in leading to the Oregon proposal.[48] The participation of informed health care professionals—including nurses—in such forums is an indispensable part of the process. As Capuzzi and Bowden's account of nurse involvement in the development of the Oregon proposal indicates (Section 4), expert testimony from nurses about (1) the difficulties their patients had in gaining access to care, (2) the nurse's roles in the health care system, and (3) the nature and cost-effectiveness of nursing care contributed significantly to democratic deliberation about rationing.[49] Citizens and politicians need to understand the realities of health care—the limitations as well as the promises, the values of palliation as well as of attempts to cure, the costs as well as the benefits. They must also come to grips, as must health professionals themselves, with what is perhaps the greatest barrier to devising a contractually justified rationing system—a denial, deeply rooted in our culture, of limits imposed by the human condition

"There is," Daniel Callahan points out in his challenging account of the limits of medical progress, "a hard philosophical truth at which we have avoided looking, one that must be radically disquieting for any hopeful beliefs about the possibility of some ultimate efficiency. It is simply the burden of mortality: *Illness, decline, aging, and death can only be forestalled, kept at bay, never permanently vanquished.*"[50] Until the culture and those shaping and shaped by it acknowledge limits to what health care can achieve, the network of problems, to which a contractually justified system of rationing provides the most plausible answer, will continue to be ignored. Health care professionals are well placed to bring this "hard truth" to the attention of the public and will, in this capacity, make a vital contribution to the eventual development of a more just and efficient health care system.

Nursing care plays a special role in this connection. To withhold further (marginally beneficial) efforts to cure certain patients in the name of a contractually justified system of health care rationing does not justify or require abandoning them. On the contrary, patients denied highly expensive, only marginally effective, curative treatments would generally have a need and a right to various forms of palliative care and emotional support that *must* be included as part of an ethically justified basic minimum to which everyone would have access. "At the center of caring," writes Callahan,

> should be a commitment never to avert its eyes from, or wash its hands of, someone who is in pain or is suffering, who is disabled or incompetent, who is retarded or demented; that is the most fundamental demand made upon us. It is also the one commitment a health care system can almost always make to everyone, *the one need that it can reasonably meet.* Where the individual need for cure is infinite in its possibilities, the need for caring is much more finite—there is always something we can do for each other. The possibilities of caring are, in that respect, far more self-contained than the possibilities of curing. That is why their absence is inexcusable.[51] (emphasis added)

The need for caring enters debates over rationing in two ways. First, the need for caring is increasingly sacrificed by the present system as the quest for cure, regardless of cost or likelihood of success, consumes an increasing percentage of the health care dollar. One motivation, then, for seeking a justifiable rationing policy is to assure that the resources for meeting this vital need for caring are adequate and fairly distributed. Second, in designing such a policy we must see to it that the sort of caring under consideration is available to all, regardless of ability to pay.

No other health professionals know as much about, or are as skilled in, meeting the patient's round-the-clock, combined needs for physical, emotional, and spiritual care as nurses. Given the central role of such caring in any rationing scheme and the fact that withholding very expensive, marginally beneficial efforts to cure may require redoubled efforts at caring, nurses assume a correspondingly central role in deliberation over and experiments in health care rationing. As Barbara Redman, former Executive Director of the American Nurses Association, once pointed out:

> Nurses see who needs care, who is getting care and who is not. We see it every day and all through the night; in our emergency departments and trauma

centers, in our hospital wards and ICUs; in nursing homes and mental health centers; in the streets, schools and workplaces of our communities.

Nurses have something important to say about health care reform, and *now* is the time to say it. It is not only our right, but our obligation to speak out. We must speak out forcefully and with one voice about the terrible inequities and inconsistencies in our nation's health policy; about the nearly 37 million Americans without adequate health insurance, prevented from access to appropriate and affordable care; about the barriers that discriminate and disenfranchise our most vulnerable populations—the unborn and very young, the very old, those with chronic illnesses, the working poor, and those whose skin color, ethnic or life-style backgrounds are different from the majority; and about what we believe must be done to correct this growing national travesty.[52]

The problems—"the growing national travesty"—are worse now than they were when Redman spoke. Those without access to adequate health insurance, for example, now number 47 million rather than 37. And the special knowledge and expertise of nurses are still indispensable to the enormously complex, but unavoidable, social, and political task of turning the ideal of an ethically justified system of health care rationing into a just and caring reality.

7. THE EXPANDING SCOPE OF NURSING ETHICS

We conclude with a case that dramatically illustrates the expanding scope of ethics in health care. It is not a new case, but the issues it raises are instructive and still with us.

7.4 Ending Life Support Against the Family's Wishes

In 1989, 86-year-old Helga Wanglie tripped on a scatter rug in her hallway and fractured her right hip. A month after undergoing surgery for her hip, she developed breathing problems and was placed on a respirator. For five months, she remained fully conscious and alert, writing notes to her doctors and her husband, since the respirator prevented her from speaking. A week after being weaned from the respirator and transferred to a long-term care institution, her heartbeat and respiration suddenly stopped. By the time she could be resuscitated, she had undergone severe brain damage and was subsequently determined to be in a persistent vegetative state. She had, in other words, suffered a total and permanent loss of consciousness.

Eight months later, the question was whether, and if so how long, treatment should be continued. Led by its medical director, the hospital wanted to terminate Mrs. Wanglie's life support. Yet the family vehemently objected. Mrs. Wanglie, her husband said in an interview, is the daughter of a Lutheran

---

(Continued)

minister "and she has strong religious convictions. We talked about this a year ago. If anything happened to her, she said, she wants everything done. She told me, 'Only He who gave life has the right to take life.' It seems to me they're trying to play God. Who are they to determine who's to die and who's to live? I take the position that as long as her heart is beating there's life there."[53]

This case, as the newspaper reports emphasized, placed a new twist on a familiar problem. Often, it has been the family that wants treatment withdrawn in cases like this and the nurses, physicians, and hospital who object. Here, however, the roles were reversed. The family wanted treatment continued, and it was the caretakers who wanted to terminate treatment. It is not difficult to imagine why health professionals found such treatment medically futile and ethically questionable. The conflict between the physicians and the family was settled in court about 18 months after the accident. The judge decided in favor of the family, appointing Mrs. Wanglie's husband as her legal guardian. A few days after the court's decision, however, Mrs. Wanglie died of multiple organ failure.

The case raises many complex issues that we cannot pursue here. Our main concern, in line with the subject of the chapter, is with the cost of Mrs. Wanglie's care and whether it was borne by a larger social group. Mrs. Wanglie lived for about 18 months after the accident and her medical expenses came to about $800,000, which were paid in full by Medicare and by a supplemental insurer. Though we do not know exactly how much was spent after Mrs. Wanglie was diagnosed as totally and permanently unconscious, the question is: Was this a just and efficient use of shared funding? Were there other claims to medical care that, under a just and efficient rationing scheme, would have had a stronger claim to those dollars? Should private insurance companies or Medicaid or Medicare continue to underwrite such forms of life-extending treatment while the sort of basic needs identified in Section 2 are routinely denied to large portions of the population? More generally, should we, as a nation, be spending, as we do, between about $1.25 billion and $2.5 billion per year for patients who are not, and will never again be, conscious? These questions will soon become unavoidable, if they are not already.[54]

This chapter outlines a framework for thinking about such matters—a framework based upon fairness, contractualist justification, and respect for persons. It directs us to ask the following kinds of questions: What are the competing, unmet health care needs of the relevant population (members of a prepaid health plan or those covered by a private insurance plan, Medicaid, or Medicare)? How important are these needs to the relevant population when compared with sustaining permanently unconscious patients for as long as they or their families may wish? Are health care resources genuinely limited? If so, would members of the population be likely to give informed, unforced, general agreement to a policy that would pay for the care of patients like Mrs. Wanglie after she was diagnosed as permanently unconscious but not, for example, high quality long-term care for those suffering from Alzheimer's disease or other mental disabilities?

Our concern in this chapter is not to settle these complex questions but rather to show that matters of overall cost, efficiency, and justice can no longer be separated from more individualized ethical considerations. As payment for health care becomes increasingly shared or social, conceptions of nursing ethics that focus entirely on individual patients will, as Leonard M. Fleck has cogently argued, prove to be much too narrow:

> If the demands of justice are to be taken seriously, if we are to have just health care policies and a just health care system, then nurses will have to be advocates of such policies. They will have to participate intelligently and vigorously in the broad moral and political conversations that will shape future health care policy. *This is not an optional aspect of the nurse's role.*[55] (emphasis added)

With this, we heartily agree, and it has been the aim of this chapter to provide a foundation for such an expanded conception of nursing ethics.

Appendix A

The International Council of Nurses Code of Ethics for Nurses

PREAMBLE

Nurses have four fundamental responsibilities: to promote health, to prevent illness, to restore health and to alleviate suffering. The need for nursing is universal.

Inherent in nursing is respect for human rights, including cultural rights, the right to life and choice, to dignity and to be treated with respect. Nursing care is respectful of and unrestricted by considerations of age, colour, creed, culture, disability or illness, gender, sexual orientation, nationality, politics, race or social status.

Nurses render health services to the individual, the family and the community and co-ordinate their services with those of related groups.

THE ICN CODE

The ICN Code of Ethics for Nurses has four principal elements that outline the standards of ethical conduct.

An international code of ethics for nurses was first adopted by the International Council of Nurses (ICN) in 1952. It has been revised and reaffirmed at various times since, most recently with this review and revision completed in 2005. Reprinted by permission

Elements of the Code

1. Nurses and people

The nurse's primary professional responsibility is to people requiring nursing care.

In providing care, the nurse promotes an environment in which the human rights, values, customs and spiritual beliefs of the individual, family and community are respected.

The nurse ensures that the individual receives sufficient information on which to base consent for care and related treatment.

The nurse holds in confidence personal information and uses judgement in sharing this information.

The nurse shares with society the responsibility for initiating and supporting action to meet the health and social needs of the public, in particular those of vulnerable populations.

The nurse also shares responsibility to sustain and protect the natural environment from depletion, pollution, degradation and destruction.

2. Nurses and practice

The nurse carries personal responsibility and accountability for nursing practice, and for maintaining competence by continual learning.

The nurse maintains a standard of personal health such that the ability to provide care is not compromised.

The nurse uses judgement regarding individual competence when accepting and delegating responsibility.

The nurse at all times maintains standards of personal conduct which reflect well on the profession and enhance public confidence.

The nurse, in providing care, ensures that use of technology and scientific advances are compatible with the safety, dignity and rights of people.

3. Nurses and the profession

The nurse assumes the major role in determining and implementing acceptable standards of clinical nursing practice, management, research and education.

The nurse is active in developing a core of research-based professional knowledge.

The nurse, acting through the professional organization, participates in creating and maintaining safe, equitable social and economic working conditions in nursing.

4. Nurses and co-workers

The nurse sustains a co-operative relationship with co-workers in nursing and other fields.

The nurse takes appropriate action to safeguard individuals, families and communities when their health is endangered by a co-worker or any other person.

Suggestions for Use of the ICN Code of Ethics for Nurses

The ICN Code of Ethics for Nurses is a guide for action based on social values and needs. It will have meaning only as a living document if applied to the realities of nursing and health care in a changing society.

To achieve its purpose the Code must be understood, internalized and used by nurses in all aspects of their work. It must be available to students and nurses throughout their study and work lives.

Applying the Elements of the ICN Code of Ethics for Nurses

The four elements of the ICN Code of Ethics for Nurses: Nurses and people, nurses and practice, nurses and the profession, and nurses and co-workers, give a framework for the standards of conduct. The following chart[1] will assist nurses to translate the standards into action. Nurses and nursing students can therefore:

Study the standards under each element of the Code.

Reflect on what each standard means to you. Think about how you can apply ethics in your nursing domain: practice, education, research or management.

Discuss the Code with co-workers and others.

Use a specific example from experience to identify ethical dilemmas and standards of conduct as outlined in the Code. Identify how you would resolve the dilemmas.

Work in groups to clarify ethical decision making and reach a consensus on standards of ethical conduct.

Collaborate with your national nurses' association, co-workers, and others in the continuous application of ethical standards in nursing practice, education, management and research.

Appendix B

The Patient Care Partnership: Understanding Expectations, Rights, and Responsibilities

When you need hospital care, your doctor and the nurses and other professionals at our hospital are committed to working with you and your family to meet your health care needs. Our dedicated doctors and staff serve the community in all its ethnic, religious, and economic diversity. Our goal is for you and your family to have the same care and attention we would want for our families and ourselves.

The sections explain some of the basics about how you can expect to be treated during your hospital stay. They also cover what we will need from you to care for you better. If you have questions at any time, please ask them. Unasked or unanswered questions can add to the stress of being in the hospital. Your comfort and confidence in your care are very important to us.

WHAT TO EXPECT DURING YOUR HOSPITAL STAY

High-Quality Hospital Care

Our first priority is to provide you the care you need, when you need it, with skill, compassion and respect. Tell your caregivers if you have concerns about your care or if you have pain. You have the right to know the identity of doctors, nurses, and others involved in your care, and you have the right to know when they are students, residents, or other trainees.

Reprinted with permission of the American Hospital Association, copyright 2003.

A Clean and Safe Environment

Our hospital works hard to keep you safe. We use special policies and procedures to avoid mistakes in your care and keep you free from abuse or neglect. If anything unexpected and significant happens during your hospital stay, you will be told what happened, and any resulting changes in your care will be discussed with you.

Involvement in Your Care

You and your doctor often make decisions about your care before you go to the hospital. Other times, especially in emergencies, those decisions are made during your hospital stay. When decision making takes place, it should include:

Discussing your medical condition and information about medically appropriate treatment choices. To make informed decisions with your doctor, you need to understand:
   The benefits and risks of each treatment.
   Whether your treatment is experimental or part of a research study.
   What you can reasonably expect from your treatment and any long-term effects it might have on your quality of life.
   What you and your family will need to do after you leave the hospital.
   The financial consequences of using uncovered services or out-of-network providers.

Please tell your caregivers if you need more information about treatment choices.

Discussing your treatment plan. When you enter the hospital, you sign a general consent to treatment. In some cases, such as surgery or experimental treatment, you may be asked to confirm in writing that you understand what is planned and agree to it. This process protects your right to consent to or refuse a treatment. Your doctor will explain the medical consequences of refusing recommended treatment. It also protects your right to decide if you want to participate in a research study.

Getting information from you. Your caregivers need complete and correct information about your health and coverage so that they can make good decisions about your care. That includes:
   Past illnesses, surgeries, or hospital stays.
   Past allergic reactions.
   Any medicines or dietary supplements (such as vitamins and herbs) that you are taking.
   Any network or admission requirements under your health plan.

Understanding your health care goals and values. Your may have health care goals and values or spiritual beliefs that are important to your well-being. They will be taken into account as much as possible throughout your hospital stay. Make sure your doctor, your family and your care team know your wishes.

Understanding who should make decisions when you cannot. If you have signed a health care power of attorney stating who should speak for you if you become unable to make health care decisions for yourself, or a "living will" or "advance directive" that states your wishes about end-of-life care, give copies to your doctor, your family and your care team. If you or your family need help making difficult decisions, counselors, chaplains and others are available to help.

Protection of Your Privacy

We respect the confidentiality of your relationship with your doctor and other caregivers, and the sensitive information about your health and health care that are part of that relationship. State and federal laws and hospital operating policies protect the privacy of your medical information. You will receive a Notice of Privacy Practices that describes the ways that we use, disclose and safeguard patient information and that explains how you can obtain a copy of information from our records about your care.

Preparing You and Your Family for When You Leave the Hospital

Your doctor works with hospital staff and professionals in your community. You and your family also play an important role in your care. The success of your treatment often depends on your efforts to follow medication, diet and therapy plans. Your family may need to help care for you at home.

You can expect us to help you identify sources of follow-up care and to let you know if our hospital has a financial interest in any referrals. As long as you agree that we can share information about your care with them, we will coordinate our activities with your caregivers outside the hospital. You can also expect to receive information and, where possible, training about the self-care you will need when you go home.

Help with Your Bill and Filing Insurance Claims

Our staff will file claims for you with health care insurers or other programs such as Medicare and Medicaid. They also will help your doctor with needed documentation. Hospital bills and insurance coverage are often confusing. If you have questions about your bill, contact our business office. If you need help understanding your insurance coverage or health plan, start with your insurance company or health benefits manager. If you do not have health coverage, we will try to help you and your family find financial help or make other arrangements. We need your help with collecting needed information and other requirements to obtain coverage or assistance.

While you are here, you will receive more detailed notices about some of the rights you have as a hospital patient and how to exercise them. We are always interested in improving. If you have questions, comments, or concerns, please contact: [Local Hospital Contact].

Appendix C

Cases for Analysis

A.1 Refusing the Physician Researcher

Matthew Burns, head nurse at a large university medical center, was not certain that Dr. Hemphill's oncology research was best for the patients involved. Matthew tried to consider the research from Dr. Hemphill's point of view, which, he reasoned, included concern for the overall results, Hemphill's reputation as an oncologist and researcher, and funding. When Matthew examined the research from his own point of view, he focused on the sufferings of individual patients. He questioned whether the patients should have consented to spend their last months undergoing experimental chemotherapy since the treatments did not seem to help and often made patients sicker. He could support the research and the patients' participation only because he knew there was no cure for them and because he believed that oncology research was vital.

According to Matthew, "Dr. Hemphill insisted on having things his way. Staff nurses on the oncology unit were not paid by him and did not work for him, but he asked us to do many things that I could not okay. For instance, he wrote orders for the nurses to give a certain medication straight IV push, a medication that was not included in the overall hospital policy as approved for IV push by nurses. I had to consider what would happen to any of the nurses if they went against the policy, which was designed, I think, to protect them. I also had to be supportive of nursing administration policy in order to remain head nurse." Matthew believed, as well, that his staff wanted him to tell them to follow hospital policy rather than Dr. Hemphill's orders.

When he told the doctor that the nurses could not give the medication IV push, the doctor asked him to deviate from the policy and not to tell anyone he was doing so. Matthew refused. Dr. Hemphill's solution was to hire his own nurse to give the medication, which created problems for the staff nurses. Adding to the general tension was Matthew's belief that Dr. Hemphill was trying to make his life miserable so that he would quit, and the doctor might be able to work with someone he could manipulate. Nevertheless, the doctor's efforts to make Matthew uncomfortable by embarrassing him

(Continued)

on rounds in front of physicians, nurses, and patients failed to cause him to resign, and both Dr. Hemphill and Matthew worked to the end of the research period

A.2 Summer Employee

Sarah, a junior nursing student, has recently started a summer job in a rural area near her parents' house. She is working at Restwood Nursing Home. The staff for the evening shift consists of only nurse aides. Sarah does not know of any RN, LPN, or Certified Medication Aide on duty during her shift. Sarah also learns that the nurse aides are trained with a short instruction from day staff LPNs on how to pass medications.

Sarah questions this procedure. After a little research, she finds out that state law does not allow a nurse aide without certification as a medication aide to pass medications. Sarah also wonders if the doctors are aware that staff carrying out their orders have such a low level of training.

She asks Becky, another staff member from her shift, why aides who are not Certified Medication Aides are passing medications to the clients. Becky explains, "We cannot get any RNs or LPNs to work the evening shift here. That leaves no one to pass medication on this shift, so an aide ends up doing this. It just happens that none of the present evening shift aides have done the state certification program." Sarah also questions Becky to see if the doctors are aware of this procedure. "Yes," Becky answers, "the doctors are aware of who is passing the medication, and they agree with our ways. Because if we did not do this, we would not have a nursing home for all these old people. Where would all these older people live, since most of their families either cannot take care of them or else they don't want to?" (This case has been adapted from one prepared for our Ethical Issues in Nursing course by Beth Carrington.)

A.3 Too Many Medicines

Connie Delinger, community health nurse for six years, knew that Grace Weiss, a 78-year-old widow who lived alone, preferred to handle her own affairs. On a previous visit, Connie had encouraged Mrs. Weiss to speak to her doctor about the large number of prescription medications she took routinely. Later, Mrs. Weiss told Connie that the doctor had said she was doing the right thing—she was taking her medicine. Connie was not convinced that Mrs. Weiss had told her doctor clearly that she was taking at least ten different medications. Connie could see, as she had seen before, that the numerous drug containers filled a small cake pan. Connie carefully examined each container and immediately recognized "two different heart medications that did essentially the same thing." Connie now realized that Mrs. Weiss was totally confused about the purpose of her various medications. "It was probable," Connie reasoned, "that Mrs. Weiss was being abused by medication, and her doctor didn't really know what was happening to her." However, when Connie said that she would like to check the medicines with the pharmacy, Mrs. Weiss balked: the physician had very recently said that she was doing the right thing. Connie thought that Mrs. Weiss probably did not want her to do anything that might call attention to the fact that she needed help. Nevertheless, Connie chose to ignore Mrs. Weiss' protests, called the pharmacist, obtained a review of the medications, and then called Mrs. Weiss' doctor. The office nurse could hardly believe that such an array of medications had been ordered, but at Connie's insistence she arranged for Mrs. Weiss to show the doctor all her medications. Mrs. Weiss was perturbed at Connie for setting up the appointment, but she agreed to go since the doctor was expecting her.

A.4 Birth Control

Aretha Washington is a public health nurse in an urban County Health Department. Among her case load of 15 to 20 families are high-risk infants and children and potential or actual child abuse and neglect families. During a home visit, Aretha learned that Sheila Long was having leg pains and had been getting refills on her birth control prescriptions. Given Sheila's medical history and possible side effects from birth control pills, Aretha thought that Sheila should contact her doctor for evaluation. Aretha also thought that the physician would take Sheila off the pill and substitute a potentially less effective form of birth control. Knowing Sheila, Aretha expected that Sheila would like nothing so well as the pill.

Aretha thought, "This woman has to take the pill; I really don't want her to have any more kids. I don't think it's right for children to be born when they are not wanted. Also, Sheila has the right not to have to bear children she doesn't want. But what are the consequences of that? Should she stay on the pill and possibly endanger her life? Should she try something that may not be as effective and possibly have an unwanted child?"

Aretha could see advantages and disadvantages both with Sheila's continuing on the pill and changing to another form of contraception which, though possibly safer, might also be likely to be less effective. Aretha had to decide whether to discuss this problem with Sheila, and, if so, whether she should encourage her to opt for one alternative rather than another.

A.5 Aides' Sit-Down Strike

Ronna Smith is one of two registered nurse team leaders in the Pinecrest Care Center north wing, which serves one hundred geriatric patients who require skilled nursing care. Adequate staffing requires 13 aides on the north wing, but on Sunday Ronna arrived at 6:30 to find she was short-staffed again. For the past four months, she had had an adequate staff fewer than ten days. Lights were blinking, food was ready for breakfast, and the seven

(Continued)

aides scheduled to work announced that they were not staying. To prove their point, they sat in the staff lounge.

The aides were at the breaking point; they were infuriated by minimum wages and the task of caring for one hundred people with only seven or even fewer aides. Aware that they could not do an adequate job and tired of everyone's complaints, they had met repeatedly with the administration but had made no progress.

Ronna called her director, who told her to "try to be a motivating leader," but Ronna thought, "How am I going to motivate anyone when I feel pretty unmotivated myself?" She knew the patients needed help from more aides than the administration had hired, and she felt sorry for the patients, the aides, and herself. Even while on the phone, she could hear the patients calling impatiently for help. She quickly told the director she must come to the center and, with the other team leader, attempted to answer the blinking lights and calls for help from the patients.

The director came, and, after failing to convince the aides to return to work, she called the departmental administrator, who finally arrived after almost an hour's delay. After three hours, the sit-down strike ended with a promise of time-and-a-half for the day and with another meeting between the aides and administration scheduled for Monday. At that meeting, all the aides received a fifteen-cent hourly raise and the promise that when the north wing was short-staffed in the future, each would receive a seven-dollar bonus for the day.

Ronna was not satisfied because she believed that paying more for the same inadequate level of service would not help patients or nursing staff. After work on Monday, she contemplated resigning. After Ronna married four months ago, she took the nursing home job because she could get day work and no shift rotation. However, she was offered $1.50 less per hour than at the local hospital and was told that the nursing home did not pay differentials for weekends or shifts because nurses were hired for the shift they selected. On the other hand, she believes that she has developed professionally in this, her first nursing home job; she has learned much about older people, finds her care of geriatric patients rewarding, likes the responsibility, and works well with the doctors, especially the woman who cares for most of the patients. She has learned, however, that few nurses stay for more than a year and that many aides stay less than a month. The nursing director repeatedly hires people as aides who have no prior experience and minimal training, so that consequently the team leaders must teach them on the job. Ronna resents the lost time she has spent on those who have quit after the first week or two of orientation. She has talked repeatedly to the nursing director and administrator about the low pay scale for aides and nurses, hiring minimally qualified people, consequent high turnover rates, and detrimental effects on the patients' welfare, only to be told that because the center is new and takes a while to grow, they are sorry but, at present, aides' and nurses' wages can not be raised.

Ronna seriously doubts that the short-staffing problem will be resolved merely because the administration made some concessions to the aides. After seeing how drastically the many helpless patients were affected by even a three-hour sit-down strike (no one ate until after 9:30), she does not believe that she and the other registered nurse should use a strike in trying to change pay scales and hiring policies. Yet talking has been useless, and if she leaves, some other nurse will take the job, and the cycle will only continue. Ronna now wonders whether she would be ethically justified if she joined the aides to exert pressure on an administration that has refused to respond to the nurses' suggestions and complaints but has responded promptly to the aides' sit-down-strike.

A.6 Compliance Issue

Nora Horner, staff nurse on a general medical unit in a large urban private hospital, and Mrs. Barton, a 73-year-old retired schoolteacher hospitalized with a diagnosis of congestive heart failure, look upon Mrs. Barton's fluid intake differently. Nora sees that Mrs. Barton should stay within moderate amounts of fluid intake, and she tries to encourage that goal. Mrs. Barton, who is oriented and talkative, agrees with Nora's explanations, but she drinks fluids excessively, especially when her friends visit. In describing Mrs. Barton, Nora says that "The guidelines are just not important to her, or she doesn't see what fluids do to her. Maybe she doesn't care." After attempting to reason with Mrs. Barton and to understand the reasons for her failure to stop drinking fluids excessively, Nora tried teasing and finally scolding her to gain her cooperation, but without success. Finally, Nora explained to Mrs. Barton's friends the reasons for discouraging excessive fluid intake and gained their cooperation in keeping her bedside intake record accurate so that Mrs. Barton would be prompted to drink moderate amounts. Nonetheless, Nora wondered whether she was morally justified in acting behind Mrs. Barton's back.

A.7 Removal of Tracheostomy Tubes

At 7:55 a.m. Mary Kowalski was about to give report when she heard patients yelling "Nurse, Nurse!" She and two other nurses rushed to the room and saw Mrs. Audrey Johnson turning blue. Her tracheostomy tubes, in place a few minutes earlier, were on the table, and she had a large new dressing with an Ace bandage around her neck. After they quickly cut everything off and reinserted the tubes, the other nurses stayed with Mrs. Johnson, who was extremely upset, while Mary left to get another set of tubes and ties. As she passed the nurses' station and saw the two physicians who, without informing the nurses, had removed Mrs. Johnson's tracheostomy tubes and applied the dressings, she said, "We're putting the tube back in; she can't breathe." Mary remembers that neither moved and one said, "Oh, she

(*Continued*)

obstructed, huh." When she returned to the room, a very frightened Mrs. Johnson would not let the nurses leave her to attend report until someone else would sit with her.

According to Mary, "After the crisis was over, the two physicians proceeded to chew us out because we didn't know where the obturator was for the trach tube. They missed the point of the whole incident. They didn't tell us they were doing it, and they picked a very bad time because there were only three of us working that night. When we went to report, there was nobody left."

Mary does not want to be someone the physicians can "walk right over," keep ignorant of information important for safe nursing care, or blame when things don't go right. To her, the doctors had just "yanked out the tube" and walked out, expecting that the nurses—being women—"would clean up their mess." When the situation developed into a crisis, they found fault with the nurses over the obturator.

The nurses first told the physicians how they felt and discussed the incident with the assistant head nurse, who was coming on duty at the time, and who was also the otology clinician. A few days later, however, the same doctors did essentially the same thing. In that situation, however, a nurse observed them and informed the rest of the nursing staff. Mary thinks that the incident concerning Mrs. Johnson should be prevented from happening repeatedly. She has talked with her coworkers, "trying to figure out what to do, and the answer keeps coming up as zero."

A.8 A Suggestion Is Rejected

As charge nurse of a 32-bed orthopedic unit, MacKenzie Bowles is used to working with nurse discretion medical orders, to asking physicians for particular medications, and to questioning treatments. She thinks her interdisciplinary relationships with health care providers are generally good, especially with some of the surgeons who, as she describes them, "are very open to hearing your points." But her relationship with Dr. John Olsen is different.

John was treating Mr. Floyd Trapp for an orthopedic problem when MacKenzie asked him to arrange a medical consultation. The doctor who came was Mr. Trapp's general practitioner. He had discontinued Mr. Trapp's hypertension medication earlier, and after seeing him in the hospital, had not reordered the medication. MacKenzie continued to be concerned, however, because "Mr. Trapp was still running a fairly high blood pressure plus having some other symptoms." She told John about Mr. Trapp's continuing problems and asked if he would consider another medical consultant who was associated with the hospital. In response, John asserted that he was the doctor, that he would take care of the consults, and that MacKenzie should take care of nursing matters.

After he left, MacKenzie wondered, "Was there another way that I could have said it but didn't? Could I have done it differently?" She had tried, as she usually did with all health care workers, "to phrase questions so they would be non-threatening." Should she try to find another way to get a medical consult for Mr. Trapp?

A.9 Request to Be Excused

Josie Chakos, a newly immigrated Filipino surgical scrub nurse, has told her supervisor, Sue Taylor, that she absolutely cannot participate in sterilization procedures. The previous week she had been caught by surprise when, immediately after a caesarean delivery, the surgeon had proceeded to ligate the fallopian tubes of the young mother. Even though the mother had requested the operation, this did not satisfy Josie since she is strongly opposed to sterilization on religious grounds. Josie now says that she cannot participate in any caesarean delivery because doing so may well lead to a similar situation.

Sue is unsure how to deal with Josie's request to be excused from future participation in caesarean surgeries, some of which may well include similar unscheduled procedures. On the one hand, she would like to respect and accommodate Josie's religious views. On the other hand, she thinks that doing so would involve a number of problems; juggling staff assignments would be time-consuming and take away from other duties; other nurses would probably resent what they would perceive as special treatment; and, given the hospital's emphasis on cost containment, accommodating Josie would require some additional costs without appreciably improving services. Is there a morally acceptable compromise solution that might address Josie's concerns and limit problems to the unit and hospital? (Case created for this text.)

A.10 Refusal to Begin a Research Procedure

An 82-year-old woman is referred to the hospital research unit for consideration in a therapeutic research protocol that may improve her physical condition. The research physician discusses the study with the woman and her husband and, as she is interested in participating, the patient reads over the informed consent document, and the physician questions her afterward to assess her comprehension of the material. The physician is satisfied that the patient understands, and she schedules her for the study.

Two days later, the patient arrives on the research unit to begin the study but is confused and unable to remember why she is there or any of the information provided in the informed consent that she had agreed to and signed previously.

After talking with the patient, the nurse refuses to begin the infusion and contacts the research physician. She arrives and orders that the procedures begin according to the study schedule, stating she will take responsibility for

(Continued)

the decision. (This case was prepared by Catherine McGrath-Miller, M.S., Research Volunteer Services Coordinator, Bronson Clinical Investigation Unit, Kalamazoo, Michigan.)

A.11 Confidentiality and an Attempted Suicide

In a particular metropolitan area, public health nurses employed by the County Health Department are organized in teams of four nurses. In the field, the nurses practice independently, but they arrange meetings to collaborate on difficult cases, such as that of the Cass family. LeeAnn Cass, pregnant at age 16, planned to keep her baby after delivery. Her father believed that he could not afford a separate apartment for LeeAnn and that she must, therefore, stay with the family. Mrs. Cass, age 38, feared that LeeAnn's presence in the home—and the baby's—would upset the family, especially LeeAnn's three younger sisters. Mrs. Cass had been having anxiety with each of her menstrual periods and recurrent urinary tract infections.

Susan Statler, a public health nurse and one of several professionals involved with the Cass family, learned that Mrs. Cass had attempted suicide by taking an overdose of a tranquilizer. One team member urged Susan to pass that information to the physician since she legally could do so. Susan did not want to risk alienating Mrs. Cass by breaking her confidentiality unless it was absolutely necessary. She knew that Mrs. Cass' psychotherapist, a psychiatric social worker, was aware of her suicide attempt. Susan had not discussed with Mrs. Cass whether all the professionals involved with her, including the physician, knew of her suicide attempt. One of her colleagues argued that if the physician knew about it, he would probably prescribe fewer or different tranquilizers as a limited form of protection for Mrs. Cass.

Within a few days, Susan discussed with Mrs. Cass the question of informing the physician about Mrs. Cass' attempted suicide, but Mrs. Cass rejected the suggestion that she herself inform him or that Susan tell him. Mrs. Cass saw no value in doing so and did not want to discuss personal problems with the physician since she was already doing so with her therapist.

Susan and her nursing team never agreed as to the correct course of action, and Susan did not tell the physician.

A.12 Candor and Hope

Wendy Barrett, a senior-level nursing student, sees her clients—mainly elderly persons with chronic or terminal illnesses—in their own homes. Over the course of the last month 69-year-old Sam Richardson has become one of Wendy's favorite people. Mr. Richardson suffers from prostate cancer that has metastasized to his spine. Weak and in pain, he is nonetheless alert and able to move about in his home with the aid of a walker. He is very conscientious about taking medications and complying with Wendy's suggestions.

His wife is equally conscientious and provides his 24-hour care (e.g., fixing meals, bathing and dressing him, and so on).

On her last visit just as Wendy was leaving, Mrs. Richardson had asked when Sam would start getting better. The couple knew that Mr. Richardson had cancer, but Wendy's suspicions were now confirmed: They did not fully understand that his condition was worsening and that death was impending. She strongly believes that if the couple were to face up to Mr. Richardson's prognosis, they would give up hope and his care would quickly deteriorate, and this would result in an earlier death.

Wendy did not have time to discuss Mr. Richardson's prognosis with his wife on her last visit. Her next visit is scheduled for tomorrow. Although she has tried to put the question out of her mind, she can no longer do so. How candid should she be, she wonders, about Mr. Richardson's prognosis? (This case is based on a situation reported by Andrea Taylor when she was a student in the College of Nursing, Michigan State University.)

A.13 Medical Supplies

Vicky LaPorte, a Visiting Nurses' services supervisor, is concerned about nursing care costs. Vicki has assigned Tiffanya Johnson, a nurse with two years' experience, to Jin Hua, a 58-year-old woman who was discharged from the local hospital the previous day. To prepare for her visit to Jin, Tiffanya has collected from the VNS supply room some medical supplies, including some nonstick dressings and a 500 ml bottle of normal saline that she plans to use in Jin's care. Tiffanya knew from previous experience that the hospital probably had not sent home adequate medical supplies to cover Jin's first week at home.

Tiffanya also knew that Jin's care was reimbursed by Medicaid. In addition, she believed that the supplies she selected were routinely reimbursed so she did not waste her time reading the posted computer printout that listed which supplies are reimbursed by Medicaid without prior authorization.

After the visit Tiffanya learned that neither the particular type of nonstick dressings she selected nor the 500 ml size bottle of normal saline was covered by Medicaid. Had she substituted a different type of dressing and chosen a 1000 ml size bottle (knowing that she would waste half), Medicaid would have reimbursed VNS for the supplies. Being aware of these restrictions, Tiffanya initiated a prior authorization process to cover medical supplies she would need in Jin's future care.

Vicki is concerned about Tiffanya's failure to check which supplies were covered, but she is also concerned about the amount of time nurses like Tiffanya must spend in learning the special nuances of reimbursement. Vicki wonders who should pay for VNS supplies not routinely reimbursed. Should Tiffanya be charged for the cost (or some of the cost) of the unauthorized supplies she used? Should the hospital, which routinely does not send an

(Continued)

adequate first week of medical supplies, be charged? Should VNS increase its charges to all patients to cover non-reimbursed medical supplies?(Case provided by Lois Hauver, RN, Visiting Nurses' Services of Greater Lansing.)

A.14 Strike Vote

Thomas Hames is debating whether to vote in support of a nursing strike in 17 hospitals in his metropolitan area. The two major issues over which the union would strike are:

1. A layoff clause in the contract proposed by the hospitals. The union maintains that if layoffs are needed, staff reductions should proceed according to seniority; that is the least senior registered nurse is to be laid off first, then those with somewhat more seniority, and so on. The hospitals want to reduce staff by cutting the hours of specific nurses, with each hospital free to determine which nurse and the extent of his or her reduction in hours on the basis of total nursing hours needed for various services of the hospital. The union is concerned that the hospitals may take advantage of this to lay off more-experienced (and expensive) nurses and to replace them with less-experienced (and less expensive) nurses.
2. The duration of training across specialty areas. Such training is designed to allow nurses trained in one specialty (e.g., pediatrics) to function in another (e.g., intensive care). The union wants a four-week training period. The hospitals want a two-week training period. The union maintains that two weeks is too little time for even a senior nurse to safely make the transition from one specialty to another.

Thomas Hames wonders what he should do. Is a vote for going on strike justified: and, if not, what should he do if the majority, in fact, votes to go on strike? (Case created for this text.)

A.15 Who Gets a Transplant?

Diane Alff, 40-year-old nursing manager of an intensive care unit, has been a member of the team caring for Lana Oberstar during the final days of her life. Seventeen-year-old Lana was a victim of an auto accident caused by an intoxicated driver. In the hours immediately following admission, Marge Oberstar, Lana's mother, discussed with the physician and her minister her decision to donate Lana's organs for transplant should Lana die. Soon thereafter, the physician told Marge that Lana had died. A few minutes later, as Diane sat holding Marge's hand, Marge told Diane about Lana's short life. She ended by saying that at least with modern technology, some other young person could be saved with Lana's organs. Then she faced Diane and asked, "They wouldn't take anything to save a drunk, would they?"

Diane knows that the state transplant committee has discussed whether persons whose alcoholism has destroyed their livers ought to receive liver transplants. The media has carried statements by national experts in bioethics and summaries of research that support making liver transplants available to such persons if, after careful medical and psychological evaluation, they are judged as likely to keep the new liver as long as a recipient whose liver failure was not caused by alcohol. Further, the media have reported that former alcoholics have received liver transplants in the state. What should Diane say? (Case created for this text.)

A.16 Sexually Active Adolescent

Mrs. Teresa Velasco, school nurse, is assigned to four elementary schools, two middle schools, and one high school, which results in a full, busy schedule. This week Charlotta Smith, a 9th grader, asked Ms. Velasco how best to prevent another urinary tract infection. Charlotta reported that her mother had recently taken her to an urgent care clinic and that she had just finished taking all of a prescribed antibiotic. She told Mrs. Velasco that clinic staff told her she had "honeymoon disease." Charlotta didn't want to catch that painful disease again.

Hearing "honeymoon disease," Mrs. Velasco suspected that Charlotta was sexually active, and after a few more questions, Charlotta confirmed her suspicions. Ms. Velasco believes that premarital sex is wrong and has terrible consequences for both individuals and society; therefore, she told Charlotta that staying away from the boys was the way to prevent recurrence.

Mrs. Velasco also believes that she has a duty to fight promiscuity whenever possible. To stay true to her own values, she decided to say nothing to Charlotta that the girl might construe as condoning or encouraging her sexual activities. Therefore, she did not mention a standard preventative measure to avoid urinary tract infection, voiding both before and after sexual intercourse.

Can Mrs. Velasco's refusal to give Charlotta complete information be justified? (Case created for this text.)

A.17 An Obese Nurse

When Sabrina Glenn, a staff nurse with three years' experience, joined a small group of coworkers in the hospital cafeteria, she met Harriet Stearns, a staff nurse who worked in the university's endocrinology clinic. During the meal, Sabrina tried to calculate Harriet's weight while Harriet quickly ate two hamburgers, two orders of French fries, and cherry pie a la mode as the rest of the group finished small lunches . To Sabrina, Harriet appeared not merely overweight, but obese. Each time thereafter that Sabrina saw Harriet, she wondered if Harriet could actually do her job. Sabrina believed that an obese nurse implicitly communicated disdain for the importance of diet and exercise. Surely some overweight patients would simply ignore an obese nurse's guidance about diet and health issues.

(Continued)

Sabrina recognized as well that her ideas about obesity and potentially compromised nursing care went beyond Harriet. She saw too many nurses well on their way to being overweight and thought that the problem could only grow. She asked herself: Since I'm not overweight, is this just my problem? Do I have any obligation to bring this issue to the nursing administration's attention? Should the university hospital try to foster good health among all nurses through an institutional plan that encourages (and potentially rewards) staff members to exercise, control weight, and pursue a healthy lifestyle? If an institutional "good health" plan is considered, will I have an obligation to participate in committees charged with organizing and overseeing its conception and application? (Case created for this text.)

A.18 Which Housing?

Summit Group Home, community-based housing for developmentally disabled adults, provides Residential Care Facility Services and Home and Community-based Services to nine men and nine women. A combination of federal, state, and county monies supports each resident. During the day, all residents attend Fourco, a well-run facility where they have a variety of classes, lunch, time to socialize, and scheduled work for which they are paid. Some clients attend classes on shopping, meal planning, cooking, and other skills to prepare them for living with one or two other persons under limited supervision in an apartment or house. Such a change of housing for an individual from Summit Group Home reduces costs for that person.

Shirley Theda is a 31-year-old woman who was diagnosed with Down syndrome at birth. She moved to Summit Group Home three years ago when her widowed mother entered a nursing home; she has gotten along well at Summit and at Fourco. She is small with short, naturally curly blond hair, blue eyes, and a ready smile. She is friendly, gives people she knows hello-and-goodbye hugs, and has good social skills. For example, at the end of an informal slide show, Shirley surprised the guest speaker by rising from her seat and announcing, "Now let's give a hand in thanks," and by leading the applause.

Shirley's interdisciplinary team, which establishes her service plan, is considering whether she should move to an apartment where two other developmentally disabled women live, and where a third person is needed to fill the unit. Various team members have supported the move. Linda McCray, a social worker and Case Manager of Southeast State Case Management, pointed to other individuals with Down syndrome who have developed many skills once thought to be beyond them. She argued that increased client independence, in addition to being good for individuals, requires less supervision and is a positive way to reduce costs. The Administrator of Fourco reported that Shirley had some housekeeping skills when she arrived at Fourco and has tried hard to learn more. When asked whether she wanted to move into an apartment, Shirley, also a member of the interdisciplinary team, smiled broadly and answered, "O.K."

The Resident Director of Summit Group Home, Lisa Robinson, agrees that Shirley can successfully carry out routine housekeeping and some meal preparation tasks. Lisa, however, opposes the plan to change Shirley's housing. So does Emma Singh, a registered nurse, Shirley's Case Manager, and a member of Shirley's interdisciplinary team. Both Lisa and Emma are worried about Shirley's decisions in social situations, and they point out that although Shirley has been taught repeatedly not to talk to strangers, she almost always smiles and says hello to everyone. Emma believes that while the rush to find a third roommate is based in part on an idealistic goal, its stronger impetus is the stressed budget, and not what is best for Shirley.

All professional team members agree that whenever possible clients ought to move to less expensive housing. All agree that Shirley probably has the minimal skills to live in an apartment, help with household chores and microwave cooking, and to shower, dress, and be ready to attend Fourco Monday through Friday. In summary, Linda, Case Manager of Southeast State Management, said that Shirley shouldn't be prevented from becoming more independent, an important next step in her development. Emma Singh, however, as Shirley's Case Manager, stressed that lack of continuous supervision during evenings and weekends would present a safety problem. She asserted that Shirley was not "street wise" and offered more than a usual target, given her small size, pretty hair, and trusting smile, especially after she had seen a person a few times. Finally, Emma concluded: "Think about a different person, perhaps your own little five-year-old. Would you allow her out on the streets after dark just to save money?"

What should the team decide about changing Shirley's housing? (Case based on information from Patricia Doak, registered nurse.)

A.19 Wake Up Call—MRSA

Four days after collapsing in her home, Phyllis Taggert, a 76-year-old retired elementary schoolteacher, died in the Intensive Care Unit of complications from a "hospital acquired" MRSA (methicillin-resistant *Staphylococcus aureus*) bladder infection. In the six months preceding her death, she had been treated in her physician's family practice clinic, in a local urology clinic, in the state university urology clinic, and in a local urgent care clinic, but she was never hospitalized. She had gone out for her routine Saturday morning breakfast with her husband on the day she was stricken.

Julia Green, one of Phyllis's intensive care nurses, graduated from a baccalaureate nursing program two years ago and is aware of increasing numbers of patients with MRSA. Thinking of Phyllis's sudden death, her family's loss, and the care that she and other providers gave to Phyllis, Julia thinks

(*Continued*)

she should view the whole situation as a "wake up call," and should try to do something about the spread of MRSA.

But, she asks herself, in addition to using my best infection control techniques and encouraging other health care workers to do the same, what, if anything, ought I to do? Should I make a fuss about Phyllis's death to raise awareness of the problem? Or would publicity about MRSA hurt my hospital, which provided her with good care during her last few days? Would it hurt the string of offices and clinics that treated her? Should I try to get this hospital as well as other hospitals and clinics in this state to specifically address MRSA? What about trying to get hospitals to follow successful control programs used elsewhere, such as surveillance programs used in the Netherlands and Denmark? Should I try to involve lawmakers? (Case created for this text and based upon an actual situation in 2007.)

A.20 Insurance Issue

Very soon after Ted Larkin, a 64-year-old accountant with pancreatic cancer, learned that he was a suitable candidate for a Whipple Operation, a complicated surgery offering a slim chance of survival from an otherwise fatal disease, he also learned from his internist that local surgeons rarely attempted the operation. Given their area's sparse population, the medical community saw few people with pancreatic cancer, and many fewer who were diagnosed early enough to benefit from the surgery.

Ted discussed with Helen Morse, the registered nurse employed in his internist's practice, the importance of finding a hospital where a surgeon performed the operation frequently because experienced surgeons who often do special, complicated surgeries increase the odds of success and lower complication rates in such surgeries.

Following Helen's urging, Ted asked his internist to locate such a hospital, and he found a well-known cancer center in a neighboring state would do Ted's surgery.

To Ted's enquiries about his insurance coverage with Mega Health Plan, Mega replied that it would not pay for such treatment at an out-of-state hospital. The rejection letter included the names of five approved local surgeons. Ted told Helen he believed the insurance company had calculated that it was cheaper to let him die than to pay a cancer center for a special surgery that offered only a slim chance of success. He added he wanted to fight the cancer and take that slim chance. But, he said, the fight would cost him everything. He figured a credit card was the only way he could pay the $5000 cancer center hospital deposit and that the actual bill would take his small house and savings. He discussed with her whether she thought he ought to go ahead and have the surgery.

Ted decided to seek treatment at the out-of-state cancer center. After the operation, he owed $80,000, which Mega Health Plan refused to pay. While he was recovering, and still worrying about his cancer, Helen and others encouraged him to fight the insurance company. He learned that the five local surgeons Mega had listed had performed a total of only five surgeries for pancreatic cancer in the past five years. Armed with that data and information concerning successful Whipple operations performed at large cancer centers, Ted, nevertheless, lost two appeals to Mega over the next year

Next, Ted went to a state review board. He represented himself because he could not afford a lawyer, and he brought a gastroenterologist for support. Mega Health Plan sent two lawyers, a doctor, and a nurse to defend its refusal to pay. Ted won.

Mega Health Plan then paid his medical bills. The company also announced it would allow more patients to be treated at high volume centers, if evidence supported better outcomes. In the end, Ted won two fights: the cancer fight—after five years he learned he was cured—and the insurance fight. (This fictitious case is based on information in Denise Grady, "Doing Battle with the Insurance Company in a Fight to Stay Alive," *New York Times,* July 29, 2007, Web. February 13, 2009.)

A.21 Who Ought to Pay?

Lucas Cruz graduated from the local community college nursing program and completed his BSN through a college outreach program in his hometown. He is employed in the local community hospital where he knows many patients and their extended families. When conversing throughout the past year with Mrs. Tompkins, a hospital volunteer, Lucas has recognized that Mrs. Tompkins is becoming more forgetful of recent events. She has started missing changed assignments in the volunteer schedule after agreeing to those changes. Lucas has also noticed that Mrs. Tompkins, although she laughs pleasantly at her own forgetfulness, often substitutes a made-up word for one she seems not to remember. Last week Mrs. Tompkins lost her car again in the hospital parking lot. Lucas wonders whether Mrs. Tompkins is in an early stage of Alzheimer's disease.

Their conversation today concerned Mrs. Tompkins's 18-year-old grandson who has been accepted at their prestigious state university. Mrs. Tompkins described with pleasure her intention to pay for her grandson's education. She already has some money for him in an education savings program, but the total will not cover four years of study. She said that since she lives with her daughter and has social security to keep her going, she is giving her grandson her savings.

Lucas doesn't know how large Mrs. Tompkins's savings are, but he assumes that the grandson's college education may require the total amount. If Lucas's suspicions are correct that Mrs. Tompkins is afflicted with Alzheimer's disease or some other debilitating condition, Mrs. Tompkins may need that money herself to meet the high costs of nursing home care.

Later Lucas thought about possible complications when an elderly person gives away assets, and he thought someone ought to be giving Mrs. Tompkins

(*Continued*)

and her family up-to-date financial advice. Lucas is aware that if in the next several years Mrs. Tompkins needs more care than her daughter can provide at home, and she applies for Medicaid to pay nursing home bills, the "look back" period is five years; that is, if she has given her money to her grandson during that period, that gift could delay her own eligibility for Medicaid assistance.

Lucas knows he should not give financial advice, but he thinks that he should encourage Mrs. Tompkins to see her health care provider about her forgetfulness. If she is facing Alzheimer's disease, a diagnosis could lead to support and help for her and her family. That help could include financial planning.

Lucas privately questions whether Mrs. Tompkins ought to give her grandson her savings, even though graduating from college without a large debt could greatly help him in the future. If it is possible to do both—arrange her affairs so she can give her grandson a large gift and qualify for Medicaid assistance in the next few years without delays or difficulties—is it right to do so? The Medicaid budget in their state is stressed, and many people need assistance. Would it be more justifiable for Mrs. Tompkins to forgo giving away her savings, and to pay her own long-term nursing costs for as long as possible before asking for public assistance? Who should pay for the high nursing care costs of Alzheimer's disease? Who should pay for the high costs of education? How are these conflicting claims of old and young to be reconciled in our society? (This fictitious case is based on information in Tom Lauricella, "Nursing Homes, Medicaid and Your Assets," *Wall Street Journal*, July 22, 2007, Web. February 13, 2009).

NOTES

Chapter 1

1. This case is based on a clinical incident in 2002.

2. International Council of Nurses, *The ICN Code of Ethics for Nurses, icn.ch,* ICN, 2006, Web. February 6, 2009. [Subsequent references to or quotations from the ICN Code can be found in Appendix A.]

3. Talk of the Town, *New Yorker,* July 3, 1978, p. 19.

4. American Nurses Association (ANA), *Code for Nurses with Interpretive Statements* (Washington, D.C.: American Nurses Association, 2001), *nursingworld.org,* ANA, n.d., Web. February, 2009. [Subsequent references to or quotations from the ANA Code can be found through the ANA Web site, *nursingwold. org.*]

5. Robert M. Veatch, *A Theory of Medical Ethics* (New York: Basic Books, 1981), p. 107. For the entire argument against the legitimacy of professional codes for adjudicating most ethical disagreements in health care, see pp. 79–107.

6. See also, Catherine M Breen, Amy P. Abernethy, Katherine H. Abbott, and James A. Tulsky, "Conflict Associated with Decisions to Limit Life-Sustaining Treatment in Intensive Care Units," *Journal of General Internal Medicine* 16 (May 2001): 283–289, *pubmedcentral,* PubMed Central, n.d., Web. February 15, 2009. Researchers reported a significant conflict in which "One nurse considered quitting to avoid facing the same situation again." One could assume that the nurse who reported this nursing care situation was required to act in ways inconsistent with her ethical framework. For a discussion of "moral distress," that is, conflicting feelings resulting from internal conflicts that nurses' develop when their actions differ from their beliefs, see Ruth M. Kleinpell, "Ethical Dilemmas Can Lead to 'Moral Distress' in the ICU," *NurseWeek* 7 (January 10, 2005), *nursingspectrum.com,* Nurse Week, n.d., Web. February 15, 2009.

7. John Stuart Mill, *On Liberty* (New York: Liberal Arts Press, 1956), p. 45.

8. Sarah Dock, "The Relation of the Nurse to the Doctor and the Doctor to the Nurse," *American Journal of Nursing* 17 (1917): 394. Cited in Marjorie J. Stenberg, "The Search for a Conceptual Framework as a Philosophic Basis for Nursing Ethics: An Examination of Code, Contract, Context, and Covenant," *Military Medicine* 144 (January 1979): 10.

9. Stenberg, "Search for a Conceptual Framework," p. 8.

10. C. K. Hofling et al., "An Experimental Study in Nurse–Physician Relationships," *Journal of Nervous and Mental Disease* 143 (1966): 171–180.

11. Ibid., p. 176.

12. Ibid., p. 177.

13. "Executive Summary of Secretary's Commission on Nursing Report," *Nursing Economic$* 7 (January–February 1989): pp. 57–58.

14. Milisa Manojlovich, and Barry DeCicco, "Healthy Work Environments, Nurse–Physician Communication, and Patients' Outcomes," *American Journal of Critical Care* 16 (November 2007): 536–543, *ajcc.aacnjournals.org*, AACN, n.d., Web. February 15, 2009.

15. Theodora Sirota, "Nurse/Physician Relationships Survey Report," *Nursing2008* 38 (July 2008): 28–31, *nursingcernter.com,* Nursing Center, n.d., Web. February 15, 2009.

16. Gerald Dworkin, "Autonomy and Behavior Control," *Hastings Center Report* 6 (February 1976): 24.

17. For an example of a nurse manager who facilitates participation in ethical inquiry among her staff, see Janet M. Cromer, "Medical Ethics at Emerson," *boston.com*, *The Boston Globe*, January 17, 2008, Web. February 15, 2009. For an example of a position statement recommending that nurses "participate in interdisciplinary ethics committees and ethics rounds," see The New York State Nurses Association, "Role of the Registered Professional Nurse in Ethical Decision-Making," *nysna.org*, NYSNA, n.d., Web. August 30, 2008.

Chapter 2

1. This case is based on an actual event.

2. Saint Augustine, *The City of God*, tr. by John Healey (London: J. M. Dent & Sons, 1945, first published 426), Book I, Chapters 18–26, pp. 22–32.

3. St. Thomas Aquinas, *Summa Theologica*, Vol. 3, tr. by Fathers of the English Dominican Province (Westminster, MD: Christian Classics, 1981, first published around 1274), 2–2, Questions 64–65, pp. 1459–1469.

4. John Stuart Mill, *Utilitarianism* (London: Longmans, Green, and Co., 1907, first published 1861), pp. 9f., 24.

5. Immanuel Kant, *Grounding for the Metaphysics of Morals*, tr. by James W. Ellington, 3rd ed. (Indianapolis, IN: Hackett Publishing, 1993, first published1785), p. 35.

6. Quoted in William E. Phipps, "Christian Perspectives on Suicide," *Christian Century* 102 (October 30, 1985): 971.

7. Ibid.

8. Ibid., p. 973.

9. More recently the celebrated British orchestra conductor Sir Edward Downes, 85, and his wife Joan, 84, ended their lives together with physician assistance in Switzerland. Their children were with them as they drank a lethal potion before lying on adjacent beds and holding hands. "'After 54 happy years together, they decided to end their own lives rather than continue to struggle with serious health problems,' said the adult children in a prepared statement." *New York Times*, July 14, 2009.

10. Bernard Williams, "A Critique of Utilitarianism," in J. J. C. Smart and Bernard Williams, eds., *Utilitarianism: For and Against* (Cambridge: Cambridge University Press, 1973), p. 149.

11. Bonnie Steinbock, John Arras, and Alex John London, *Ethical Issues in Modern Medicine*, 7th ed. (New York: McGraw-Hill, 2009), p. 9.

12. Stuart Hampshire, *Morality and Conflict* (Cambridge, MA.: Harvard University Press, 1983), pp. 143–144.

13. This section and section 5 draw, in part, on Martin Benjamin, "Between Subway and Spaceship: Practical Ethics at the Outset of the Twenty-First Century," *Hastings Center Report* (July–August 2001): 24–31; and Martin Benjamin, *Philosophy & This Actual World: An Introduction to Practical Philosophical Inquiry* (Lanham, MD: Rowman & Littlefield, 2003), pp. 112–131.

14. In recent years, a number of philosophers have come to endorse some form of moral pluralism. See, for example, Thomas Nagel, "The Fragmentation of Value," in Thomas Nagel, ed., *Mortal Questions* (Cambridge: Cambridge University Press, 1979); Charles Taylor, "The Diversity of Goods," in Amartya Sen and Bernard Williams, eds., *Utilitarianism and Beyond* (Cambridge: Cambridge University Press, 1982); Bernard Williams, *Ethics and the Limits of Philosophy* (Cambridge, MA: Harvard University Press, 1985); Charles Larmore, *Patterns of Moral Complexity* (Cambridge: Cambridge University Press, 1987); Martha Nussbaum, *The Fragility of Goodness: Luck and Ethics in Greek Tragedy* (Cambridge: Cambridge University Press, 1987); Isaiah Berlin, "On the Pursuit of the Ideal," in Henry Hardy, ed., *The Crooked Timber of Humanity* (Princeton, NJ: Princeton University Press, 1990); and Michael Stocker, *Plural and Conflicting Values* (New York: Oxford University Press, 1992.

15. Following Joshua Cohen, John Rawls draws this distinction in *Political Liberalism* (New York: Columbia University Press, 1993), p. 36.

16. Ibid., pp. 36–37.

17. Berlin, "On the Pursuit of the Ideal," p. 12.

18. Rawls, *Political Liberalism*, pp. 56–58.

19. Kristin Luker, *Abortion and the Politics of Motherhood* (Berkeley, CA: University of California Press, 1984), pp. 158–191.

20. Helga Kuhse, " 'Yes' to Caring—but 'No' to a Nursing Ethics of Care," in *Caring: Nurses, Women and Ethics* (Oxford: Blackwell Publishers, 1997), p. 142.

21. Ibid., pp. 146–147.

22. See, for example, Jean Watson, *Asssessing and Measuring Caring in Nursing and Health Science,* 2nd ed. (New York: Springer, 2008); Ann Marriner Tomey and Martha Raile Alligood, eds. *Nursing Theorists and Their Work* (St. Louis, MO: Mosby, 2006).

23. Virginia Held, "Feminist Transformations of Moral Theory," *Philosophy and Phenomenological Research* 50 (1990): 344.

24. The expression "reflective equilibrium" comes from John Rawls, *A Theory of Justice* (Cambridge, MA: Harvard University Press, 1971). It is a way of reasoning in ethics that can be traced, historically, at least as far back as Aristotle, *Nicomachean Ethics*, 1094v, 12-1096a, 10, bk. 1, ch. 3–4. For a fuller explanation, see Martin Benjamin, *Philosophy & This Actual World* (Lanham, MD: Rowman & Littlefield, 2003), pp. 112–123.

25. Ad Hoc Committee of the Harvard Medical School, "A Definition of Irreversible Coma," *Journal of the American Medical Association* 205 (August 1968): 337–340.

26. Aristotle, *Nicomachean Ethics,* 1094b, 12–28, bk1, ch. 3.

27. Hilary Putnam, "Pragmatism and Moral Objectivity," in James Conant, ed., *Words and Life* (Cambridge, MA: Harvard University Press, 1994), p. 177n.

28. K. Danner Clouser, "Medical Ethics: Some Uses, Abuses, and Limitations," *New England Journal of Medicine* 293 (August 21, 1975): 387.

29. P. H. Nowell-Smith, "Religion and Morality," in Paul Edwards, ed., *Encyclopedia of Philosophy* 7 (New York: Macmillan and Free Press, 1967), p. 153.

30. See, for example, Alan Donagan, *The Theory of Morality* (Chicago, IL: University of Chicago Press, 1977), especially pp. 1–9, 57–66; and R. M. Hare, *Freedom and Reason* (Oxford: Oxford University Press, 1963), especially pp. 86–111, 157–185.

31. See, for example, Don Marquis, "Why Abortion Is Immoral," *Journal of Philosophy* 86 (Number 4, April, 1989): 183–202. This article is widely reprinted in contemporary bioethics anthologies.

32. See, for example, Judith Jarvis Thomson, "A Defense of Abortion," *Philosophy & Public Affairs* 1 (Fall, 1971): 47–66. This article is widely reprinted in contemporary bioethics anthologies.

Chapter 3

1. By "parentalism" we mean what is conventionally referred to in the literature as "paternalism." But since women are no less capable than men of occupying the "paternal" or "father knows best" role in their dealings with others, we prefer the sexually neutral term.

2. This case was provided by Peg Jones Wright, BSN, ACSW, Infant Mental Health and Family Therapist, Lansing, Michigan.

3. An important distinction can be drawn between "parentalism" *as a social practice* having certain roles and expectations governing the behavior of patients and health care professionals in the total health care system and parentalism *as a justification for particular acts* of manipulation or coercion on the part of health care professionals. Unless otherwise indicated, we use the term "parentalism" in the second sense.

4. James F. Childress, "Paternalism and Health Care," in Wade L. Robison and Michael S. Pritchard, eds., *Medical Responsibility: Paternalism, Informed Consent, and Euthanasia* (Clifton, NJ: Humana Press, 1979), p. 18.

5. As Charles Fried puts it, "Even if the ends are the patient's own ends, to treat him as a means to them is to undermine his humanity insofar as humanity consists in choosing and being able to judge one's own ends, rather than being a machine which is used to serve ends, even one's own ends." Charles Fried, *Medical Experimentation: Personal Integrity and Social Policy* (Amsterdam: North Holland, 1974), p. 101.

6. Ibid., p. 95.

7. This revision is based upon a case initially provided by Bruce Walters while a student in the College of Human Medicine at Michigan State University; see also Centers for Disease Control and Prevention, "Falls in Nursing Homes," *cdc.gov*, last modified: 10 June 2008, CDC, Web. February 6, 2009.

8. See Bruce Miller, "Autonomy and the Refusal of Lifesaving Treatment," *Hastings Center Report* 11 (August 1981): 22–28.

9. H. L. A. Hart, *Law, Liberty, and Morality* (New York: Vintage, 1966), pp. 32–34.

10. John Stuart Mill, *On Liberty* (New York: Library of Liberal Acts, 1956), p. 117. Emphasis added.

11. Childress, "Paternalism and Health Care," p. 24.

12. Gerald Dworkin, "Paternalism," *Monist* 56 (January 1972): 76f.

13. Kirsten Li in Case 3.2 might thus be criticized for not having worked harder to obtain consent from Professor Neff, during his lucid periods, to his being

restrained, if necessary, in the future. The case, as presented, suggests that she may have been more concerned with securing his family's consent than his own.

14. Ultimately this condition must be modified to account for subjects who will never recover their capacity for rational reflection.

15. Case based upon information from Deneen Gallagher, Ingham County Communicable Disease Nurse, Lansing, Michigan.

16. This revised case is based upon one provided by Bruce Walters while a student in the College of Human Medicine at Michigan State University.

17. This revised case is based on a case provided by Dorothea Milbrandt, while Vice-President for Nursing, Ingham Medical Center, Lansing, Michigan, and Marilyn Rothert, while Director for Lifelong Education, College of Nursing, Michigan State University.

18. Lawrence Stern, "Freedom, Blame, and the Moral Community," *Journal of Philosophy* 71 (February 14, 1974): 75.

19. Ibid., p. 74.

20. Raymond Williams, *Keywords* (New York: Oxford University Press, 1976), p. 156.

21. Stern, "Freedom, Blame, and the Moral Community," p. 76.

22. For an account of eight such ways, see Roderick M. Chisholm and Thomas D. Feehan, "The Intent to Deceive," *Journal of Philosophy* 74 (March 1977): 143–159.

23. Irving M. Copi and Carl Cohen, *Introduction to Logic*, 13th ed. (Upper Saddle River, NJ: Pearson/Prentice-Hall, 2008), p. 163.

24. Martin Benjamin, "Moral Agency and Negative Acts in Medicine" in Wade L. Robison and Michael S. Pritchard, eds., *Medical Responsibility* (Clifton, NJ: Humana Press, 1979), pp. 169–180.

25. In fact some years ago one of us (M.B.) was in the same position as the patient in this case. Knowing that he had a choice in the matter and having insufficient evidence for being rushed into undertaking the risks of an angiogram, he declined to consent to the procedure. More than five years after this event he has yet to undergo angiography and remains active with annual visits to a (different) cardiologist. This example, in a different, now dated situation, was originally suggested to us by Anthony Shaw, "Dilemmas of Informed Consent in Children, *New England Journal of Medicine* 289 (October 25, 1973): 885.

26. Sissela Bok, *Lying: Moral Choice in Public and Private Life* (New York: Pantheon, 1978), 26f.

27. Alan Donagan, *The Theory of Morality* (Chicago, IL: University of Chicago Press, 1977), p. 89.

28. Bok, *Lying*, p. 223.

29. International Council of Nurses, *The ICN Code of Ethics for Nurses, icn. ch,* ICN, 2006, Web. February 6, 2009.

30. American Hospital Association, *Patient Care Partnership,* aha.org, AHA, 2003, Web. February 6, 2009.

31. American Nurses Association (ANA), *Code for Nurses with Interpretive Statements* (Washington, D.C.: American Nurses Association, 2001), p. 8.

32. Lewis Thomas, *The Lives of a Cell* (New York: Viking 1974), pp. 81–86.

33. Bok, *Lying*, p. 63.

34. Howard Brody, *Placebos, and the Philosophy of Medicine* (Chicago, IL: University of Chicago Press, 1980), pp. 25–44, 96–114.

35. ANA, *Code for Nurses with Interpretive Statements*, p. 12.

36. Ibid.

37. This case is a variation of one reported in Kathleen A. Mahon and Sally J. Everson, "Moral Outrage—Nurse's Right or Responsibility: Ethics Rounds for Nurses," *Journal of Continuing Education* 10 (Number 3, 1979): 4.

38. ANA, *Code for Nurses with Interpretive Statements*, p. 12.

39. This fictitious case was revised for this edition.

40. See Jennifer M. Lee, Marc F. Botteman, Lars Nicklasson, David Cobden, Chris L. Pashos, "Needlestick Injury in Acute Care Nurses Caring for Patients with Diabetes Mellitus: A Retrospective Study," *Current Medical Research and Opinion* 21 (Number 5, 2005): 741–747, *cme.medscape.com,* Medscape, October 6, 2005, Web. February 6, 2009.

41. David K. Henderson, "HIV Postexposure Prophylaxis in the 21st Century," *Emerging Infectious Diseaes* 7 (March–April 2001): 2, *cdc.gov,* last reviewed December 22, 2001, CDC, March–April, 2001, Web. February 6, 2009; see also Susan Q. Wilburn, "Needlestick and Sharps Injury Prevention," *Online Journal of Issues in Nursing* 9 (September, 2004): 3, *nursingworld.org,* ANA, September 30, 2004, Web. February 6, 2009.

42. This case analysis focuses on the United States of America because the authors assume that students, nurses, and teachers in other parts of the world are familiar with their own professional codes of nursing ethics or the International Code and can apply our analysis to their own countries.

43. Based on a case reported by Barbara Sibbald, "Right to Refuse Work Becomes Another SARS Issue," *cmaj.ca,* Canadian Medical Association, July 22, 2003, Web. February 6, 2009; see also Carly Ruderman, C. Shawn Tracy, Cecile M. Bensimon, Mark Bernstein, Laura Hawryluck, Randi Zlotnik Shaul, and Ross E. G. Upshur, "On Pandemics and the Duty to Care: Whose Duty? Who Cares?" *BCM Medical Ethics* 7 (2006): 5, *biomedcentral.com,* Biomed Central, April 20, 2006, Web. February 6, 2009.

44. ANA, *Code for Nurses with Interpretive Statements*, p. 7.

45. Florence Nightingale, *Notes on Nursing: What It Is and What It Is Not* (Philadelphia, PA: J.B. Lippincott, facsimile of first edition, 1859), pp. 19–20.

46. American Nurses Association, *Position Statement: Risks and Responsibility in Providing Nursing Care-6/21/06, nursingworld.org,* ANA, n.d., Web. February 6, 2009.

47. Leslie Brennan and the editors, "The Battle against AIDS: A Report from the Nursing Front," *Nursing 88* 18 (April 1988): 60–64; "Nursing News, Nursing Attitudes," *Nursing 88* (September 1988): 10.

48. ANA, *Position Statement: Risks and Responsibility in Providing Nursing Care-6/21/06.*

49. Ibid.

50. American Nurses Association, *HIV/AIDS Nursing: Scope and Standards of Practice* (Silver Spring, MD, 2007), pp. 1–3.

51. Centers for Disease Control and Prevention, "Are Health Care Workers at Risk of Getting HIV on the Job?" *cdc.gov,* last modified: January 22, 2007, CDC, Web. February 6, 2009.

52. Times Health Guide, "Severe Acute Respiratory Syndrome SARS," *The New York Times,* January 29, 2007, Web. February 11, 2009.

53. Cathryn Murphy, "The 2003 SARS Outbreak: Global Challenges and Innovative Infection," *The Online Journal of Issues in Nursing, nursingworld.org,* ANA, January 31, 2006, Web. February 6, 2009.

54. Ibid.

55. Daniel K. Sokol, "Virulent Epidemics and Scope of Healthcare Workers' Duty of Care," *Emerging Infectious Diseases, cdc.gov*, CDC, August 2006, Web. February 6, 2009.

56. Laura A. Stokowski, "Nurses and Pandemic Influenza: Are We Ready?" *medscape.com*, Medscape, March 14, 2007, Web. February 10, 2009.

57. Sokol, "Virulent Epidemics and Scope of Healthcare Workers' Duty of Care."

58. Ibid.

59. "Anna Pou." *Wikipedia, The Free Encyclopedia, wikipedia.org,* Wikipedia, October 16, 2008, Web. February 7, 2009.

60. Joseph Goldstein, Anna Freud, and Albert J. Solnit, *Before the Best Interests of the Child* (New York: The Free Press, 1979), p. 5.

61. Ibid., p. 21.

Chapter 4

1. George Rosen, *From Medical Police to Social Medicine: Essays on the History of Health Care* (New York: Science History Publications, 1974), p. 296.

2. Catherine P. Murphy, "The Moral Situation in Nursing," in Elsie L. Bandman and Bertram Bandman, eds., *Bioethics and Human Rights* (Boston, MA: Little, Brown, 1978), p. 315.

3. Joann Ashley, *Hospitals, Paternalism, and the Role of the Nurse* (New York: Columbia University, Teachers College Press, 1976), pp. 8–15.

4. Beatrice J. Kalisch and Philip A. Kalisch, "An Analysis of the Sources of Physician-Nurse Conflict," *Journal of Nursing Administration* 7 (January 1977): 52.

5. Marjorie J. Stenberg, "The Search for a Conceptual Framework as a Philosophic Basis for Nursing Ethics: An Examination of Code, Contract, Context, and Covenant," *Military Medicine* (January 1977): 52.

6. Kalisch and Kalisch, "Sources of Physician-Nurse Conflict," pp. 51–52.

7. Murphy, "Moral Situation in Nursing," p. 315.

8. Leonard I. Stein, "The Doctor-Nurse Game," *American Journal of Nursing* 68 (January 1968): 101–105.

9. Patricia A. Prescott and Sally A. Bowen, "Physician-Nurse Relationships," *Annals of Internal Medicine* 103 (July 1985): 129.

10. Ibid.

11. Leonard I. Stein, David T. Watts, and Timothy Howell, "The Doctor-Nurse Game Revisited," *New England Journal of Medicine* 322 (February 22, 1990): 546–549.

12. Sondra Vazirani, Ron D. Hays, Martin F. Shapiro, and Marie Cowan, "Effect of a Multidisciplinary Intervention on Communication and Collaboration Among Physicians and Nurses," *American Journal of Critical Care* 14 (January 2005): 71–77, *medscape.com*, Medscape, March 24, 2005, Web. February 11, 2009.

13. See also Suzanne Gordon, *Nursing Against the Odds: How Health Care Cost Cutting, Media Stereotypes, and Medical Hubris Undermine Nurses and Patient Care* (Ithaca, NY: Cornell University Press, 2005), pp. 55–75.

14. Ada Jacox, "Role Restructuring in Hospital Nursing," in Linda H. Aiken and Susan Gortner, eds., *Nursing in the 1980s: Crises, Opportunities, Challenges* (Philadelphia, PA: J. B. Lippincott, 1982), p. 78; see also, H. Tristram Engelhardt,

Jr., "Physicians, Patients, Health Care Institutions—and the People in Between: Nurses," in Anne H. Bishop and John R. Scudder, Jr., eds., *Caring, Curing, Coping: Nurse Physician Patient Relationships* (Tuscaloosa, AL: University of Alabama Press, 1985), pp. 63–67.

15. Luci Young Kelly, *The Nursing Experience: Trends, Challenges, and Transitions* (New York: MacMillan, 1987), pp. 63–67.

16. Bonnie Bullough, "The Law and the Expanding Nursing Role," American *Journal of Public Health* 66 (March 1976): 249–254; Darlene M. Trandel-Korenchuck and Keith M. Trandel-Korenchuck, "How State Laws Recognize Advanced Nursing Practice," *Nursing Outlook* 26 (November 1978): 713–719; Clare LaBar, *Statutory Definitions of Nursing Practice and Their Conformity to Certain ANA Principles* (Kansas City, MO: American Nurses Association, 1984), pp. 1, 42, 51.

17. Mary Ann Lavin, Geralyn Meyer, and Judith H. Carlson, "A Review of the Use of Nursing Diagnosis in U.S. Nurse Practice Acts," *Nursing Diagnosis* (April–June, 1999), *findarticles.com*, Bnet Business Network, n.d., Web. February 11, 2009.

18. American College of Nurse Practitioners, "What is a Nurse Practitioner," *acnpweb.org*, ACNP, n.d., Web. February 18, 2008.

19. Ibid.

20. See Olivia A. Clarin, "Strategies to Overcome Barriers to Effective Nurse Practitioner and Physician Collaboration," *Journal for Nurse Practitioners* 3 (September, 2007): 538–548, *medscape.com*, Medscape, October 30, 2007, Web. February 11, 2009.

21. This case is based upon information from physical therapists Marsha Holsinger and Linda Coats, Mt. Pleasant, Iowa, May 15, 2007.

22. According to a nonpartisan policy research organization, "Medicine overall remains one of the most well-paid professions in the United States: At least half of all patient care physicians earned more than $170,000 in 2003, and physician average net income was about $203,000 ... Although surgical specialists have lost ground to inflation since the mid-1990s, they remain the highest earning of all physicians, with average incomes of $272,000 in 2003—29% higher than medical specialists and 86% higher than primary care physicians." Center for Studying Health System Change, "Physicians Lose Ground in Real Income Between 1995 and 2003," hschange.com, Health System Change, June 22, 2006, Web. February 11, 2009.

23. Example salary ranges: Registered Nurse (RN), $30,000 to $65,000; Licensed Practical Nurse (LPN), $25,000 to $50,000; Nurse Practitioner (NP), $50,000 to $80,000; Medical Technician, $25,000 to $55,000; Physical Therapist $40,000 to $70,000, reported in "Find a Healthcare Career in the San Diego Area, Job Descriptions & Salaries, *signonsandiego.com*, San Diego Union-Tribune, n.d., Web. March 1, 2008.

24. Jill Rollet and Sarah Lebo, "2007 Salary Survey Results: A Decade of Growth," *advanceweb.com*, *ADVANCE* for Nurse Practitioners, n.d., Web. March 6, 2008. The survey reported "that the average nurse practitioner salary rose 8.8% over the past 2 years, from $74,812 in 2005 to $81,397 in 2007. The increase is an impressive 55% over the decade."

25. Kalisch and Kalisch, "Sources of Physician-Nurse Conflict," p. 53.

26. Beth T. Ulrich, Ramón Lavandero, Karen A. Hart, Dana Woods, John Leggett, and Diane Taylor, "Critical Care Nurses' Work Environments: A Baseline

Status Report," *Critical Care Nurse* 26 (October 2006): 46–57, *ccn.aacnjournals. org, Critical Care Nurse*, n.d., Web. February 11, 2009.

27. For a discussion of the ideologies of domesticity and professionalism in nursing, see Linda Hughes, "Professionalizing Domesticity: A Synthesis of Selected Nursing Historiography," *Advances in Nursing Science* 12 (July, 1990): 25–31.

28. Lucie Young Kelly, *Dimensions of Professional Nursing*, 3rd ed. (New York: Macmillan, 1975), p. 169.

29. American Nurses Association, *Facts About Nursing*, 1986–1987 (Kansas City, MO: American Nurses Association, 1987), p. 24.

30. American Nurses Association, "About Nursing," *nursingworld.org*, ANA, n.d., Web. May 8, 2008.

31. See "What Can You Do to Shape a Better Image of Nursing? Take Action with Our Plan to Remedy the Nursing Image," *nursingadvocacy*, Center for Nursing Advocacy, n.d., Web. March 8, 2008; see also Bernice Buresh and Suzanne Gordon, *From Silence to Voice: What Nurses Know and Must Communicate to the Public*, 2nd ed. (Ithaca, NY: Cornell University Press Center, 2006).

32. Carol A. Garant, "The Process of Effecting Change in Nursing," *Nursing Forum* 17 (1978): 158.

33. See Coalition for Patients Rights, "Healthcare Professionals Urge Cooperative Patient Care; Oppose SOPP & AMA Resolution 814," *patientsright-scoalition.org*, Coalition for Patients Rights. January 15, 2008, Web. February 11, 2009. Organizations that have signed on to the joint statement: American Academy of Nurse Practitioners (AANP - Nurse Practitioners), American Association for Marriage and Family Therapy (AAMFT), American Association of Colleges of Nursing (AACN - Colleges), American Association of Critical-Care Nurses (AACN - Critical Care), American Association of Naturopathic Physicians (AANP - Naturopathic Physicians), American Association of Nurse Anesthetists (AANA), American Association of Occupational Health Nurses, Inc. (AAOHN), American Association of Acupuncture and Oriental Medicine (AAAOM), American Chiropractic Association (ACA), American College of Nurse-Midwives (ACNM), American College of Nurse Practitioners (ACNP), American Nephrology Nurses Association (ANNA), American Nurses Association (ANA), American Occupational Therapy Association (AOTA), American Physical Therapy Association (APTA), American Psychological Association (APA), American Psychiatric Nurses Association (APNA), American Speech-Language Hearing Association (ASHA), Association of Nurses in Aids Care (ANAC), Association of PeriOperative Registered Nurses (AORN), Association of Rehabilitation Nurses (ARN), Association of Schools of Allied Health Professions (ASAHP), Association of Women's Health, Obstetric and Neonatal Nurses (AWHONN), California Optometric Association (COA), Emergency Nurses Association (ENA), Hospice and Palliative Nurses Association (HPNA), Integrated Health Policy Consortium (IHPC), National Association of Clinical Nurse Specialists (NACNS), National Association of Nurse Practitioners in Women's Health (NPWH), National Association of Pediatric Nurse Practitioners (NAPNAP), National League for Nursing (NLN), National Nursing Centers Consortium (NNCC), National Organization of Nurse Practitioner Faculties (NONPF), Oncology Nursing Society (ONS), Preventive Cardiovascular Nurses Association (PCNA), Wound Ostomy and Continence Nurses Society (WOCN).

34. Bonnie Moore Randolph and Clydene Ross-Valliere, "Consciousness Raising Groups," *American Journal of Nursing* 79 (May 1979): 922–924; Angel Barron

McBride, "Editorial: Nursing and the Women's Movement," *Image: The Journal of Nursing Scholarship* 16 (Summer 1984): 66; see also Sheila Bunting and Jacquelyn C. Campbell, "Feminism and Nursing: Historical Perspectives," *Advances in Nursing Science* 12 (July 1990): 11–24; and Carole A Shea, "Feminism: A Failure in Nursing?" in Joanne Comi McCloskey and Helen Kennedy Grace, eds., *Current Issues in Nursing*, 3rd ed. (St. Louis, MO: C. V. Mosby, 1990), pp. 448–454.

35. See Dorothea F. Orem, *Nursing: Concepts of Practice* (New York: McGraw-Hill, 1971), pp. 47–50, 115.

36. From a case collected by Leah L. Curtin, Acting Director, National Center for Nursing Ethics (NCNE), Cincinnati, Ohio. It is one of 60 documented cases collected by NCNE.

37. Not only what a nurse says but the way in which she says it is important. While not advocating continuation of the doctor–nurse game, the authors recognize the need for nurses to be highly skillful in talking with certain physicians, especially those who cling to outmoded or stereotypical views of nursing.

38. This recommendation is based in part on a suggestion to authors from Betty Meyer, RN, CCRN, May 16, 1989. In the actual situation, Cheryl did choose to ask a third resident, who, after listening to her reasons, told her that she was correct and canceled the feeding order. Cheryl did not say why she did not try to ask her nursing supervisor.

39. This case was revised for this edition; for one physician's defense of an outlook similar to that attributed here to Dr. Rhodes, see Richard C. Bates, "It's Our Right to Pull the Plug," *Medical Economics* 54 (May 16, 1977): 163–166.

40. See also David Orentlicher, "The Supreme Court and Physician-Assisted Suicide: Rejecting Assisted Suicide but Embracing Euthanasia," *New England Journal of Medicine* 337 (October 23, 1997): 1236–1239; For a review from Belgian health professionals of the nurse's role in terminal sedation, see Patricia Claessens, Ellen Genbrugge, Rita Vannuffelen, Bert Broeckaert, Paul Schotsmans, and Johan Menten, "Palliative Sedation and Nursing: The Place of Palliative Sedation Within Palliative Nursing Care" *Nursing Journal of Hospice and Palliative Nursing* 9 (March/April 2007): 100–106, *medscape.com*, Medscape, December 6, 2007, Web. February 11, 2009.

41. For an illuminating account of the elements of patient autonomy, see Bruce L. Miller, "Autonomy and the Refusal of Lifesaving Treatment," *Hastings Center Report* 11 (August 1981): 22–28. Most accounts of autonomy in biomedical ethics focus on patient autonomy. We have benefited from Miller's analysis and we have drawn on parts of it in developing our account of ethical autonomy as it applies to heath care professionals. See also David L. Jackson and Stuart Youngner, "Patient Autonomy and 'Death with Dignity,'" *New England Journal of Medicine* 301 (August 23, 1979): 404–408.

42. Based on a case described by Sister A. Teresa Stanley, "Is It Ethical to Give Hope to a Dying Person?" *Nursing Clinics of North America* 14 (March 1979): 69–71.

43. Ibid., p. 75

44. Jolene L. Tuma, "Professional Misconduct" (Letter), *Nursing Outlook* 25 (September 1977): 546.

45. Sally Gadow, "Existential Advocacy: Philosophical Foundation of Nursing," in Stuart F. Spicker and Sally Gadow, eds., *Nursing: Images and Ideals, Opening Dialogue with the Humanities* (New York: Springer, 1980), pp. 90–91.

46. Stanley, "Is It Ethical to Give Hope to a Dying Person?" p.78.

47. Ibid., pp. 75–76.

48. Three years after Mrs. Tuma's license was suspended, she won a reversal of the suspension ruling when the state's Supreme Court made a unanimous decision in her favor. See http://biotech.law.lsu.edu/cases/pro_lic/Tuma_v_Board_of_Nursing.htm, viewed May 5, 2008. Although licensed, she did not immediately resume practice because she felt it "unwise," given the climate of her local medical-nursing community. The junior college did not reinstate her. "Nurse Upheld in Idaho Court Case," *Concern for Dying* 5 (Fall 1979): 7.

49. See Coalition for Patients Rights, "Healthcare Professionals Urge Cooperative Patient Care; Oppose SOPP & AMA Resolution 814."

50. This revision is based on an actual situation.

51. See Mila Ann Aroskar, "Establishing Limits to Professional Autonomy: Whose Responsibility?" in Nora K. Bell, ed., *Who Decides? Conflicts of Rights in Health Care* (Clifton, NJ: Humana Press, 1982), pp. 67–78; for a brief review of the emergence of collaboration and interprofessional teamwork in health care, see Theresa J. K. Drinka and Phillip G. Clark, *Health Care Teamwork: Interdisciplinary Practice and Teaching* (Westport, CT: Auburn House, 2000), pp. 6–9.

52. John Ladd, "Some Reflections on Authority and the Nurse," in Spicker and Gadow, eds., *Nursing: Images and Ideals*, 171f.

53. Ibid., p. 172.

54. Samuel Gorovitz, "Can Physicians Mind Their Own Business and Still Practice Medicine?" in Bell, ed., *Who Decides? Conflicts of Rights in Health Care*, p. 89f.

55. See Christine Mitchell, "Integrity in Interprofessional Relationships," in George J. Agich, ed., *Responsibility in Health Care* (Dordrecht: D. Reidel, 1981), pp. 163–184.

56. American Association of Critical-Care Nurses, "AACN Position Statement: Moral Distress," aacn.org, AACN, Jan. 2006, Web. 9 Feb. 2009; See also Pauline W. Chen, "When Doctors and Nurses Can't Do the Right Thing," *New York Times*, The New York, February 5, 2009. Web. February 7, 2009.

57. Arthur Kuflik, "Morality and Compromise," in J. Roland Pennock and John W. Chapman, eds., *Compromise in Ethics, Law, and Politics: Nomos XXXI* (New York: New York University Press, 1979), p. 49.

58. Ibid., p. 51.

59. Isaiah Berlin, *Four Essays on Liberty* (Oxford: Oxford University Press, 1969), p. 1.

60. For a more thorough analysis of these considerations, see Martin Benjamin, *Splitting the Difference: Compromise and Integrity in Ethics and Politics* (Lawrence, KS: Univerity Press of Kansas, 1990).

61. This revised case is based upon information from a practicing nurse.

62. John Rawls, *A Theory of Justice* (Cambridge, MA.: Harvard University Press, 1971), pp. 368–371.

63. This fictitious case was revised for this volume; see The American College of Obstetricians and Gynecologists, update Committee Opinion #360, "Sex Selection," (February, 2007), http://www.acog.org/from_home/publications/ethics/co360.pdf.

64. James F. Childress, "Appeals to Conscience," *Ethics* 89 (1978–1979): 316–317.

65. Bernard Williams, "A Critique of Utilitarianism," in J. J. C. Smart and Bernard Williams, eds., *Utilitarianism For and Against* (Cambridge: Cambridge University Press, 1973), pp. 115–117.

66. Childress, "Appeals to Conscience," pp. 318–321.

67. The child's parents deny the Holocaust occurred and decorate their home with swastikas. Larry McShane, "Happy Birthday, Adolf Hitler! Boy with nazi name denied ShopRite cake," *NYdailynews.com, New York Daily News*, December 16, 2008. Web. February 9, 2009.

68. Herbert Fingarette, *Self-Deception* (London: Routledge and Kegan Paul, 1969) especially pp. 138–139.

69. This case was revised for this edition.

70. Regulations concerning advance directive and DNR orders vary from state to state. For two examples, see Bradley Geller, "Advance Directives: Planning for Medical Care in the Event of Loss of Decision-Making Ability," *www.michbar.org*, State Bar of Michigan, n.d., Web. May 10, 2008; and Jack R. Puffenberger, Lucas County [Ohio] Probate Court Judge, "Do Not Resuscitate (DNR) Orders," *lucas-co-probate-ct.org*, Lucas Couty Probate Court, October 1, 2003, Web. February 11, 2008.

71. Robert M. Veatch, *Death, Dying, and the Biological Revolution: Our Last Quest for Responsibility* (New Haven, CT: Yale University Press, 1976), pp. 116–163; Jackson and Youngner, "Patient Autonomy and 'Death with Dignity,'" pp. 404–408.

72. The rule was supported by opponents of abortion including the United States Conference of Catholic Bishops and the Catholic Health Association, which represents Catholic hospitals. It was opposed by the National Association of Chain Drug Stores, the American Hospital Association, and the American Medical Association, among others. David Stout, "Medical 'Conscience Rule' Is Issued," *New York Times,* New York Times, 19 December 19, 2008, Web. February 9, 2009.

73. Stout, "Medical 'Conscience Rule' Is Issued."

74. The seven states were Connecticut, California, Illinois, Massachusetts, New Jersey, Oregon, and Rhode Island. "7 States Sue Government Over U.S. Abortion Rule," *New York Times*, New York Times, January 16, 2009. Web. February 9, 2009.

75. Planned Parenthood Federation of America and the National Family Planning Reproductive Health Association quickly acted to file parallel lawsuits against the rule, and several members of the House of Representatives introduced legislation aimed at preventing the rule's implementation. "7 States Sue Government Over U.S. Abortion Rule."

76. David Templeton, "11th-Hour Abortion Rule Draws 200K Protests," *Sun Times*, January 5, 2009, *freerepublic.com*, Free Republic, January 6, 2009, Web. February 14, 2009.

77. David Stout, "Obama Moves to Undo 'Conscience' Rule for Health Workers," *New York Times*, New York Times, February 27, 2009, Web. February 27, 2009.

78. "7 States Sue Government Over U.S. Abortion Rule."

79. Edmund D. Pellegrino, "The Ethics of Team Care: Some Notes on the Morality of Collective Decision Making" (presented to the American Cancer Society, second National Conference on Cancer Nursing, St. Louis, Missouri, May 9,1977), p. 6.

80. This case is based on an actual situation.

81. Pellegrino, "The Ethics of Team Care: Some Notes on the Morality of Collective Decision Making," pp. 7–8.

82. Ibid., p. 9.

83. The notion of an act that is excusable, though not justifiable, is important in a wide variety of contexts in ethics and the law. People who violate laws or moral principles under conditions of duress may be excused for what they do, even though their actions cannot, strictly speaking, be justified. A harried parent, for example, who loses his or her temper and yells at a persistently cranky or annoying child, may be excused for what he or she does even though it cannot be justified. So too, if a nurse "loses her cool" after her reasonable attempts to correct a situation have been unsuccessful, her exasperated outburst, though perhaps not justified and even counterproductive, may under the circumstances be excused.

Chapter 5

1. Case based upon information from a rural community hospital director of nursing.

2. Robert E. Riegel, *American Women: A Story of Social Change* (Rutherford, NJ: Fairleigh Dickinson University Press, 1970), p. 182; U.S. Department of Health and Human Services, "The Registered Nurse Population: Findings from the 2004 National Sample Survey of Registered Nurses," *bhpr.hrsa.gov,* Heath Resources and Services Administration, n.d., Web. February 12, 2009.

3. Vern V. Bullough and Bonnie Bullough, *The Care of the Sick: The Emergence of Modern Nursing* (New York: Prodist, 1978), p. 192; for an example, see Joy Curtis, "Final Progress Report: Minority Project in Nursing, 1972–1977, A Study Related to the Admission, Counseling, Program Planning and Instruction of Minority Students Who Have Indicated an Interest in Nursing," supported by NU 00003–05 ORD 17603, Division of Nursing, United States Public Health Service, Department of Health, Education, and Welfare, Michigan State University, 1977; see also J. A. Sutherland, M. J. Hamilton, and N. Goodman, "Affirming At-Risk Minorities for Success (ARMS): Retention, Graduation, and Success on the NCLEX-RN," *Journal of Nursing Education* 46 (August 2007): 347–353.

4. Davina J. Gosnell, "The 1965 Entry Into Practice Proposal – Is It Relevant Today?" *Online Journal of Issues in Nursing,* 7 No. #2, *Nursingworld.org*, ANA, May 31, 2002, Web. February 12, 2009.

5. Florence Nightingale, *Notes on Nursing: What It Is and What It Is Not* (Philadelphia, PA: J. B. Lippincott, facsimile of first edition, 1859), p. 6; Virginia Henderson and Gladys Nite, *Principles and Practice of Nursing* (New York: Macmillan, 1978), pp. 15–36; Ann Marriner Tomey and Martha Raile Alligood, eds., *Nursing Theorists and Their Work*, 6th ed. (St. Louis, MO: Mosby/Elsevier, 2006).

6. The ANA reported that "over 2.4 million of the nation's 2.9 million RNs were employed in 2004, about one-quarter of them on a part-time basis," ANA, "About Nursing," *Nursingworld.org,* ANA, n.d., Web. May 8, 2008.

7. Phil McPeck, "Membership in Nursing Associations Offers RNs a Strong Professional Voice, Opportunities for Growth ," *Nurseweek*, NurseWeek, October 29, 2001. Web. February 12, 2009.

8. Note, too, the distinction between caring *about* and caring *for* (Chapter 2, Section 4) in this case. While Lisa may care about her patients no less than any of the other nurses, she is less able than they to safely and effectively care for them.

9. ANA, "About Nursing."

10. Dee Ann Gillies, *Nursing Management: A Systems Approach*, 2nd ed. (Philadelphia, PA: W. B. Saunders, 1989), pp. 232–235; Marian Keels Bennett and Janice Parks Hylton, "Modular Nursing: Partners in Professional Practice," *Nursing Management* 21 (March 1990): 20–24; Jean Ann Seago, "Chapter 39. Nurse Staffing, Models of Care Delivery, and Interventions," in Kathryn M. McDonald, *Making Health Care Safer: A Critical Analysis of Patient Safety Practices, Evidence Report/Technology Assessment Number 43,* (University of California at San Francisco—Stanford University Evidence-based Practice Center, July 20, 2001), *ahrq.gov,* Agency for Healthcare Research and Quality, n.d., Web. February 12, 2009; see also Roberta Kaplow and Kevin D. Reed, "The AACN Synergy Model for Patient Care: A Nursing Model as a Force of Magnetism" *Nursing Economics* (Jan–Feb. 2008): 17–25, *Medscape.com,* Medscape, April 23, 2008, Web. February 13, 2009.

11. American Nurses Association (ANA) and the National Council of State Boards of Nursing (NCSBN), "Joint Statement on Delegation,"(2005), ncsbn.org, NCSBN, n.d., Web. February 13, 2009.

12. Ibid.

13. American Nurses Association (ANA), *Code for Nurses with Interpretive Statements* (Washington, D.C.: American Nurses Association, 2001), p. 12. See also, National Federation of Practical Nurses, Inc., "Nursing Practice Standards for the Licensed Practical /Vocational Nurse," (Garner, NY: NFLPN, Adopted 1961 and revised 1979), *nflpn.org,* NFLPN, n.d., Web. June 1, 2008.

14. Being wronged differs from being harmed. Someone can be wronged without being harmed (e.g., being slandered and no one you know ever finding out about it or being slandered after you are dead when no physical or psychological harm results) and someone can be harmed without being wronged (e.g., being accidentally or inadvertently physically or psychologically harmed). It is possible most of Lisa's mistakes did not lead to harm to patients. Still, if the mistakes were due to negligence on her part, patients were wronged (even if not actually or literally harmed).

15. S. I. Benn, "Abortion, Infanticide and Respect for Persons" in Joel Feinberg, ed., *The Problem of Abortion*, 2nd ed. (Belmont, CA.: Wadsworth, 1984), p. 141.

16. R. S. Peters, "Respect for Persons," in James Rachels, ed., *Understanding Moral Philosophy* (Encino, CA: Dickenson, 1976), pp. 205–209.

17. ANA, *Code for Nurses with Interpretive Statements*, p. 22.

18. Ibid., p. 10.

19. Ibid., p. 7.

20. Margaret Adams, "The Compassion Trap," in Vivian Gornick and Barbara K. Moran, eds., *Women in Sexist Society: Studies in Power and Powerlessness* (New York: New American Library, 1971), pp. 555–575.

21. Joann Ashley, *Hospitals, Paternalism, and the Role of the Nurse* (New York: Columbia University, Teachers College Press, 1976), pp. 16–18.

22. This case was prepared by Linda Rowell, RN, BSN, while she was a student at Michigan State University.

23. Sissela Bok, *Secrets: On the Ethics of Concealment and Revelation* (New York: Pantheon Books, 1982), pp. 119–124.

24. In the actual case, Jerome's coworker did not discuss his behavior with the supervisor, and Jerome's problems continued for nearly a year before their cause—a deepening addiction to a tranquilizer—resulted in his being dismissed from the hospital.

25. This revision was written for this edition.

26. Herbert Morris, "Persons and Punishment," in Rachels, ed., *Understanding Moral Philosophy*, pp. 210–227.

27. For an interesting review of a pioneering study of baby-blinding and interviews with persons blinded during the first weeks of life, see David Brown, "Establishing Proof," *Washington Post, washingtonpost.com*, Washington Post, April 19, 2005, Web. February 13, 2009.

28. See Ronald Dworkin, *Taking Rights Seriously* (Cambridge, MA: Harvard University Press, 1977), pp. 206–222.

Chapter 6

1. This fictitious case was written for this edition.

2. American Nurses Association, *Code of Ethics with Interpretive Statements* (Washington, D.C.: American Nurses Association, 2001), *Nursingworld.com*, ANA, 2005, Web. February 17, 2009.

3. John Ladd, "The Ethics of Participation," in J. Roland Pennock and John W. Chapman, eds., *Participation in Politics* (New York: Lieber-Atherton, 1975), p. 121.

4. Amitai Etzioni, *Participation in Politics* (Englewood Cliffs, NJ: Prentice-Hall, 1964), p. 3.

5. See Elena O. Siegel, Heather M. Young, Pamela H. Mitchell, and Sarah E. Shannon, "Nurse Preparation and Organizational Support for Supervision of Unlicensed Assistive Personnel in Nursing Homes: A Qualitative Exploration," *The Gerontologist* 48 (2008): 453–463, *gerontologist.gerontologyjournals.org*. The Gerontologist, 2008, Web. February 17, 2009.

6. The historical summary that follows is drawn from Philip A. Kalisch and Beatrice J. Kalisch, *American Nursing: A History*, 4th ed. (Philadelphia, PA: Lippincott, 2004), pp. 427–433; Vern L. Bullough and Bonnie Bullough, *The Care of the Sick: The Emergence of Modern Nursing* (New York: Prodist, 1978), pp. 205–212; and Catherine Ecock Connelly, Lois Kuhn, Roanne Muldoon, and Nancy Adams Wieker, "To Strike or Not to Strike: A Debate on the Ethics of Strikes by Nurses," *Supervisor Nurse* 10 (January 1979): 52, 56.

7. Murtha Cullina, "NLRB Decides When Charge Nurses are Supervisors for Purposes of Unionization (Again)," *hg.org*, HG.org, October 11, 2006, Web. February 17, 2009; see also, American Nurses Association, "ANA Rejects NLRB Decision to Block Nurses' Freedom to Unionize," *nursingworld.org*, ANA, October 3, 2006, Web. February 17, 2009.

8. William N. Nelson, "Special Rights, General Rights and Social Justice," *Philosophy & Public Affairs* 3 (Summer 1979): 52, 56.

9. See, for example, Michigan Nurses Association, "New Contract at West Shore Medical Center Includes Staffing Language for RNs," *minurses.org*, Michigan Nurses Association, September 25, 2008, Web. February 17, 2009.

10. For a discussion of different solutions to nursing shortages, see Karen W. Budd, Linda S. Warino, and Mary Ellen Patton, "Traditional and Non-Traditional

Collective Bargaining: Strategies to Improve the Patient Care Environment," *Online Journal of Issues in Nursing* 9 (Jan. 2004), *medscape.com,* Medscape, November 3, 2004, Web. February 18, 2009.

11. See Ellen Fox, Sarah Myers, and Robert A. Pearlman, "Ethics Consultation in United States Hospitals: A National Survey," *American Journal of Bioethics* 7 (February 2007): 13–25.

12. "Terri Schiavo case," *wikipedia.org,* Wikipedia, February 10, 2009, Web. February 17, 2009.

13. This is an updated and revised version of a case originally reported by Lynell Mickelsen, "The Ordeal of Residency," *Detroit Free Press,* May 5, 1985.

14. See Kevin B. O'Reilly, "Willing, but Waiting: Hospital Ethics Committees," *ama-assn.org,* AMA, January 28, 2008, Web. February 17, 2009.

15. Dolly Katz, "MD Suspended from Operating Room," *Detroit Free Press,* October 12, 1984.

16. ANA, "Whistleblowing/Patient advocacy. Protections for Nurses," *nursingworld.org,* ANA, 2007. Web. February 17, 2009.

17. Sissela Bok, *Secrets: On the Ethics of Concealment and Revelation* (New York: Pantheon, 1982), p. 214.

18. Ibid., p. 212.

19. Ibid., p. 213.

20. George Annas, "Baby Doe Redux: Doctors as Child Abusers," *Hastings Center Report* 13 (October 1983): 26.

21. Leah Curtin, "The Babies Doe: Common Sense and Common Decency," *Nursing Management* 14 (December 1983): 26.

22. Federal regulations concerning handicapped newborns have since been revised. Nurses are no longer explicitly placed in an institutionalized whistle-blowing role.

23. Bok, *Secrets*, p. 227.

24. See, for example, Debra Wood, "Whistle-Blowing Nurse Gets Fired, Sues Employer," *nurse.zone.com,* Nurse Zone, 2008, Web. November 25, 2008.

25. See, for example, Patricia Murphy, "Deciding to Blow the Whistle," *American Journal of Nursing* (September 1981): 1691f.

26. Myron Glazer, "Ten Whistleblowers and How They Fared," *Hastings Center Report* 13 (December 1983): 33–41; see S. McDonald and K. Ahern, "Professional Consequences of Whistleblowing by Nurses," *Journal of Professional Nursing* 16 (November–December 2000), *ncbi.nlm.nih.gov,* PubMed, n.d., Web. February 17, 2008; see also Vicki D. Lachman, "Whistleblowers: Troublemakers or Virtuous Nurses?" *Dermatology Nursing* 20 (2008): 390–393, *medscape.com,* Medscape, November 25, 2008, Web. February 17, 2009.

27. Bok, *Secrets,* p. 221.

28. Ibid.

29. ANA, "Whistleblower Protection," *nursingworld.org,* ANA, 2008, Web. February 17, 2009.

30. ANA, "Whistleblowing/Patient Advocacy. Protections for Nurses."

31. For a useful summary of relevant considerations, see Alfred G. Feliu, "Thinking of Blowing the Whistle?" *American Journal of Nursing* 83 (November 1983): 1541f., see also ANA, "Toward an Ethical Defense of Whistle Blowing" *nursingworld.org,* ANA, Fall 2001, Web. February 17, 2009.

32. Anne Wilkinson, Neil Wenger, and Lisa R. Shugarman, "Literature Review on Advance Directives," U. S. Department of Health and Human Services (June 2007), *aspe.hhs.gov,* HHS, n.d., Web. February 23, 2009.

33. Ibid.

34. This case has been adapted from one reported by Janice Olson, "To Treat or to Allow to Die: An Ethical Dilemma in Gerontological Nursing," *Journal of Gerontological Nursing* 7 (March 1981): 154lf.

35. See, for example, Bruce L. Miller, "Autonomy and the Refusal of Lifesaving Treatment, *Hastings Center Report* 11 (August 1981): 22–28; and David L. Jackson and Stuart Youngner, "Patient Autonomy and 'Death with Dignity,'" *New England Journal of Medicine* 301 (August 23, 1979): 404–408.

36. Physician Orders for Life-Sustaining Treatment Paradigm, *ohsu.edu,* Center for Ethics in Health Care, Oregon Health & Science University, 2008, Web. February 17, 2009; See also, S. E. Hickman, C. P. Sabatino, A. H. Moss, and J. Nester Wehrle, "The POLST (Physician Orders for Life-Sustaining Treatment) Paradigm to Improve End-of-Life-Care: Potential State Legal Barriers to Implementation," *Journal of Law, Medicine and Ethics* 36 (2008): 119–140; J. L. Meyers, C. Moore, A. McGrory, J. Sparr, and M. Ahern, "Use of the Physician Orders for Life-Sustaining Treatment (POLST) Form to Honor the Wishes of Nursing Home Residents for End of Life Care: Preliminary Results of a Washington State Pilot Project," *Journal of Gerontological Nursing* 30 (2004): 37–46; and T. A. Schmidt, S. E. Hickman, S. W. Tolle, and H. S. Brooks, "The Physician Orders for Life-Sustaining Treatment (POLST) Paradigm: Oregon Emergency Medical Technicians' Practical Experiences and Attitudes," *Journal of the American Geriatrics Society* 52 (2004): 1430–1434.

37. POLST, "The National POLST Paradigm Initiative Task Force Newsletter," *ohsu.edu,* Oregon Health & Science University, September 2008, Web. February 17, 2009.

38. See Jane E. Brody, "Putting Muscle Behind End-of-Life Wishes," *New York Times,* New York Times, February 24, 2009. Web. February 24, 2009.

39. POLST, "The National POLST Paradigm Initiative Task Force," *ohsu.edu,* Oregon Health & Science University, n.d., Web. February 16, 2009.

40. Valerie C. Danesh, Donna Malvey, and Myron D. Fottler, "Hidden Workplace Violence: What Your Nurses May Not Be Telling You," *Health Care Manager* 27 (October/December 2008): 357–363, *ncbi.nlm.nih.gov,* Pub Med, n.d., Web. February 17, 2009; for an unhidden example of violence, see "Mich. Nursing Home: Patient Hit Nurse with Hammer," *chicagotribune.com,* Chicago Tribune, February 16, 2009, Web. February 17, 2009.

41. This fictitious case is based on information from David Tuller, "Nurses Step Up Efforts to Protect Against Attacks." *New York Times,* New York Times, July 8, 2008, Web. February 17, 2009.

42. See U.S. Department of Labor Occupational Safety & Health Administration, "Hospital eTool: Emergency Department (ED) Module," *osha.gov,* OSHA, November 12, 2008, Web. December 27, 2008.

43. *New York Times,* September 23, 1984 and March 20, 1985.

44. In certain situations, however, complications for professional providers can occur. For an example of legal problems experienced by a physician who as a parent disconnected his child's ventilator, see "Father Acquitted in Death of His

Premature Baby," *New York Times,* New York Times, February 3, 1995. Web. February 16, 2009.

Chapter 7

1. This case is based upon an editorial by Lucie S. Kelly, "When Nurses Ration Patient Care," *Nursing Outlook* 33 (May/June 1985): 123.

2. Mila Ann Aroskar, "The Interface of Ethics and Politics in Nursing," *Nursing Outlook* 35 (November/December 1987): 269.

3. Ibid.

4. See, for example, Nancy L. Falk and Elizabeth S. Chong, "Beyond the Bedside: Nurses a Critical Force in the Macroallocation of Resources," *Online Journal of Issues in Nursing* 13 (Number 2, May 2008), *nursingworld.org*, ANA, May 2008, Web. February 18, 2009.

5. Problems in diagnosis and poor nursing home records make it difficult to determine exact figures. Joy Hirsch, "Raising Consciousness," *The Journal of Clinical Investigation* 115 (May 2005): 1102–1103.

6. This case is based on several contemporary reports and Daniel Callahan, *Setting Limits: Medical Goals in an Aging Society with "A Response to my Critics"* (Washington: Georgetown University Press, 2003); and Leonard M. Fleck, *Just Caring: Health Care Rationing and Democratic Deliberation* (New York: Oxford University Press, 2009).

7. "National Health Expenses Fact Sheet," Centers for Medicare & Medicaid Services, *cms.hhs.gov*, HHS, last modified: 01/06/2009, Web. February 21, 2009.

8. Ibid.

9. Ibid.

10. Robert M. Sade, "Is There a Right to Health Care?" *New England Journal of Medicine* 285 (December 2, 1971): 1288–1292.

11. Norman Daniels, *Just Health Care* (New York: Oxford University Press, 1985), pp. 36–58.

12. James Roosevelt, Jr., "Breaking the Cycle of Waste in Healthcare," *Boston Globe* (October 22, 2008).

13. Dartmouth Institute for Health Policy & Clinical Practice, "Improving Quality and Curbing Health Care Spending: Opportunities for the Congress and the Obama Administration," (December 2008): i.

14. Reed Abelson, "Medicare Spending Still Varies Widely by Region," *New York Times,* New York Times, February 26, 2009. Web. February 26, 2009.

15. Ibid. p. ii.

16. Leonard M. Fleck, *Just Caring: Health Care Rationing and Democratic Deliberation* (New York: Oxford University Press, 2009), p. x.

17. Daniel Callahan, *What Kind of Life: The Limits of Medical Progress* (New York: Simon and Schuster, 1990), p. 63.

18. Ibid., p. 64f.

19. Ichiro Kawachi, "Why the United States Is Not Number One in Health," in James A. Morone and Lawrence R. Jacobs, eds., *Healthy, Wealthy, and Fair: Health Care and the Good Society* (New York: Oxford University Press, 2005), p. 20.

20. Ibid., pp. 29–33.

21. DeNavas-Walt, C. B. Proctor, and J. Smith, "Income, Poverty, and Health Insurance in the United States: 2007," *U.S. Census Bureau* (August 2008).

22. National Coalition on Health Care, "Health Insurance Costs," *nchc.org*, NCHC, n.d., Web. February 21, 2009.

23. President's Commission for the Study of Ethical Problems in Medicine and Biomedical and Biobehavioral Research, *Securing Access to Health Care*, vol. 1 (Washington, D.C.: U.S. Government Printing Office, 1983), p. 111.

24. Ibid., p. 20.

25. *New York Times*, January 3, 2008.

26. We are grateful to Carl Cohen of the University of Michigan for having called this to our attention.

27. Victor R. Fuchs, "The 'Rationing' of Medical Care," *New England Journal of Medicine* 311 (December 13, 1984): 1572.

28. Committee for Counting the Medically Indigent, "1986 Health Insurance Coverage Survey," Description of Findings (Portland, OR, 1986).

29. Ralph Crawshaw et al., "Oregon Health Decisions: An Experiment with Informed Community Consent," *Journal of the American Medical Association* 254 (December 13, 1985.)

30. Bruce Jennings, "A Grassroots Movement in Bioethics," *Hastings Center Report* 18 (June/July 1988): special supplement. See also the collection of articles assembled by Jennings under the heading "Grassroots Bioethics Revisited: Health Care Priorities and Community Values," *Hastings Center Report* 20 (September/October 1990): 3213–3216.

31. Timothy Egan, "Oregon Seeks to Revive Health Care 'Rationing' Plan," *New York Times* (August 14, 1992).

32. Jonathan Oberlander, Theodore Marmor, and Lawrence Jacobs, "Rationing Medical Care: Rhetoric and Reality in the Oregon Health Plan," *Canadian Medical Association Journal* 164 (May 29, 2001): 1584.

33. Jennifer Fisher Wilson, "Oregon Surpasses Struggles of Early Reform and Develops a Road Map for Future Success," *Annals of Internal Medicine* 149 (July 15, 2008): 149.

34. Ibid.

35. Cecilia Capuzzi and Jeanne Bowden, "Rationing Health Care: The Oregon Story," in Diana J. Mason, Judith K. Leavitt, and Mary W. Chaffee, eds., *Policy & Politics in Nursing and Health Care*, 4th ed. (Philadelphia, PA: W. B. Saunders, 2002): p. 302.

36. Ibid., p. 309.

37. This oversimplified case has been constructed especially for this book.

38. The distinction between something's being unfortunate and its being unfair is cogently drawn by H. Tristram Engelhardt, Jr., "Allocating Scarce Medical Resources and the Availability of Organ Transplantation," *New England Journal of Medicine* 311 (July 5, 1984): 66–71.

39. Paul T. Menzel, *Strong Medicine: The Ethical Rationing of Health Care* (New York: Oxford University Press, 1990), p. 10. "In something very close to the detail hypothesized here," Menzel adds in an endnote, "Group Health Cooperative of Puget Sound considered heart and liver transplants in 1985–1986. The outcome of their long and complex process was board of trustees approval of coverage for heart transplants and for liver transplants in children with biliary atresia but not coverage of liver transplants for adults."

40. Thomas Scanlon, "Contractualism and Utilitarianism," in Amartya Sen and Bernard Williams, eds., *Utilitarianism and Beyond* (Cambridge: Cambridge University Press, 1982), p. 110.

41. Menzel, *Strong Medicine*, p. 10.

42. See Norman Daniels, *Am I My Parents' Keeper?* (New York: Oxford University Press, 1988), for an argument to the effect that in choosing among rationing systems we must consider how each will affect us over the course of an entire life span.

43. Ibid.

44. Norman Daniels, "Why Saying No to Patients in the United States is So Hard: Cost Containment, Justice, and Provider Autonomy," *New England Journal of Medicine* 314 (May 22, 1986): 1380–1383.

45. William B. Schwartz and Henry J. Aaron, "The Achilles Heel of Health Care Rationing," *New York Times*, July 9, 1990.

46. Fleck, *Just Caring: Health Care Rationing and Democratic Deliberation.* See, especially, Chapter 5, "Rational Democratic Deliberation: Scope and Structure." (New York: Oxford University Press, 2009).

47. There is nothing about such a system, we should note, that precludes the availability of higher levels of health care or more amenities for those with the desire and financial resources to pay for them, out-of-pocket or with additional insurance. The similarity with access to education is again instructive. That the system aspires to provide access to a decent minimum of education for all, regardless of ability to pay, does not preclude access to higher levels of education (private schools) for those who value and can pay for them.

48. Jennings, *A Grassroots Movement in Bioethics.*

49. Capuzzi and Bowden, p. 302.

50. Callahan, *What Kind of Life*, p. 100.

51. Ibid., p. 145.

52. Barbara Redman, "Mobilizing Nurses for Health Care Reform," *The American Nurse* (January 1991): 4.

53. *New York Times*, January 10, 1991.

54. We leave it to the reader to imagine the conversation about this set of questions that might take place among Livia, Ursula, and Renee of Chapter 2, Section 1.

55. Leonard M. Fleck, "Decisions of Justice and Health Care," *Journal of Gerontological Nursing* 13 (March 1987): 45.

Appendix A

1. ICN Code, pp. 5–9.

SUGGESTIONS FOR FURTHER READING

(This list is designed to supplement sources identified in the text. Therefore footnoted works have been omitted.)

1. Philosophical Analysis and Reasoning

Browne, M. Neil, and Keeley, Stuart M. *Asking the Right Questions.* 9th ed., Upper Saddle River, NJ: Prentice-Hall, 2010.

Govier, Trudy. *A Practical Study of Argument.* 7th ed., Belmont, CA: Wadsworth, 2009.

Ruggiero, Vincent Ryan. *Thinking Critically about Ethics.* 7th ed., New York: McGraw-Hill, 2008.

——. *The Art of Thinking.* 9th ed., New York: Longman, 2009.

Weston, Anthony, *A 21st Century Ethical Toolbook.* 2nd ed., New York: Oxford University Press, 2007.

——. *A Rulebook for Arguments.* 4th ed., Indianapolis, IN: Hackett Publishing, 2008.

2. Ethical Theory

Becker, Lawrence C., and Becker, Charlotte B., eds. *Encyclopedia of Ethics.* 2nd ed., New York: Routledge, 2001.

Cahn, Steven M. *Exploring Ethics: An Introductory Anthology.* New York: Oxford University Press, 2008.

Daniels, Norman. *Justice and Justification: Reflective Equilibrium in Theory and Practice.* Cambridge: Cambridge University Press, 1996.

Lindemann, Hilde. *An Invitation to Feminist Ethics.* New York: McGraw-Hill, 2006.

Pojman, Louis P., and Tramel, Peter, eds. *Moral Philosophy: A Reader.* 4th ed., Indianapolis, IN: Hackett Publishing, 2009.

Rachels, James, and Rachels, Stuart. *The Elements of Moral Philosophy.* 6th ed., New York: McGraw-Hill, 2009.

Singer, Peter. *Practical Ethics.* 2nd ed., New York: Cambridge University Press, 1999.

Smart, J. J. C., and Williams, Bernard. *Utilitarianism: For and Against.* Cambridge: Cambridge University Press, 1973.

3. Bioethics

Andre, Judith. *Bioethics as Practice*. Chapel Hill, NC: University of North Carolina Press, 2002.

Beauchamp, Tom L., and Childress, James F. *Principles of Biomedical Ethics*. 6th ed., New York: Oxford University Press, 2008.

Brody, Howard. *Stories of Sickness*. 2nd ed., New York: Oxford University Press, 2003.

——.*The Future of Bioethics*. New York: Oxford University Press, 2009.

Buchanan, Allen, Brock, Dan W., Daniels, Norman, and Wikler, Daniel. *From Chance to Choice: Genetics and Justice*. Cambridge: Cambridge University Press, 2000.

Eckenwiler, Lisa A., and Cohn, Felicia G., eds. *The Ethics of Bioethics: Mapping the Moral Landscape*. Baltimore, MD: Johns Hopkins University Press, 2007.

Jonsen, Albert, Siegler, Mark, and Winslade, William, eds. *Clinical Ethics: A Practical Approach to Ethical Decisions in Clinical Medicine*. 6th ed., New York: McGraw-Hill, 2006.

Levine, Carol, ed. *Taking Sides: Clashing Views on Bioethical Issues*. 12th ed., New York: McGraw-Hill, 2008.

Lindemann, Hilde, Verkerk, Marian, and Walker, Margaret Urban, eds. *Naturalized Bioethics: Toward Responsible Knowing and Practice*. Cambridge: Cambridge University Press, 2008.

Mappes, Thomas A., and DeGrazia, David, eds. *Biomedical Ethics*. 6th ed., New York: McGraw-Hill, 2006.

McGee, Glenn, ed. *Pragmatic Bioethics*. 2nd ed., Cambridge, MA: MIT Press, 2003.

Momeyer, Richard W. *Confronting Death*. Bloomington, IN: Indiana University Press, 1988.

Nelson, James Lindemann. *Hippocrates' Maze*. Lanham, MD: Rowman & Littlefield, 2003.

Pence, Gregory. *Medical Ethics: Accounts of the Cases That Shaped and Define Medical Ethics*. 5th ed., New York: McGraw-Hill, 2007.

Post, Stephen Garrard, ed. *Encyclopedia of Bioethics*. 3rd ed., New York: Macmillan Reference, 2004.

Quill, Timothy E., and Battin, Margaret P., eds. *Physician-Assisted Dying: The Case for Palliative Care and Patient Choice*. Baltimore, MD: Johns Hopkins University Press, 2004.

Scully, Jackie Leach. *Disability Bioethics: Moral Bodies, Moral Difference*. Lanham, MD: Rowman & Littlefield, 2008.

Singer, Peter, and Viens, A. M. eds. *The Cambridge Textbook of Bioethics*. Cambridge: Cambridge University Press, 2008.

Steinbock, Bonnie, ed. *The Oxford Handbook of Bioethics*. New York: Oxford University Press, 2007.

Steinbock, Bonnie, Arras, John D., and London, Alex John, eds. *Ethical Issues in Modern Medicine: Contemporary Readings in Bioethics*. 7th ed., New York: McGraw-Hill, 2009.

Tomlinson, T. "Caring for Risky Patients: Duty or Virtue?" *Journal of Medical Ethics*, 34 (2008): 458–462.

Van De Veer, Donald. *Paternalistic Interference.* Princeton, NJ: Princeton University Press, 1986.

Wolf, Susan M., ed. *Feminism & Bioethics: Beyond Reproduction.* New York: Oxford University Press, 1996.

4. The Nursing Context

Aiken, Linda H. "Improving Quality Through Nursing." In Mechanic, David, Rogut, Lynn, Colby, David, and Knickman, James, eds. *Policy Challenges in Modern Health Care.* New Brunswick, NJ: Rutgers University Press, 2005.

American Association of Colleges of Nursing. "News Watch." *aacn.nche.edu*, AACN. Updated monthly. Web. February 23, 2009.

American Nurses Association. *Guidance for Providing Care Under Altered Conditions: A Review of Standards, Guidelines and Competencies during Emergencies and Disasters.* Silver Spring, MD: American Nurses Association, 2008.

——. *Guide to the Code of Ethics for Nurses: Interpretation and Application.* Silver Spring, MD: American Nurses Association, 2008.

——. *Nursing: Scope and Standards of Practice.* Silver Springs, MD: American Nurses Association, 2004.

——. *A Social Policy Statement. 2nd ed.* Silver Springs, MD: American Nurses Association, 2003.

Amnesty International. *Ethical Codes and Declarations Relevant to Health Professionals: An Amnesty International Compilation of Selected Ethics and Human Rights Texts.* 4th ed., London: Amnesty International, 2000.

Aroskar, Mila, Moldow, D. Gay, and Good, Charles. "Nurses' Voices: Policy, Practice and Ethics." *Nursing Ethics,* 11 (May 2004): 266–276.

Ashley, Jeri. "Pain Management: Nurses in Jeopardy." *Oncology Nursing Forum,* 35 (2008): E70–E75.

Austin, Wendy. "Nursing Ethics in an Era of Globalization." *Advances in Nursing Science,* 24 (December 2001): 1–18.

——. "The Ethics of Everyday Practice: Healthcare Environments as Moral Communities." *Advances in Nursing Science,* 30 (January/March 2007): 81–88.

Bandman, Elsie L., and Bandman, Bertram. *Nursing Ethics Through the Life Span.* 4th ed., Upper Saddle River, NJ: Prentice Hall, 2002.

Bell, Jennifer and Breslin, Jonathan. "Healthcare Provider Moral Distress as a Leadership Challenge." *JONA'S Healthcare Law, Ethics, and Regulation,* 10 (Oct./Dec. 2008): 94–97.

Bishop, Anne H., and Scudder, John R. *Nursing Ethics: Holistic Caring Practice.* 2nd ed., Sudbury, MA: Jones and Bartlett, 2001.

Bosek, Marcia Sue DeWolf, and Savage, Teresa A. *The Ethical Component of Nursing Education: Integrating Ethics into Clinical Experience.* Philadephia, PA: Lippincott Williams and Wilkins, 2007.

Burkhardt, Margaret A, and Nathaniel, Alvita K. *Ethics and Issues in Contemporary Nursing. 3rd ed.*, Clifton Park, NY: Thomson Delmar Learning, 2008.

Chaska, Norma L. *The Nursing Profession: Tomorrow's Vision.* Thousand Oaks, CA: Sage Publications, 2001.

Cowen, Perle Slavik, and Moorhead, Sue. *Current Issues in Nursing*. 7th ed., St. Louis, MO: Mosby, 2006.

Davis, Anne J., Arosker, Mila A., Liaschenko, Joan, and Drought, Theresa. *Ethical Dilemmas and Nursing Practice*. 4th ed., Stamford, CT.: Appleton & Lange, 1997.

Department of Health and Human Services, *The Future Supply of Long-term Care Workers in Relation to the Aging Baby Boom Generation Report to Congress*. Washington, DC: Department of Health and Human Services, 2003.

Fry, Sara T., and Johnstone, Megan-Jane. *Ethics in Nursing Practice: A Guide to Ethical Decision Making*. Osney Mead, Oxford; Malden, MA: Blackwell Science, 2002.

Fry, Sara T., and Veatch. Robert M. *Case Studies in Nursing Ethics*. 2nd ed., Sudbury, MA: Jones and Bartlett, 2000.

Goodridge, Donna, Duggleby, Wendy, Gjevre, John, and Rennie, Donna. "Caring for Critically Ill Patients with Advanced COPD at the End of Life: A Qualitative Study." *Intensive and Critical Care Nursing*, 24 (2008): 162–170 .

Halvorsen, Kristin, Forde, Reidun, and Nortredt, Per. "Professional Challenges of Bedside Rationing in Intensive Care." *Nursing Ethics*, 15 (2008): 715–728.

Hanna, Debra R. "Moral Distress: The State of the Science." *Research and Theory for Nursing Practice: An International Journal*, 18 (Number 1 2004): 73–93.

Helft, Paul, et al. "Facilitated Ethics Conversations: A Novel Program for Managing Moral Distress in Bedside Nursing Staff." *JONA'S Healthcare Law, Ethics, and Regulation*, 11 (January/March 2009): 27–33.

Maddox, Peggy J. "Ethics and the Brave New World of E-Health." *Online Journal of Issues in Nursing* 6 (November 21, 2002). *Nursingworld.org*, ANA. Web. 16 Feb. 2009.

McBride, Angela Barron. *Nursing and Philanthropy: An Energizing Metaphor for the 21st Century*, Conference Proceedings. Indianapolis, IN: Sigma Theta Tau International Honor Society of Nursing, Center Nursing Press, 2000.

Monsen, Rita Black, ed. *Genetics and Ethics in Health Care: New Questions in the Age of Genomic Health*. (Co-published with the International Society of Nurses in Genetics). Silver Springs, MD: American Nurses Association, 2009.

Nursing Ethics: An International Journal for Health Care Professionals (March 1994 to present).

Pinch, Winifred J. Ellenchild, and Haddad, Amy M., eds., *Nursing and Health Care Ethics: A Legacy and a Vision*, Silver Spring, MD: American Nurses Association, 2008.

Pierce, Jessica, and Jameton, Andrew. *The Ethics of Environmentally Responsible Health Care*. New York: Oxford University Press, 2003.

Purtilo, Ruth B. *Ethical Dimensions in the Health Professions*. 4th ed., Philadelphia, PA: W. B. Saunders, 2005.

Ratner, Terry, ed. *Reflections on Doctors: Nurses' Stories about Physicians and Surgeons*. New York: Kaplan, 2008.

Redman, Barbara. "When Is Patient Education Unethical?" *Nursing Ethics*, 15 (2008): 813–820.

Sandelowski, Margarete. *Devices and Desires: Gender, Technology, and American Nursing* (Studies in Social Medicine). Chapel Hill, NC: University of North Carolina Press, 2000.

Silva, Mary Cipriano, and Ludwick, Ruth. "What Would You Do? Ethics and Infection Control." *Online Journal of Issues in Nursing*, 11 (November 6, 2006). *Nursingworld.org.* ANA Web. February 16, 2009 .

Sorrell, Jeanne M. "Ethics in Healthcare Organizations: Struggling with New Questions." *Online Journal of Issues in Nursing*, 13 (August 20, 2008). *Nursingworld.org.* ANA Web. February 16, 2009.

Tschudin, Verena, ed. *Approaches to Ethics: Nursing Beyond Boundaries.* Boston, MA: Harcourt, 2003.

——. *Ethics in Nursing: The Caring Relationship.* 3rd ed., Boston, MA: Butterworth-Heinemann, 2003.

Tschudin, Verena, and Davis, Anne J., eds. *The Globalisation of Nursing.* Abingdon, U.K.: Radcliffe, 2008.

World Health Organization. *Ethical Considerations in Developing a Public Health Response to Pandemic Influenza.* Geneva: World Health Organization, 2007.

INDEX